BARRON'S

PCAT

Pharmacy College Admission Test

5TH EDITION

Marie A. Chisholm-Burns, Pharm.D., MPH, FCCP, FASHP
Professor and Head, Department of Pharmacy Practice and Science
University of Arizona College of Pharmacy
Tucson, Arizona

Contributing Authors:

Alan Wolfgang, Ph.D.
Assistant Dean for Student Affairs
The University of Georgia College of Pharmacy
Athens, Georgia

Mark A. McCombs, M.S.
Senior Lecturer, Department of Mathematics
University of North Carolina at Chapel Hill
Chapel Hill, North Carolina

Suzanne Carpenter, M.S.
Associate Professor of Chemistry
Armstrong Atlantic State University
College of Science and Technology
Savannah, Georgia

Henry R. Bose, Jr., Ph.D.
Mary Betzner Morrow Centennial Chair
in Molecular Genetics and Microbiology
Director, School of Biological Sciences
The University of Texas at Austin
Austin, Texas

Monica Ali, Ph.D., R.Ph.
Emerita Professor of Chemistry
Oxford College of Emory University
Oxford, Georgia

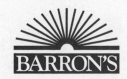

BARRON'S

All inquiries should be addressed to:
Barron's Educational Series, Inc.
250 Wireless Boulevard
Hauppauge, NY 11788
www.barronseduc.com

ISBN: 978-0-7641-4618-3

Library of Congress Catalog Card No.: 2011931235

Contents

Introduction

For many colleges and schools of pharmacy, grades achieved in college pre-pharmacy courses, and Pharmacy College Admission Test (PCAT) scores are the most important criteria used to evaluate students for admission. Therefore, it is very important for you to perform your very best on the PCAT. The PCAT was developed to provide college admission committees with comparable information about the academic abilities of applicants in designated areas.

This study guide can be very useful in preparing you for the PCAT, and for pharmacy education in general. When used properly and in combination with other materials, this guide will enhance your chances in the applicant pool of a college or school of pharmacy. All chapters are written by practicing pharmacists and/or educators (professors or instructors) with extensive experience in the admission procedures of U.S. pharmacy schools. In addition, each of the chapter authors has special expertise in the designated subject; this will further help you do your best on the PCAT.

This guide should help focus your review by outlining and reviewing subjects that are currently included on the PCAT. In addition, this guide can be very useful in the early stages of your pre-pharmacy education by pointing out the areas that will be covered on the PCAT. Thus, you will be able to prioritize topics for studying, a step that will aid you in achieving your desired score.

Remember, your pre-pharmacy courses are designed to serve as the foundation for your pharmacy education, and the PCAT is intended to determine your grasp of this material and your ability to apply it during your continued education. To be successful on the PCAT, it is important that you not only understand the material in a particular course, but that you can also apply it in your future program of higher education. If you take your pre-pharmacy courses with this in mind, the PCAT should be less difficult.

Use this and any other study guide as just that—a guide to what and how to study. The chance that the same exact questions contained in this text will be on the exam you take is remote; however, the likelihood that the same material will be covered is great. When reviewing a particular question, don't just look for the sentence or phrase that "answers the question"; study the topic and refresh your understanding of the material. Pay particular attention to facts that are related but differ in a "testable" way. For example, do you remember the terms *mitosis* and *meiosis*? You may remember these words and perhaps know that they have something to do with cell propagation, but that is not enough. If the multiple-choice answers to a question on the PCAT include descriptions of both mitosis and meiosis, you must

As of July 2011, the PCAT will be administered in computer-based format only. Modifications to the sections will also be made for the 2012–2013 cycles. Please see page 38 for a description of these changes.

be able to distinguish between the terms to select the correct answer, or risk receiving no more credit than someone who never took a biology course.

This book reviews all sections of the PCAT (as of 2011) and therefore serves as a good focal point to begin studying for the exam. Please keep in mind, however, that this is a guide; its purpose is not to review all required pre-pharmacy courses, but rather to aid you in studying for the PCAT. For optimal performance, it is strongly suggested that you use this guide along with your pre-pharmacy coursework to prepare for the PCAT.

FORMAT AND USE OF THIS BOOK

The format of this book is user-friendly. Chapter 1 covers general information about the pharmacy profession, pharmacy school admissions, and pharmacy education. In Chapters 2 and 3, general information on the PCAT and specific test-taking strategies and tactics are presented, respectively. Six chapters addressing verbal ability, biology, chemistry, quantitative ability, reading comprehension, and essay writing follow. Also, each chapter (with the exception of the essay chapter) has a set of questions with full explanatory answers to test, review, and enhance your knowledge of the various subjects. The chapter on writing your PCAT essay contains helpful tips on writing effectively. Finally, so you can practice taking the exam and evaluate your skills, two sample PCATs with full explanatory answers are provided in Chapters 10 and 11.

Planning for a Career in Pharmacy

CHAPTER 1

A CAREER IN PHARMACY

Over the last few decades, pharmacy practice has undergone significant changes. Since the 1960s, the pharmacy profession has branched out in many directions other than traditional pharmacy settings (community and hospital). Once you have graduated from pharmacy school and have successfully passed a pharmacy state board licensure examination, career opportunities in pharmacy are great. These opportunities include, but are not limited to, community pharmacy (chain and independent), hospital pharmacy, pharmaceutical industry, government agencies, geriatric pharmacy, clinical pharmacy, pharmacy services, managed-care pharmacy, pharmaceutical research, pharmacy and medical education, nuclear pharmacy, and other specialty areas.

Job opportunities are immense for a person who earns a degree in pharmacy. In addition, postgraduate training or graduate education provides an excellent opportunity for continuing your pharmacy education and thereby enhancing your career opportunities in this field. Although career counseling is best done in a pharmacy program, the purpose of this section is to familiarize you with several pharmacy careers (see the list that follows). Once accepted into a pharmacy school, you should inquire further about career opportunities in pharmacy.

Examples of Career Opportunities in Pharmacy

Academia
  Administration
  Biological Science
  Clinical Pharmacy
  Continuing Education
  Experiential Education
  Medicinal Chemistry
  Pharmaceutics
  Pharmacy Administration
  Pharmacy Practice

Administration
  Continuing Education
  Professional Relations
Business
  Administration
  Management
  Marketing
  Sales
Chain (Community)
  Apothecary
  Franchise
  Home Health Care
  Long-term Care

Clinical
  Adult Medicine
  Ambulatory Care
  Clinical Coordinator
  Clinical Manager
  Critical Care
  Drug Information
  Family Medicine
  Geriatrics
  Infectious Disease
  Internal Medicine
  Nutrition
  Oncology
  Pain Management
  Pediatrics
  Pharmacokinetics
  Poison Control
  Psychiatry
  Surgery
  Transplantation
Computer Technology
Consultant
  Clinical Pharmacy
  Home Health Care
  Long-term Care
Drug Information
Federal
  Alcohol, Drug Abuse, and
    Mental Health
  Armed Services
  Clinical Pharmacy
  Drug Enforcement Administration
  Food and Drug Administration
  Health Administration
  Health Care Financing
  Indian Health Services
Hospital
  Administration
  Clinical Pharmacy
  Inventory Control
  Staff

Independent
  Clinical Pharmacy
  Franchise
  Home Health Care
  Long-term Care
Industry
  Regulatory Affairs
  Medical Communication
  Medication Safety
Mail-Order Pharmacy
Managed Care Pharmacy
Nuclear Pharmacy
Pharmacy Associations
Research and Development
  Biological Sciences
  Clinical Outcomes
  Informatics
  Medicinal Chemistry
  Pharmaceutical Research
  Pharmaceutics
  Pharmacogenomics
  Pharmacognosy
  Pharmacology
  Pharmacy Administration
  Pharmacy Practice
State
  Board of Pharmacy
  Clinical Outcomes
  Department of Consumer
    Affairs
  Department of Health
Technical/Scientific
  Drug Information
  Manufacturing
  Postmarketing Surveillance
  Product Control
Veterans Administration Facilities

IMPORTANT CONSIDERATIONS IN PLANNING YOUR PHARMACY EDUCATION

On the following page is a flowchart that displays some general guidelines to help you in planning your pharmacy education and completing the admission process at a U.S. college/school of pharmacy. For additional information, refer to the pre-pharmacy advisor at the institution where you are taking your pre-pharmacy required courses and the college/school of pharmacy you wish to attend. The information given in this chapter should not replace or supersede information obtained from your pre-pharmacy advisor or the college/school of pharmacy in which you would like to continue your education.

Pre-Pharmacy Curricula

You should be familiar with the requirements of each of the institutions to which you wish to apply. Many students who apply to pharmacy school have more than the minimum pre-pharmacy course requirements and/or have attended college for more than two years. The pre-pharmacy required coursework may be able to be completed within two years (of course, this depends on the individual requirements of the pharmacy school); however, there are some schools that require more than two years of coursework. Obviously, the pre-pharmacy curricula at each school may vary, but there are typically some similarities that will give you an idea of the type of courses required. Below is an outline detailing the subject areas covered by many pre-pharmacy curricula. Please note: additional coursework may be required and the courses listed below may or may not be required at many schools of pharmacy; therefore, it is imperative to check with the school of pharmacy for its exact pre-pharmacy requirements.

PRE-PHARMACY CURRICULUM OUTLINE

- Humanities and Fine Arts Courses
  - English—two courses or one year.
  - Literature—one course.
  - Speech—one course.
- Social Science Courses
  - History—one or more courses.
  - Political Science—one course. This may be covered with an additional History course.
  - Economics—one course.
  - Other Social Science elective—one course (e.g., Sociology, Psychology, Anthropology, or additional History courses).
- Math and Science Courses
  - Pre-Calculus—one course. Some programs may only require Calculus courses, but prerequisites may be required of some post-secondary applicants.
  - Calculus/Analytical Geometry—one or two courses.
  - Statistics—one course.

Remember

The information provided in this book regarding the PCAT is current at the time of the book's writing; for the most recent PCAT updates and information, please refer to the official PCAT website at *www.pcatweb.info.*

PHARMACY SCHOOL APPLICANT GUIDELINES

Identify pharmacy school(s) of interest.
Important considerations that may help you
in the identification process include:
- school's geographical location;
- your program preference;
- cost and scholarship availability;
- school's reputation; and
- academic requirements for admission.

Identify what pre-pharmacy courses are required.
- This information will vary between different
  pharmacy schools.
- Since many pre-pharmacy courses are sequential,
  it is important to focus on the scheduling of courses.
- As soon as possible, make an appointment
  to consult with the pre-pharmacy advisor
  at your school.

Take pre-pharmacy courses.
- It is important to make the best grades and
  get the best background possible in these
  courses. Keep materials from courses as they
  may be helpful to study for the PCAT.

**Apply to pharmacy school(s) and/or
PharmCAS (*www.pharmcas.org*).**
Check with your pre-pharmacy advisor
concerning the most appropriate
time to apply.
- Apply as early as possible and when
  appropriate, considering when you will
  be finished with pre-pharmacy requirements.
- If faculty or personal references are
  required, select professors and others who
  know you well, will provide a good
  reference, and will send it in *on time*.
- If the school utilizes PharmCAS, check to
  see if supplemental forms are required.

Register to take the PCAT.
Allow yourself the opportunity to take
the PCAT more than once; check with
your pre-pharmacy advisor and the
PCAT website (*www.pcatweb.info*)
for scheduling and registration.
Check with the pharmacy school(s)
concerning policy on taking the PCAT
more than once and how multiple
PCAT scores are considered in the
admission process.

**Complete the application
process and await status letter.**
Make sure you follow up if you
are offered admission. You will
need to confirm and may have
to provide a tuition deposit.

**Most pharmacy schools
require an interview.**
- Check with the school(s).
- If required, plan and
  prepare for the interview.

**Is the PCAT required by
the pharmacy school(s)
to which you are applying?**

YES

NO

- Biological Sciences–two courses or one year with labs. Some programs may require Anatomy and Physiology as a pre-pharmacy course.
- Chemistry–four courses or two years. These courses include General Chemistry and Organic Chemistry with labs.
- Physics–up to two courses or one year. Physics is not required by some programs.

Each institution's program will have its own pre-pharmacy course requirements; you should obtain this information directly from the desired school. Many colleges and universities offer pre-professional advising programs to assist students in course selection. Utilize these advisors and the recruitment and admission staff of your desired pharmacy program as important resources. Since many programs only accept students once a year, if you do not complete the pre-pharmacy curriculum by the designated time, it may delay acceptance by an entire academic year. If you have previously completed coursework for which you expect to receive credit, in lieu of some specific pre-pharmacy prerequisites, verify whether the course will satisfy requirements early in your application process.

Doctorate of Pharmacy Degree Curricula

DOCTORATE OF PHARMACY DEGREE ("2+4" PROGRAM)

Each school or college of pharmacy has a list of courses that are considered prerequisites to the pharmacy professional program. For many schools, the pre-pharmacy prerequisites can take two years or longer to complete. The pre-pharmacy curriculum, along with the four-year professional curriculum, comprises what is called a "2+4" professional doctor of pharmacy degree program. Some programs require eighty or more hours of pre-pharmacy coursework, and may even require applicants to have earned a bachelor's degree; thus, it could take considerably longer than two years to complete the pre-pharmacy requirements for those schools. There is at least one variation to this model (see "0+6" Program below).

DOCTORATE OF PHARMACY DEGREE ("0+6" PROGRAM)

One of the variations to the "2+4" program is the "0+6" program. This program allows students to be accepted directly into the school or college of pharmacy where they will complete the pre-pharmacy core as part of a six-year academic program. Most of these programs also consider applicants to the professional program; however, if the student is accepted, he or she will enter at the beginning of the third year of the program.

PharmCAS

The Pharmacy College Application Service (PharmCAS) is a centralized application service designed to assemble, process, and distribute applicants' information. Some pharmacy programs utilize this service to gather admission data from applicants, advisors, and other sources. The system is similar to those used by other professional programs such as medical schools, law schools, and veterinary medicine programs.

TIP

Familiarize yourself with PharmCAS by obtaining information from their online site, *www.PharmCAS.org.*

The PharmCAS system has been used by some schools since the early 2000s application cycle, but is not used by all pharmacy programs. The information presented here is current as of the preparation of this edition of the book.

PharmCAS is designed to be a comprehensive application system providing a mechanism to distribute information about an applicant to one or more participating pharmacy schools. According to the information detailed on the PharmCAS website, the system operates to benefit applicants, participating pharmacy schools, and advisors of pre-pharmacy students. Information for each participating school is provided on the PharmCAS site. Listed below are some examples of the information that is provided:

1. application deadlines
2. transcript submission requirements
3. pre-pharmacy requirements
4. recommendation submission procedures
5. any special or additional requirements for specific schools

Non-participating schools—those NOT participating in PharmCAS—are listed and links to various school websites are provided. Be aware that PharmCAS participating schools may still require that supplemental application data be submitted directly to the school to which the student is applying.

As of 2011, the application fee for an individual to submit an application to a single participating school is $150. There is a graduated fee scale to apply for more than one school. For example, to apply for a second school, an additional $50 is required. The PharmCAS website contains the most current information.

The PharmCAS website lists several sources of instructions. Applicants are encouraged to familiarize themselves with the "Step-by-Step" checklist, PharmCAS Application Instructions, and Applicant Code of Conduct. Visit the PharmCAS website at *www.PharmCAS.org.*

In addition to various supplemental materials that may be required by schools participating in PharmCAS, applicants must submit transcript request forms to the registrar of each U.S. and Canadian college or university they have attended. A requirement in the 2010–2011 application cycle is the provision for Letters of Reference to be submitted via PharmCAS. There are currently three categories of Letter of Reference procedures for participating schools: (1) No letters of reference; (2) Letters submitted directly to the school (and not to PharmCAS); and (3) Letters submitted (either electronically via e-mail or on paper) to PharmCAS, which are then distributed to the applicant's specified schools. Again, the applicant should consult the PharmCAS website for specific instructions for the program or programs in which he or she is interested.

Some participating pharmacy programs offer an "Early Decision" process via the PharmCAS system. As of the 2010–2011 application cycle, the early decision application deadline is September 3. The PharmCAS website indicates that an applicant must contact the schools offering early decision to obtain information regarding early decision guidelines. Additionally, if you are offered admission as an early decision application participant, you are obligated to accept that offer AND you will not be permitted to apply to another PharmCAS institution. PharmCAS institutions that participate in the early decision process will announce those choices by a date selected annually.

Part of the application process for PharmCAS requires that the applicant enter all coursework and grades using personal transcripts or grade reports. These entries are verified by PharmCAS upon receipt of official copies of your transcripts. Additional copies of your official transcripts may be required by the institution(s).

Students who have completed college-level work at foreign institutions must contact the schools to which they are applying, or get specific information from the school's website. Usually, foreign transcripts must be submitted to a service that specializes in this type of evaluation. Individual schools vary in their procedures for accepting credit toward the completion of pre-pharmacy coursework from non-U.S. accredited programs.

Applicants who submitted and paid for an application to PharmCAS in the pervious cycle are eligible to have their application information carried over to the new cycle. Please refer to the application instructions on the PharmCAS website for further details.

The PharmCAS system offers a mechanism for an applicant to pursue a number of pharmacy programs while possibly reducing the amount of repeated materials that must be submitted. Currently, more than one-half of all pharmacy programs utilize PharmCAS. Applicants should contact each pharmacy school of interest to obtain admission requirements.

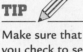

TIP

Make sure that you check to see if any additional materials are required, even if a school uses PharmCAS.

U.S. Colleges and Schools of Pharmacy Admission Requirements

Applications for admission to schools and colleges of pharmacy have increased significantly in the twenty-first century. For example, the American Association of Colleges of Pharmacy (AACP) reported an average application-to-enrollment ratio of approximately 3:1 for U.S. schools of pharmacy in 1990; however, in 2009 the average applicant-to-enrollment ratio was about 8:1. The increased number of applicants can be interpreted in many ways in terms of pharmacy practice and education, but what it means to the student applicant is certain—increased competition for acceptance into a pharmacy school.

As of 2011, there are approximately 123 schools of pharmacy with accreditation status in the U.S. The listing of schools can be found through the Accreditation Council of Pharmacy Education website (*www.acpe-accredit.org*) or through the AACP website (*www.aacp.org*). All schools of pharmacy utilize the college pre-pharmacy grade point average (GPA) in evaluating candidates for admission. In addition to the GPA, the PCAT is utilized by most pharmacy schools in selecting students. Therefore, the two main academic performance selection criteria for admission are the PCAT scores and the pre-pharmacy GPA. Most schools also conduct interviews to evaluate students for acceptance; however, whether a candidate is selected for an interview is often dependent on his or her GPA and PCAT performance.

Since acceptance into pharmacy school is very competitive, it is extremely important for you to do your best in both.

U.S. Colleges and Schools of Pharmacy

The following information represents the U.S. colleges and schools of pharmacy as reported by the Accreditation Council for Pharmacy Education (ACPE). Greater than 95% of the schools listed here have been accredited by ACPE. To obtain the most current information and accreditation status, contact the specific college or school of pharmacy in which you are interested.

Albany College of Pharmacy
Appalachian College of Pharmacy
Auburn University
Belmont University
Butler University
California Northstate College of
  Pharmacy
Campbell University
Chicago State University
College of Notre Dame
Concordia University
Creighton University
Drake University
Duquesne University
D'Youville College
East Tennessee State University
Ferris State University
Florida A&M University
Hampton University
Harding University
Howard University
Husson University
Idaho State University
Lake Erie College of Osteopathic
  Medicine
Lipscomb University
Loma Linda University
Long Island University
Massachusetts College of Pharmacy—
  Boston
Massachusetts College of Pharmacy—
  Manchester
Massachusetts College of Pharmacy—
  Worcester
Mercer University
Midwestern University—Chicago
Midwestern University—Glendale
North Dakota State University

Northeastern Ohio Universities
Northeastern University
Nova Southeastern University
Ohio Northern University
Ohio State University
Oregon State University
Pacific University
Palm Beach Atlantic University
Presbyterian College
Philadelphia College
Purdue University
Regis University
Roosevelt University
Rosalind Franklin University
Rutgers University
Samford University
Shenandoah University
South Carolina College of Pharmacy
South Dakota State University
South University
Southern Illinois University—
  Edwardsville
Southwestern Oklahoma State
  University
St. John Fisher College
St. John's University
St. Joseph College
St. Louis College of Pharmacy
State University of NY—Buffalo
Sullivan University
Temple University
Texas A&M University—Kingsville
Texas Southern University
Texas Tech University
Thomas Jefferson University
Touro College
Touro University
Union University

University of Arizona
University of Arkansas
University of California—
   San Diego
University of California—
   San Francisco
University of Charleston
University of Cincinnati
University of Colorado
University of Connecticut
University of Findlay
University of Florida
University of Georgia
University of Hawaii
University of Houston
University of Illinois
University of the Incarnate Word
University of Iowa
University of Kansas
University of Kentucky
University of Louisiana
University of Maryland
Univeristy of Maryland Eastern Shore
University of Michigan
University of Minnesota
University of Minnesota—Duluth
University of Mississippi
University of Missouri
University of Montana

University of Nebraska
University of New England
University of New Mexico
University of North Carolina
University of Oklahoma
University of the Pacific
University of Pittsburgh
University of Puerto Rico
University of Rhode Island
University of the Sciences in
   Philadelphia
University of Southern California
University of Southern Nevada
University of Tennessee
University of Texas
University of Toledo
University of Utah
University of Washington
University of Wisconsin
University of Wyoming
Virginia Commonwealth University
Washington State University
Wayne State University
West Virginia University
Western New England College
Western University of Health Sciences
Wilkes University
Wingate University
Xavier University of Louisiana

Directory of U.S. Colleges and Schools of Pharmacy (by State)

ALABAMA

Harrison School of Pharmacy
Auburn University
2316 Walker Building
Auburn University, Alabama 36849-5501
(334) 844-8348
pharmacy.auburn.edu/
Professional Degree Offered: Doctor
of Pharmacy

McWhorter School of Pharmacy
Samford University
800 Lakeshore Drive
Birmingham, Alabama 35229
(205) 726-2982
pharmacy.samford.edu
Professional Degree Offered: Doctor
of Pharmacy

ARIZONA

College of Pharmacy—Glendale
Midwestern University
19555 North 59th Avenue
Glendale, Arizona 85308
(623) 572-3215
*www.midwestern.edu/Programs_and_Admissions/
AZ_Pharmacy.html*
Professional Degree Offered: Doctor
of Pharmacy

College of Pharmacy
University of Arizona
1295 N. Martin Avenue
P.O. Box 210202
Tucson, Arizona 85721
(520) 626-1427
www.pharmacy.arizona.edu/
Professional Degree Offered: Doctor
of Pharmacy

ARKANSAS

College of Pharmacy
Harding University
915 East Market Avenue
Searcy, Arkansas 72149
(501) 279-5528
www.harding.edu/pharmacy
Professional Degree Offered: Doctor
of Pharmacy

College of Pharmacy
University of Arkansas for Medical Sciences
4301 West Markham Street, Slot 522
Little Rock, Arkansas 72205
(501) 686-5557
www.uams.edu/cop/
Professional Degree Offered: Doctor
of Pharmacy

CALIFORNIA

California Northstate College of Pharmacy
10811 International Drive
Rancho Cordova, California 95670
(916) 631-8108
www.californiacollegeofpharmacy.org
Professional Degree Offered: Doctor
of Pharmacy

School of Pharmacy
Loma Linda University
West Hall 1316
11262 Campus Street
Loma Linda, California 92350
(909) 558-1300
www.llu.edu/pharmacy\index.page
Professional Degree Offered: Doctor
of Pharmacy

College of Pharmacy
Touro University—California
1310 Johnson Lane, Mare Island
Vallejo, California 94592
(707) 638-5200
www.tu.edu/
Professional Degree Offered: Doctor
of Pharmacy

Skaggs School of Pharmacy and Pharmaceutical
Sciences
University of California—San Diego
9500 Gilman Drive, MC 0657
La Jolla, California 92093-0657
(858) 822-4900
www.pharmacy.ucsd.edu/
Professional Degree Offered: Doctor
of Pharmacy

School of Pharmacy
University of California at San Francisco
513 Parnassus Avenue
UCSF Box 0150, Room S-960
San Francisco, California 94143
(415) 476-2732
pharmacy.ucsf.edu/
Professional Degree Offered: Doctor
of Pharmacy

Thomas J. Long School of Pharmacy
and Health Sciences
University of the Pacific
3601 Pacific Avenue
Stockton, California 95211
(209) 946-2211
web.pacific.edu\x817.xml
Professional Degree Offered: Doctor
of Pharmacy

School of Pharmacy
University of Southern California
1985 Zonal Avenue
Los Angeles, California 90089-9121
(323) 442-1369
www.usc.edu/schools/pharmacy/
Professional Degree Offered: Doctor
of Pharmacy

College of Pharmacy
Western University of Health Sciences
309 E. Second Street
Pomona, California 91766-1854
(909) 469-5335
*www.westernu.edu/xp\edu/pharmacy/pharmd_
about.xml*
Professional Degree Offered: Doctor
of Pharmacy

COLORADO

School of Pharmacy
Regis University
3333 Regis Boulevard
Denver, Colorado 80221-1099
(303) 458-4344
www.regis.edu/rh.asp?page=study.pharm
Professional Degree Offered: Doctor
of Pharmacy

School of Pharmacy
University of Colorado Anschutz Medical
Campus
Mail Stop C238
Pharmacy and Pharmaceutical Sciences Building
12850 East Montview Boulevard
Aurora, Colorado 80045
(303) 724-2634
www.uchsc.edu/sop/
Professional Degree Offered: Doctor
of Pharmacy

CONNECTICUT

School of Pharmacy
St. Joseph College
229 Trumbull Street
Hartford, Connecticut 06103-0501
(860) 231-5858
www.sjc.edu
Professional Degree Offered: Doctor
of Pharmacy

School of Pharmacy
The University of Connecticut
69 North Eagleville Road, Unit 3092
Storrs, Connecticut 06269-3092
(860) 486-2129
pharmacy.uconn.edu/
Professional Degree Offered: Doctor
 of Pharmacy

DISTRICT OF COLUMBIA

College of Pharmacy, Nursing and
 Allied Health Science
School of Pharmacy
Howard University
2300 Fourth Street, Northwest
Washington, DC 20059
(202) 806-6530
www.cpnahs.howard.edu/
Professional Degree Offered: Doctor
 of Pharmacy

FLORIDA

College of Pharmacy and Pharmaceutical
 Sciences
Florida Agricultural and Mechanical University
1415 South Martin Luthur King, Jr. Boulevard
Tallahassee, Florida 32307
(850) 599-3301
pharmacy.famu.edu/
Professional Degree Offered: Doctor
 of Pharmacy

College of Pharmacy
Nova Southeastern University
3200 South University Drive
Fort Lauderdale, Florida 33328
(954) 262-1300
pharmacy.nova.edu
Professional Degree Offered: Doctor
 of Pharmacy

Lloyd L. Gregory School of Pharmacy
Palm Beach Atlantic University
901 South Flagler Drive
West Palm Beach, Florida 33416-4708
(561) 803-2000
cosmas.pba.edu/pharmacy/
Professional Degree Offered: Doctor
 of Pharmacy

College of Pharmacy
University of Florida
P.O. Box 100484
Gainesville, Florida 32610
(352) 273-6312
www.cop.ufl.edu/
Professional Degree Offered: Doctor
 of Pharmacy

GEORGIA

College of Pharmacy and Health Sciences
Mercer University
3001 Mercer University Drive
Atlanta, Georgia 30341-4415
(678) 547-6232
cophs.mercer.edu
Professional Degree Offered: Doctor
 of Pharmacy

College of Pharmacy
Philadelphia College of Osteopathic Medicine
625 Old Peachtree Road, NW
Suwanee, Georgia 30024
(678) 225-7500
www.pcom.edu/General_information/georgia/
 georgia.html
Professional Degree Offered: Doctor
 of Pharmacy

School of Pharmacy
South University
709 Mall Boulevard
Savannah, Georgia 31406
(912) 201-8120
www.southuniversity.edu/campus/pharmacy
Professional Degree Offered: Doctor
 of Pharmacy

College of Pharmacy
The University of Georgia
R. C. Wilson Pharmacy Building
Athens, Georgia 30602-2351
(706) 542-5278
www.rx.uga.edu/
Professional Degree Offered: Doctor
of Pharmacy

HAWAII

College of Pharmacy
The University of Hawaii at Hilo
200 West Kawili Street
Hilo, Hawaii 96720-4091
(808) 933-7664
pharmacy.uhh.hawaii.edu
Professional Degree Offered: Doctor
of Pharmacy

IDAHO

College of Pharmacy
Idaho State University
970 South 5th Street, Stop 8288
Pocatello, Idaho 83209-8288
(208) 282-3475
pharmacy.isu.edu/live/
Professional Degree Offered: Doctor
of Pharmacy

ILLINOIS

College of Pharmacy
Chicago State University
9501 South King Drive
206 Douglas Hall
Chicago, Illinois 60628-1598
(773) 821-2500
www.csu.edu/collegeofpharmacy/
Professional Degree Offered: Doctor
of Pharmacy

Chicago College of Pharmacy
Midwestern University
555 31st Street
Downers Grove, Illinois 60515
(630) 515-6171
www.midwestern.edu
Professional Degree Offered: Doctor
of Pharmacy

College of Pharmacy
Roosevelt University
1400 N. Roosevelt Boulevard
Schaumburg, Illinois 60173
(847) 619-7300
www.roosevelt.edu/Pharmacy.aspx
Professional Degree Offered: Doctor
of Pharmacy

College of Pharmacy
Rosalind Franklin University of Medicine and
Sciences
3333 Green Bay Road
North Chicago, Illinois 60064
(847) 578-3204
http://rosalindfranklin.edu/collegeofpharmacy/
Professional Degree Offered: Doctor
of Pharmacy

School of Pharmacy
Southern Illinois University, Edwardsville
Campus Box 2000
Edwardsville, Illinois 62026-2000
(618) 650-5150
www.siue.edu/PHARMACY/
Professional Degree Offered: Doctor
of Pharmacy

College of Pharmacy
University of Illinois at Chicago
833 South Wood Street, m/c 874
Chicago, Illinois 60612
(312) 996-7242
www.uic.edu/pharmacy/
Professional Degree Offered: Doctor
of Pharmacy

INDIANA

College of Pharmacy and Health Sciences
Butler University
4600 Sunset Avenue
Indianapolis, Indiana 46208
(317) 940-9969
www.butler.edu/cophs/
Professional Degree Offered: Doctor
of Pharmacy

School of Pharmacy and Pharmaceutical Sciences
Purdue University
575 Stadium Mall Drive
West Lafayette, Indiana 47907
(765) 494-1361
www.pharmacy.purdue.edu/
Professional Degree Offered: Doctor
of Pharmacy

IOWA

College of Pharmacy and Health Sciences
Drake University
Cline 106
2507 University Avenue
Des Moines, Iowa 50311-4505
(515) 271-2011 or 1-800-44-DRAKE (ext. 3018)
www.drake.edu/cphs
Professional Degree Offered: Doctor
of Pharmacy

College of Pharmacy
The University of Iowa
115 South Grand Avenue
Iowa City, Iowa 52242
(319) 335-8794
www.pharmacy.uiowa.edu/
Professional Degree Offered: Doctor
of Pharmacy

KANSAS

School of Pharmacy
University of Kansas
2010 Becker Drive, Room 2050
Lawrence, Kansas 66047-1620
(785) 864-3591
www.pharm.ku.edu/
Professional Degree Offered: Doctor
of Pharmacy

KENTUCKY

College of Pharamcy
Sullivan University
2100 Gardiner Lane
Louisville, Kentucky 40205
(502) 413-8640
www.sullivan.edu/pharmacy
Professional Degree Offered: Doctor
of Pharmacy

College of Pharmacy
University of Kentucky
789 South Limestone
Lexington, Kentucky 40536-0596
(859) 323-6163
pharmacy.mc.uky.edu
Professional Degree Offered: Doctor
of Pharmacy

LOUISIANA

School of Pharmacy
The University of Louisiana at Monroe
700 University Avenue
Monroe, Louisiana 71209
(318) 342-3800
rxweb.ulm.edu/pharmacy/
Professional Degree Offered: Doctor
of Pharmacy

College of Pharmacy
Xavier University of Louisiana
1 Drexel Drive
New Orleans, Louisiana 70125
(504) 520-5365
www.xula.edu/cop/index.php
Professional Degree Offered: Doctor
of Pharmacy

MAINE

School of Pharmacy
Husson University
One College Circle
Bangor, Maine 04401-2999
(207) 973-1019
www.husson.edu
Professional Degree Offered: Doctor
of Pharmacy

College of Pharmacy
University of New England
716 Stevens Avenue
Portland, Maine 04103
(207) 221-4225
www.une.edu/pharmacy.index.cfm
Professional Degree Offered: Doctor
of Pharmacy

MARYLAND

School of Pharmacy
College of Notre Dame
4701 North Charles Street
Baltimore, Maryland 21210
(410) 435-0100
*www.ndm.edu/admissions/schoolofpharmacy/
index.cfm*
Professional Degree Offered: Doctor
of Pharmacy

School of Pharmacy
University of Maryland
20 North Pine Street
Baltimore, Maryland 21201
(410) 706-7650
www.pharmacy.umaryland.edu/
Professional Degree Offered: Doctor
of Pharmacy

School of Pharmacy
University of Maryland Eastern Shore
117 Somerset Hall
Princess Anne, Maryland 21853
(410) 651-8354
www.umes.edu/pharmacy
Professional Degree Offered: Doctor
of Pharmacy

MASSACHUSETTS

School of Pharmacy—Boston
Massachusetts College of Pharmacy
and Health Sciences
179 Longwood Avenue
Boston, Massachusetts 02115-5896
www.mcphs.edu/campuses/boston
(617) 732-2800
Professional Degree Offered: Doctor
of Pharmacy

School of Pharmacy—Worcester
Massachusetts College of Pharmacy
and Health Sciences
19 Foster Street
Worcester, Massachusetts 01608-1715
www.mcphs.edu/campuses/worcester
(508) 890-8855
Professional Degree Offered: Doctor
of Pharmacy

Bouvé College of Health Sciences—School of
  Pharmacy
Northeastern University
Behrakis Health Sciences Center
360 Huntington Avenue
206 Mugar Building
Boston, Massachusetts 02115
(617) 373-3380
www.northeastern.edu/bouve/pharmacy
Professional Degree Offered: Doctor
  of Pharmacy

School of Pharmacy
Western New England College
1215 Wilbraham Road
Springfield, Massachusetts 01119
(413) 796-2113
www.wne.edu/pharmacy/home.cfm
Professional Degree Offered: Doctor
  of Pharmacy

MICHIGAN

College of Pharmacy
Ferris State University
220 Ferris Drive, PHR 105
Big Rapids, Michigan 49307
(231) 591-3780
www.ferris.edu/colleges/pharmacy/index.cfm
Professional Degree Offered: Doctor
  of Pharmacy

College of Pharmacy
The University of Michigan
428 Church Street
Ann Arbor, Michigan 48109-1065
(734) 764-7312
www.umich.edu/pharmacy/home
Professional Degree Offered: Doctor
  of Pharmacy

Eugene Applebaum College of Pharmacy
  and Health Sciences
Wayne State University
259 Mack Avenue
Detroit, Michigan 48201
(313) 577-1716
www.cphs.wayne.edu
Professional Degree Offered: Doctor
  of Pharmacy

MINNESOTA

College of Pharmacy, Duluth
University of Minnesota
232 Life Science
1110 Kirby Drive
Duluth, Minnesota 55812
(218) 726-6000
www.pharmacy.umn.edu/duluth
Professional Degree Offered: Doctor
  of Pharmacy

College of Pharmacy
University of Minnesota
5-130 Weaver-Densford Hall
308 Harvard Street, SE
Minneapolis, Minnesota 55455
(612) 624-1900
www.pharmacy.umn.edu
Professional Degree Offered: Doctor
  of Pharmacy

MISSISSIPPI

School of Pharmacy
The University of Mississippi
P.O. Box 1848
University, Mississippi 38677
(662) 915-7996
www.pharmacy.olemiss.edu/
Professional Degree Offered: Doctor
  of Pharmacy

MISSOURI

St. Louis College of Pharmacy
4588 Parkview Place
St. Louis, Missouri 63110-1088
(314) 367-8700
www.stlcop.edu
Professional Degree Offered: Doctor
of Pharmacy

School of Pharmacy
University of Missouri—Kansas City
Health Sciences Building
2464 Charlotte Street
Kansas City, Missouri 64108
(816) 235-1613
www.umkc.edu/pharmacy/
Professional Degree Offered: Doctor
of Pharmacy

MONTANA

Skaggs School of Pharmacy
The University of Montana
32 Campus Drive, 340 Skaggs Building
Missoula, Montana 59812-1512
(406) 243-4621
www.health.umt.edu/schools/pharmacy/default.htm
Professional Degree Offered: Doctor
of Pharmacy

NEBRASKA

School of Pharmacy and Health Professions
Creighton University
2500 California Plaza
Criss III, Room 151
Omaha, Nebraska 68178
(402) 280-2662
pharmacy.creighton.edu/
Professional Degree Offered: Doctor
of Pharmacy

College of Pharmacy
University of Nebraska
986000 Nebraska Medical Center
Omaha, Nebraska 68198-6000
(402) 559-4333
www.unmc.edu/pharmacy/
Professional Degree Offered: Doctor
of Pharmacy

NEVADA

College of Pharmacy
University of Southern Nevada
11 Sunset Way
Henderson, Nevada 89014
(702) 968-2007
www.usn.edu
Professional Degree Offered: Doctor
of Pharmacy

NEW HAMPSHIRE

School of Pharmacy—Manchester
Massachusetts College of Pharmacy
and Health Sciences
1260 Elm Street
Manchester, New Hampshire 03101
(603) 314-0210
www.mcphs.edu/campuses/manchester
Professional Degree Offered: Doctor
of Pharmacy

NEW JERSEY

Ernest Mario School of Pharmacy
Rutgers, the State University of New Jersey
160 Frelinghuysen Road
Piscataway, New Jersey 08854
(732) 445-2675
pharmacy.rutgers.edu/
Professional Degree Offered: Doctor
of Pharmacy

NEW MEXICO

College of Pharmacy
University of New Mexico
MSC 09 5360
1 University of New Mexico
Albuquerque, New Mexico 87131-0001
(505) 272-3241
hsc.unm.edu/pharmacy/
Professional Degree Offered: Doctor
   of Pharmacy

NEW YORK

Albany College of Pharmacy and Health Sciences
106 New Scotland Avenue
Albany, New York 12208
(888) 203-8010
www.acphs.edu
Professional Degree Offered: Doctor
   of Pharmacy

School of Pharmacy
D'Youville College
320 Porter Avenue
Buffalo, New York 14201
(716) 829-7846
www.dyc.edu/academics/pharmacy
Professional Degree Offered: Doctor
   of Pharmacy

Arnold and Marie Schwartz College of Pharmacy
   and Health Sciences
Long Island University
75 DeKalb Avenue
Brooklyn, New York 11201
(718) 488-1004
www.brooklyn.liu.edu/pharmacy/
Professional Degree Offered: Doctor
   of Pharmacy

Wegmans School of Pharmacy
St. John Fisher College
3690 East Avenue
Rochester, New York 14618
(585) 385-8430
www.sjfc.edu/pharmacy
Professional Degree Offered: Doctor
   of Pharmacy

College of Pharmacy and Allied Health
   Professions
St. John's University
8000 Utopia Parkway
Queens, New York 11439
(718) 990-6275
new.stjohns.edu/academics/undergraduate/pharmacy
Professional Degree Offered: Doctor
   of Pharmacy

Touro College of Pharmacy—New York
2090 Adam Clayton Powell Jr. Boulevard,
   5th floor
New York, New York 10027
(212) 851-1192, ext. 2500
www.touro.edu/pharmacy/
Professional Degree Offered: Doctor
   of Pharmacy

School of Pharmacy and Pharmaceutical Sciences
University of Buffalo, the State University
   of New York
129 Cooke Hall
Buffalo, New York 14260-1200
(716) 645-2825
www.pharmacy.buffalo.edu/
Professional Degree Offered: Doctor
   of Pharmacy

NORTH CAROLINA

College of Pharmacy and Health Sciences
Campbell University
P.O. Box 1090
Buies Creek, North Carolina 27506
(800) 334-4111
www.campbellpharmacy.net
Professional Degree Offered: Doctor
of Pharmacy

Eshelman School of Pharmacy
University of North Carolina at Chapel Hill
CB #7355
Chapel Hill, North Carolina 27599-7355
(919) 966-9429
www.pharmacy.unc.edu/
Professional Degree Offered: Doctor
of Pharmacy

School of Pharmacy
Wingate University
Campus Box 3087
Wingate, North Carolina 28174
(704) 233-8331
pharmacy.wingate.edu/
Professional Degree Offered: Doctor
of Pharmacy

NORTH DAKOTA

College of Pharmacy, Nursing, and
Allied Sciences
North Dakota State University
NDSU Dept. 2650
Sudro Hall, Room 123
PO Box 6050
Fargo, North Dakota 58108
(701) 231-7456
www.ndsu.nodak.edu/pharmacy/
Professional Degree Offered: Doctor
of Pharmacy

OHIO

College of Pharmacy
Northeastern Ohio Universities
4209 State Route 44
P.O. Box 95
Rootstown, Ohio 44272
(800) 686-2511
*www.neoucom.edu/audience/gradschool/pharmacy/
intro*
Professional Degree Offered: Doctor
of Pharmacy

Rudolph H. Raabe College of Pharmacy
Ohio Northern University
525 S. Main Street
Roberston-Evans Pharmacy 132
Ada, Ohio 45810
(419) 772-2275
www.onu.edu/academics/pharmacy
Professional Degree Offered: Doctor
of Pharmacy

College of Pharmacy
The Ohio State University
217 Parks Hall
500 West 12th Avenue
Columbus, Ohio 43210
(614) 292-2266
www.pharmacy.ohio-state.edu/index.cfm
Professional Degree Offered: Doctor
of Pharmacy

James L. Winkle College of Pharmacy
University of Cincinnati
3225 Eden Avenue
136 Health Professions Building
Cincinnati, Ohio 45267-0004
(513) 558-3784
pharmacy.uc.edu/
Professional Degree Offered: Doctor
of Pharmacy

College of Pharmacy
University of Findlay
300 Davis Street
Findlay, Ohio 45840
(419) 434-5327
*www.findlay.edu/academics/colleges/cphm/
    default.htm*
Professional Degree Offered: Doctor
    of Pharmacy

College of Pharmacy
The University of Toledo
Main Campus, Wolfe Hall
2801 West Bancroft Street, MS 608
Toledo, Ohio 43606
(419) 383-1904
www.utoldeo.edu/pharmacy/index.html
Professional Degree Offered: Doctor
    of Pharmacy

OKLAHOMA

College of Pharmacy
Southwestern Oklahoma State University
100 Campus Drive
Weatherford, Oklahoma 73096
(580) 774-3105
www.swosu.edu/pharmacy/
Professional Degree Offered: Doctor
    of Pharmacy

College of Pharmacy
University of Oklahoma
P.O. Box 26901
Oklahoma City, Oklahoma 73126-0901
(405) 271-6484
pharmacy.ouhsc.edu/index.asp
Professional Degree Offered: Doctor
    of Pharmacy

OREGON

College of Pharmacy
Oregon State University
203 Pharmacy Building
Corvallis, Oregon 97331-3507
(541) 737-3424
pharmacy.oregonstate.edu/
Professional Degree Offered: Doctor
    of Pharmacy

School of Pharmacy
Pacific University
222 Southeast 8th Avenue
Hillsboro, Oregon 97123
(503) 352-2218
www.pacificu.edu/pharmd/
Professional Degree Offered: Doctor
    of Pharmacy

PENNSYLVANIA

Mylan School of Pharmacy
Duquesne University
600 Forbes Avenue
Pittsburgh, Pennsylvania 15282
(412) 396-6222
www.pharmacy.duq.edu
Professional Degree Offered: Doctor
    of Pharmacy

School of Pharmacy
Lake Erie College of Osteopathic Medicine
1858 West Grandview Boulevard
Erie, Pennsylvania 16509-1025
(814) 866-6641
www.lecom.edu/school_pharmacy.php
Professional Degree Offered: Doctor
    of Pharmacy

School of Pharmacy
602-00
Temple University
3307 North Broad Street
Philadelphia, Pennsylvania 19140
(215) 707-4900
www.temple.edu/pharmacy/
Professional Degree Offered: Doctor
of Pharmacy

Jefferson School of Pharmacy
Thomas Jefferson University
130 South 9th Street
Edison Building
Philadelphia, Pennsylvania 19107
(877) 533-3247
www.jefferson.edu/jchp/pharmacy
Professional Degree Offered: Doctor
of Pharmacy

School of Pharmacy
University of Pittsburgh
Student Services
904 Salk Hall
Pittsburgh, Pennsylvania 15261
(412) 383-9000
www.pharmacy.pitt.edu/
Professional Degree Offered: Doctor
of Pharmacy

Philadelphia College of Pharmacy
University of the Sciences in Philadelphia
600 South 43rd Street
Philadelphia, Pennsylvania 19104
(215) 596-8800
www.usip.edu/pcp/
Professional Degree Offered: Doctor
of Pharmacy

School of Pharmacy
Wilkes University
Stark Learning Center
84 West South Street
Wilkes-Barre, Pennsylvania 18766
(570) 408-4298
www.wilkes.edu/pages/390.asp
Professional Degree Offered: Doctor
of Pharmacy

PUERTO RICO

School of Pharmacy
University of Puerto Rico
Medical Sciences Campus
P.O. Box 365067
San Juan, Puerto Rico 00936-5067
(787) 758-2525 ext. 5427, 5400
farmacia.rcm.upr.edu/
Professional Degree Offered: Doctor
of Pharmacy

RHODE ISLAND

College of Pharmacy
University of Rhode Island
Fogarty Hall
41 Lower College Road
Kingston, Rhode Island 02881
(401) 874-5842
www.uri.edu/pharmacy/
Professional Degree Offered: Doctor
of Pharmacy

SOUTH CAROLINA

School of Pharmacy
Presbyterian College
307 North Broad Street
Clinton, South Carolina 29325
(864) 938-3900
www.presby.edu/pharmacy
Professional Degree Offered: Doctor
of Pharmacy

South Carolina College of Pharmacy
MUSC Campus
274 Calhoun Street
MSC 141
Charleston, South Carolina 29425
(843) 792-3740
www.sccp.sc.edu
Professional Degree Offered: Doctor
of Pharmacy

South Carolina College of Pharmacy
USC Campus
715 Sumter Street
Coker Life Science Building
Columbia, South Carolina 29208
(803) 777-4151
www.sccp.sc.edu
Professional Degree Offered: Doctor
of Pharmacy

SOUTH DAKOTA

College of Pharmacy
South Dakota State University
Avera Health and Science Center 133
Box 2202C
Brookings, South Dakota 57007
(605) 688-6197
www.sdstate.edu/pha/index.cfm
Professional Degree Offered: Doctor
of Pharmacy

TENNESSEE

School of Pharmacy
Belmont University
1900 Belmont Boulevard
Nashville, Tennessee 37212-3757
(615) 460-8122
www.belmont.edu/pharmacy
Professional Degree Offered: Doctor
of Pharmacy

Bill Gatton College of Pharmacy
East Tennessee State University
P.O. Box 70414
Johnson City, Tennessee 37614-1704
(423) 439-6338
www.etsu.edu/pharmacy/
Professional Degree Offered: Doctor
of Pharmacy

College of Pharmacy
Lipscomb University
Burton Health Sciences Center, Suite 217
One University Park Drive
Nashville, Tennessee 37204
(615) 966-7160
pharmacy.lipscomb.edu
Professional Degree Offered: Doctor
of Pharmacy

School of Pharmacy
Union University
1050 Union University Drive
Box 1802
Jackson, Tennessee 38305
(731) 661-5910
www.uu.edu/academics/sop
Professional Degree Offered: Docotor
of Pharmacy

College of Pharmacy
University of Tennessee
Health Science Center
847 Monroe Avenue, Suite 226
Memphis, Tennessee 38163
(901) 448-6036
www.uthsc.edu/pharmacy
Professional Degree Offered: Doctor
of Pharmacy

TEXAS

Irma Lerma Rangel College of Pharmacy
Texas A&M Health Science Center
MSC 131, 1010 West Avenue B
Kingsville, Texas 78363
(361) 593-4272
pharmacy.tamhsc.edu
Professional Degree Offered: Doctor
   of Pharmacy

College of Pharmacy and Health Sciences
Texas Southern University
3100 Cleburne Street
Gray Hall, Room 134
Houston, Texas 77004
(713) 313-6700
www.tsu.edu/academics
Professional Degree Offered: Doctor
   of Pharmacy

School of Pharmacy
Texas Tech University Health Sciences Center
1300 Coutler, Suite 2210
Amarillo, Texas 79106
(806) 354-5457
www.ttuhsc.edu/sop/
Professional Degree Offered: Doctor
   of Pharmacy

College of Pharmacy
University of Houston
141 Science & Research Building 2
Houston, Texas 77204-5000
(713) 743-1300
pharmacy.uh.edu/index.php
Professional Degree Offered: Doctor
   of Pharmacy

Feik School of Pharmacy
University of the Incarnate Word
4301 Broadway, CPO #99
San Antonio, Texas 78209-6397
(210) 883-1000
www.uiw.edu/pharmacy/
Professional Degree Offered: Doctor
   of Pharmacy

College of Pharmacy
The University of Texas at Austin
1 University Station, A1900
Austin, Texas 78712-0120
(512) 471-1737
www.utexas.edu/pharmacy/
Professional Degree Offered: Doctor
   of Pharmacy

UTAH

College of Pharmacy
University of Utah
30 South 2000 East
Salt Lake City, Utah 84112-5820
(801) 581-6731
www.pharmacy.utah.edu/
Professional Degree Offered: Doctor
   of Pharmacy

VIRGINIA

Appalachian College of Pharmacy
1060 Dragon Road
Oakwood, Virginia 24631
(276) 498-4190 ext. 5233
www.uacp.org/
Professional Degree Offered: Doctor
   of Pharmacy

School of Pharmacy
Hampton University
Office of Student Affairs/Admissions
Hampton, Virginia 23668
(757) 727-5071
pharm.hamptonu.edu
Professional Degree Offered: Doctor
   of Pharmacy

Bernard J. Dunn School of Pharmacy
Shenandoah University
1460 University Drive
Winchester, Virginia 22601
(540) 678-4340 or (888) 420-7877
www.su.edu
Professional Degree Offered: Doctor
   of Pharmacy

School of Pharmacy
Virginia Commonwealth University/
    MCV Campus
P.O. Box 980581
410 North 12th Street, Room 500
Richmond, Virginia 23298-0581
(804) 828-3000
www.pharmacy.vcu.edu/
Professional Degree Offered: Doctor
    of Pharmacy

WASHINGTON

School of Pharmacy
University of Washington
H-362 Health Sciences Building, Box 357631
Seattle, Washington 98195-7631
(206) 543-6100
depts.washington.edu/pha/
Professional Degree Offered: Doctor
    of Pharmacy

College of Pharmacy
Washington State University
P.O. Box 646510
Pullman, Washington 99164-6510
(509) 335-5901
www.pharmacy.wsu.edu/
Professional Degree Offered: Doctor
    of Pharmacy

WEST VIRGINIA

School of Pharmacy
University of Charleston
2300 MacCorkle Avenue, Southeast
Charleston, West Virginia 25304
(304) 357-4858
pharmacy.ucwv.edu
Professional Degree Offered: Doctor
    of Pharmacy

School of Pharmacy
West Virginia University
P.O. Box 9500
Morgantown, West Virginia 26506-9500
(304) 293-5101
www.hsc.wvu.edu/sop/
Professional Degree Offered: Doctor
    of Pharmacy

WISCONSIN

School of Pharmacy
Concordia University
12800 North Lake Shore Drive
Mequon, Wisconsin 53097-2402
(262) 243-5700
www.cuw.edu/programs/pharmacy/index.html
Professional Degree Offered: Doctor
    of Pharmacy

School of Pharmacy
University of Wisconsin—Madison
777 Highland Avenue
Madison, Wisconsin 53705-2222
(608) 262-6234
www.pharmacy.wisc.edu/
Professional Degree Offered: Doctor
    of Pharmacy

WYOMING

School of Pharmacy
University of Wyoming
Health Sciences Center
Department 3375
1000 East University Avenue
Laramie, Wyoming 82071
(307) 766-6120
www.uwyo.edu/Pharmacy/
Professional Degree Offered: Doctor
    of Pharmacy

Admission Committees

The individuals who wrote the "Admission Committees" and the "Interview Process" sections of this book have served on pharmacy school admission committees for several years. Based on their experiences, they have summarized their observations of students who were successful in being accepted into a college/school of pharmacy. The following describes the purpose of the admission committee and provides tips to successfully guide you through the admission process.

The purpose of the admission committee for a pharmacy school is to select the most qualified students to enter the program. The phrase "most qualified student" will have a slightly different interpretation by each committee and may vary slightly within an institution from year to year. As soon as possible, contact the institutions in which you are interested and request materials regarding application requirements. Much of this data may be available on the school's website, and therefore it is important to review materials most schools make available on the Internet. By reviewing these materials you should be able to determine not only the requirements for the institution, but which factors are utilized to select students for admission.

The committees will use various sources of information and mechanisms to compare students to make selection decisions. You should make sure that the information requested is provided for the committee. If you have a special interest, ability, or experience that you think would be helpful in your application, include a letter or other supporting documentation in the materials you submit to the institution(s) for the committee to consider.

As important as it is for you to do well academically and to take the required courses, the practice of pharmacy requires various skills and talents that you may develop and enhance prior to attending a pharmacy school. Some of these areas include:

- Work Experience
- Verbal and Written Communication Skills
- Community Involvement/Leadership
- Entrepreneurial Ability

Some institutions will request information regarding the activities listed above as part of the applications, others may rely on recommendations to provide this information. More and more institutions are utilizing a personal interview as part of the application process to give the student a chance to present information regarding his or her personal and academic background. You should determine how to best develop and exhibit your skills in these areas, and also how to communicate this information to the pharmacy college(s)/school(s). If your current school has a career center that offers practice interviews, take advantage of that opportunity to optimize your interview skills.

Work experience provides the student with a background about the workplace in general. It also gives students a chance to develop good work habits and communication skills. Work experience in the profession of pharmacy will be an excellent way for you to understand what pharmacy is about and whether your interests and skills are compatible. Also, you will be able to find out more information about the variety of career opportunities that exist in the practice of pharmacy. Work

TIP

Provide additional information that you think is important for the committee to understand your interest in pharmacy and their program in particular.

experience in pharmacy is great, but other jobs can also be supportive and provide information about a student's interests and abilities. Work in a doctor's office, a health clinic, or hospital setting should provide the student with a background in health care issues, contact with patients, and a chance to see various health care professionals in action. Additionally, seemingly unrelated jobs in retail or food services still provide a medium for the student to develop good work skills, communication skills, and the ability to work with people. No matter what work experience you have, try to see what aspects of that job might apply to your activities as a pharmacist or pharmacy student. Make sure to communicate this effectively to the admission committee.

Communication skills are important in all aspects of a pharmacy. Students and pharmacists must be able to communicate effectively with a wide range of people. Also, they must be able to communicate about potentially complex subject matter in a manner that is effective for their audience, whether it be a patient, another student, a professor or other health care professional. Additionally, the ability to listen effectively is just as important as the ability to communicate.

Community involvement is a way for the admission committee to determine more about the character of an applicant. The practice of pharmacy requires that a person be empathetic to the needs of the patient or other professional contact. This means that a pharmacist can be most effective when he or she can "put him- or herself in the other's shoes." By showing a history of participation in organizations that show compassion by assisting others, you may be more likely to have the desired character to practice effectively and ethically. It is suggested that you show a history of participation in these types of activities, not just recent participation in one or two events to have something to place on an application or state in an interview. Make sure that you can talk about the type of activities or events you have been involved in, not just list organizations or events.

Entrepreneurship is the interest in new opportunities—not only business ventures, but also professional development and new ways of doing things. Pharmacy, like most professions, will go through various changes throughout one's career, and the ability and interest to pursue new avenues of practice assures that one will continue to be competent and competitive in practice. A committee might assess an applicant's entrepreneurial abilities through questions in the interview such as "tell me about a project you instituted or carried out with others." By asking such a question, the committee might be looking for creativity, leadership skills, and motivation.

It is important to consider the composition of the admission committee. Committees may consist of any combination of faculty members, pharmacists, non-pharmacists, alumni members, and administrative members. Be sure to think in terms of what that type of individual would want to know about you that will help them realize you will be a good pharmacy student and practitioner.

Not all students will have experience or strong backgrounds in each of the areas mentioned; however, you want to have a good mixture of skills and talents. Don't go out and try to "check-off all the boxes" just to satisfy the committee. It is important that you represent yourself completely and honestly to the committee so that your interest can best be served and the committee can assess not only what you bring to the program, but how the program will benefit your development as a pharmacist.

The Interview Process

Most schools require an interview as part of the admission process. The structure and goals of this process will vary between programs. This general information regarding interviews is meant to help you have a better idea of what to expect, and therefore be more effective in communicating your abilities and desires to the interviewers. Even if a program does not require an interview, you may have the opportunity in your contact with an institution to utilize these points to enhance your application process. Either way, one of the most positive benefits of preparing yourself for an interview is that it gives you a structured assessment of your strengths, weaknesses, and professional goals. By quantifying these at this critical time in your career, you will be sure of your goals and motivation for your chosen career path.

There are many texts providing copious information on how interviews are structured and can prepare you for this event. Most of these address the pursuit of a job in your chosen field. This fact makes their recommendations a bit more structured than might be appropriate for an academic interview for a position in a professional program. Overall, the committee or interviewer is not looking for one right person for the job. They look for a wide range of backgrounds and interests that will not only assure the students success in a rigorous academic program, but will also provide support for a variety of practice settings. Not everyone will work in a direct patient care environment for his or her whole career. As important as patient empathy is to a health care professional, some are going to be better than others and some will work in an area where this skill is not the most important one required on a case-by-case basis. There is room for diversity in pharmacy programs in every sense of the word. Thus, interviewers may evaluate candidates on a range of criteria including communication skills, critical thinking, maturity, and motivation. Just as interviewees will vary, so will the interviewers. Some will be more skilled than others and some may look at the applicant in terms of their own career choices. It is important for you to try and listen to the interviewer, and determine what is meant by the question being asked and how you should best relate your own feelings while being sensitive to the setting and the audience. One thing that comes through in the interview texts reviewed is that honesty is the best policy. If you feel that you have to compromise your interests to say what the interviewer wants to hear, you should review your choice of this institution or career pursuit.

TIP

Get as much information as possible about the program and have some good questions ready (for example, a question about points that were brought up by committee members). This shows that you are "thinking on your feet."

Overall, the greatest benefit to be gained by the interview is for the committee to see the sincerity of the interest you have in the program and a career in pharmacy. Also, it is important that you receive positive reinforcement of your goals and helpful information from the institution administering the interview.

Based on our experience, here are three of the most common topics discussed during a pharmacy application interview:

- Professional Background
- Academic Background
- Personal Background

PROFESSIONAL BACKGROUND

Basically, you have been preparing all of your life for the interview. However, you should spend some significant time before the interview making an "inventory" of your answer to the question "why pharmacy?" Here are some self-assessment questions to help prepare you for this type of discussion.

- Why have you chosen pharmacy as a career path? When did you first consider pharmacy as a career?

- Do you know anyone who is a pharmacist?

- What other careers did you consider?

- What steps have you taken to learn more about pharmacy as a profession?

- Who influenced your choice of career, and how (actively or through example)?

- Who would you consider to be your mentor? Why?

- What type of jobs have you held? What have been your likes and dislikes about those jobs? Have these jobs influenced your decision to pursue pharmacy as a career?

- What other careers or academic pursuits interest you?

- What jobs are available to pharmacists? What type of career in pharmacy interests you most?

- What will you do if you are not admitted into a school or college of pharmacy?

- Have you held any leadership positions such as in an organization or on a sports team?

- What hobbies or extracurricular activities are you involved in?

- What are your opinions on professional and community service?

- How would you describe yourself? What are your strengths and weaknesses?

- What is the most challenging personal situation you have faced? How did you cope?

- Can you provide an example of a situation in which you faced a moral or ethical dilemma? How did you confront or resolve this situation?

Pointer

Avoid yes or no answers to questions posed to you, as well as one-line answers.

Any student can come up with answers to these types of questions. Ideally, there is no right or wrong answer. What the committee should be looking for is the background information that you relate to support your answers. Understand that any answer to the questions, such as the ones above, should include an implicit explanation of why or how you arrived at that decision. This is the best way to relate to the committee the maturity of your decision-making process and career interest. It also helps minimize the problem with a difficult interviewer who may be looking for your answer to match his or her choices. If you have a good explanation of how you arrived at that decision, it validates your answer.

Be aware of the professional questions being posed to you as an applicant. The interviewers have been in their profession a long time and often can only relate to subject matter that they have come to accept as common knowledge. An example of a question being asked about a professional setting scenario is—"What would you do if a patient comes in and needs a refill for so and so and you have no refills indicated on the prescription?" The possible answers are myriad, and often the question is asked of a student who has retail pharmacy experience and has observed a pharmacist handle this situation many times. If you do not have any experience or any idea of how to answer this question, consider explaining your lack of experience in that area and that this is the type of thing you know training in the professional program will provide. Then, try to relate the question to something you are more familiar with. For example, you might respond, "It sounds like this is a question that deals with utilizing appropriate people skills and ethical behavior on the part of the pharmacist; let me tell you about a situation that I dealt with in a job where we had an employee who was involved in stealing. . . ." This allows you to put the question on your own terms and to talk about something about which you are familiar. Follow-up your description with a question as to whether that scenario related sufficiently to the professional question posed by the interviewer(s).

Ideally, you will have some pharmacy or related experiences to utilize in the interview. This not only shows your competency in areas that you have been trained, but also, that you are making your decision regarding a career choice based on personal experience. Pharmacy jobs for pre-pharmacy students can be difficult to obtain, particularly if you are in an area with a high concentration of pharmacy students. Often, students first think of retail because this practice option is so visible, but don't neglect opportunities in hospitals, clinics, long-term care facilities and many other areas where pharmacists or other healthcare professionals have the opportunity to work with interested students. Hopefully you started working in a related area as early as high school. In doing this, you may have had the opportunity to advance to a position which provides direct contact with the operation of a pharmacy. If you are unable to obtain a job in a pharmacy, you may be able to obtain relevant experience by shadowing pharmacists or volunteering in health care settings that provide pharmacy services.

ACADEMIC BACKGROUND

The nature of academic performance reported to the institution you are applying to is very quantitative. All require that transcripts be provided and often calculate a single grade point average (GPA) for ranking the applicant pool. Some interviews may be conducted "blind" in that the interviewers do not have access to the student's credentials prior to the interview. In this case, you may still bring this information into the process if they refer to your performance or discuss this as part of the interview. If academic success is a strong point in your background, by all means, include it in your discussions. Most interviewers will have had the chance to review a student's admission file before and during the interview. It is important that all available materials, transcripts, and other required information have been provided and that your application is as complete as possible. Also, the committee may ask specific questions regarding courses that you did especially well in or faced challenges. Don't try to ignore bad academic events or specific grades. Address them honestly to the committee and explain any extenuating circumstances which may have adversely affected performance in the short term. In most circumstances, you should avoid blaming the instructor in a course; it is important to take responsibility for your own performance. Point out improvements or trends which show improved effort or understanding of vital material. Talk about additional courses that you may have taken which, even though not required, might provide a benefit during the pharmacy program or in professional practice. Even courses in business, psychology, writing or education can be very applicable and helpful in one's career pursuit. Usually, high school grades or performance are not an issue, but if you had a particularly good experience in a class or with a teacher who was pivotal in your career choice or academic performance, it would be good to include this in your discussion.

Be aware of the pre-pharmacy requirements for the program and discuss how you plan to complete any remaining courses in time to begin the professional program in the desired term. If you have courses for which you hope to receive credit toward pharmacy prerequisites, check that out with the admission office before the interview. Often the interviewers are faculty who, though familiar with the requirements of the program, are not the ones to make transfer credit decisions. Thus, questions concerning transfer credit should be addressed to the admissions office.

Often you will be asked if you have applied to other pharmacy or academic programs. Again, be honest and discuss other plans you have or pursuits you have considered. Considering other programs or even other academic pursuits, which are based on the interests you have stated in the interview, should be a positive factor and show that you are a serious and mature student. However, if you detect that the interviewers feel some competitiveness toward another pharmacy program which you are considering, tell them that this shows how serious you are about your pursuit of a career in pharmacy. We believe it is a good idea to consider and apply to any program you feel you could attend and get the education that will allow you to pursue your career goals.

TIP

Don't just state that you were a member of a particular organization. Discuss what you did in it to show your leadership abilities or interest in providing service to the community.

PERSONAL BACKGROUND

The interview is a chance to put some "personality" into your application. The process prior to the time of the interview is very quantitative, with GPAs and PCAT scores often being the primary consideration that allowed you an interview. It's your responsibility to make the impression on the interviewers that you will do well in their institution and will be the type of pharmacist that they want to represent their institution. Talk not only about the experiences in your background that led you to pharmacy, but also talk about the experiences that helped you to develop a personality that will support you through the academic program and as a pharmacist. Include information about outside activities, sports, and hobbies. Include involvement in organizations in addition to academic pursuits, such as membership in service groups. Membership in honor societies should be mentioned; discuss activities or opportunities that were provided during your membership, not just that you were a member because of your grades or other academic qualities.

The various background areas overlap, each one providing important information in how you got to where you are and what type of student and person you are. Therefore, it is natural that the relationship between academics, professional pursuits, and personality will be extensions of each other.

ON-SITE ESSAY

Some schools may require that you complete an essay during your interview at the school/college. Examples of possible essay topics include:

- What are two (2) messages or themes about responsibility for personal health care and well being that you feel are important to advance to American teenagers today?
- What one or two areas of health maintenance and disease treatment should U.S. scientific research efforts and resources be directed toward during the next 10 years?
- What are some knowledge or skill requirements essential for practitioners in today's community and environment? Why?

The length of the essay and the time allotted for completion of the essay will vary by school/college. Essay evaluation criteria may include use of language, grammar, punctuation, clarity, and cohesiveness. We recommend that you take a few minutes at the beginning of the essay-writing session to prepare an outline to help guide your writing process. We also recommend that you save a few minutes at the end of the essay-writing session to review and edit your essay as necessary. Other general essay-writing tips can be found in Chapter 9.

CONCLUSION OF THE INTERVIEW

At the end of the interview make sure you summarize your interest in the program and "wrap-up" any issues regarding remaining coursework. State your plans for future academic terms, and make sure you know what the next step will be and when you can expect to hear from the committee regarding the results of your application.

TIPS FOR SUCCESSFUL INTERVIEWING

- Arrive on time for the interview. Arriving late may send the message that the interview is not a priority to you.

- Try not to appear nervous. Arriving to the interview early will give you the opportunity to adjust to the environment and may decrease your anxiety.

- Dress professionally.

- Be courteous.

- Be positive, friendly, and smile.

- Answer all questions as completely as possible.

- Speak clearly.

- Make eye contact with the interviewers.

- Don't exhibit unnecessary movements.

- Educate yourself on the institution.

- If you have questions, ask if there is enough time to ask your questions. If so, ask questions.

- If you have any additional materials that you want the committee to review, bring them with you to the interview.

- Listen attentively and learn from the interview. The information exchange should be a two-way process.

- Bring a pen and notebook to the interview. Have a list of questions that you may want to ask and make notes as appropriate.

- Don't limit yourself to one or two word answers.

Graduate Degrees in Pharmacy

Master of Science (M.S.) and Doctor of Philosophy (Ph.D.) degrees are available for pharmacy disciplines including, but not limited to, medicinal chemistry, pharmaceutics, pharmacology, pharmacy care administration, and toxicology. For more information regarding graduate programs, you should contact the specific college or school of pharmacy in which you are interested.

Postgraduate Training: Residencies and Fellowships

A graduate of a college or school of pharmacy may decide to pursue postgraduate training in a specific area of pharmacy practice or pharmacy research (see the later section, entitled "Residency and Fellowship Programs: Areas of Pharmacy Practice and Research"). Residencies and fellowships are two distinct types of postgraduate training programs. General requirements for an applicant seeking a residency or fellowship include graduating from an accredited college or school of pharmacy and an interest in and aptitude for advanced training in pharmacy. A resident or fellow receives a stipend plus benefits (insurance, vacation, etc.). The amount of the stipend and the specific benefits vary according to the individual program.

RESIDENCIES

A residency is an organized, directed postgraduate training program in a defined area of pharmacy practice. Residencies are typically one year in duration; however, some may be longer. The primary goal of a residency is to train pharmacists in a specific area of pharmacy practice. The objective of a residency is to develop competent practitioners who are able to provide pharmacy services such as clinical, drug information, pharmacotherapeutic dosing and monitoring, and administration.

A pharmacy practice residency is a general residency in pharmacy practice. In addition to pharmacy practice residencies, a host of specialized residencies exists. A specialized residency focuses on a particular niche of pharmacy practice; pediatric pharmacy, psychiatric pharmacy, and nuclear pharmacy are all examples of specialized residencies. Whether the residency is a pharmacy practice residency or a specialty residency, training typically involves structured rotations within the pharmacy department as well as medical rotations with physicians and other health care professionals. The practice experiences of residents are closely directed and evaluated by qualified practitioner-preceptors who are trained in particular areas of pharmacy practice.

The American Society of Health-System Pharmacists is the accrediting body for residencies. To obtain a list of postgraduate pharmacy practice residency programs, write to or visit:

American Society of Health-System Pharmacists
7272 Wisconsin Avenue
Bethesda, MD 20814
accred.ashp.org

FELLOWSHIPS

A fellowship is a directed, highly individualized postgraduate program, typically two years in duration, that is designed to prepare the participant to become an independent researcher. The primary goal of a fellowship is to develop competency in scientific pharmacy research. A fellow works under the close direction and instruction of a qualified researcher-preceptor. Many fellowships are affiliated with a college or school of pharmacy. To obtain a list of postgraduate fellowship programs, you can write to or visit:

American College of Clinical Pharmacy
13000 W. 87th St. Parkway
Lenexa, Kansas 66215-4530
www.accp.com

RESIDENCY AND FELLOWSHIP PROGRAMS: AREAS OF PHARMACY PRACTICE AND RESEARCH

Administration
Ambulatory Care
Cardiology
Clinical Informatics
Clinical Pharmaceutical Sciences
Clinical Pharmacology
Community Pharmacy
Critical Care
Drug Development
Drug Information
Emergency Medicine
Endocrinology
Family Medicine
Geriatrics
HIV Pharmacy
Hospice
Immunology
Infectious Disease
Internal Medicine
Managed Care
Nephrology
Neurology
Nuclear Pharmacy

Nutrition
Obstetrics-Gynecology
Oncology
Outcomes Research
Pain Management
Patient Safety
Pediatrics
Pharmacoeconomics
Pharmacoepidemiology
Pharmacogenomics
Pharmacokinetics
Pharmacometrics
Pharmacotherapy
Pharmacy Practice
Primary Care
Psychopharmacy
Pulmonary
Rheumatology
Toxicology
Translational Research
Transplantation
Women's Health

The PCAT

WHAT IS THE PCAT?

The Pharmacy College Admission Test (PCAT) is a national examination developed by PsychCorp, a brand of Pearson Education, Inc. The PCAT was developed to provide admission committees of pharmacy schools with comparable information about the academic abilities of applicants in six topic areas: verbal ability, reading comprehension, chemistry, biology, quantitative ability (math), and writing.

The exam consists of 240 multiple-choice questions and two essay topics. The stem portion of each multiple-choice question may be presented as a question, partial statement, or math equation followed by four possible answers. Only one answer is correct. Often the other choices are distractors, may contain errors, do not apply to the question, or may not be the best answer to the question. Often the distractors are taken from the same content area of study as the correct answer, so it is important to recognize specific facts, not just be familiar with topics. The PCAT score is calculated from the number of correct answers. There is NO penalty for guessing, so candidates should not leave any answers blank.

The first writing section of the PCAT was added for the 2005–2006 application cycle, and a second writing section was added beginning with the 2007–2008 application cycle. Currently, only one of the essays is graded and results reported (the other writing section is considered experimental).

According to Pearson (as posted on the PCAT website, *www.pcatweb.info*, in August 2010), as of July 2011, all candidates will take the PCAT via computer. The computer-based PCAT is the same as the paper-based PCAT in terms of content, subtests, scoring, and reporting. Refer to the PCAT website, *www.pcatweb.info*, for further details.

PCAT Contents

The following is a description of the PCAT's six scoring sections:

- **Verbal Ability.** This section consists of 48 word-pairing analogies and sentence completion questions. Thirty minutes are given to complete this section.
- **Biology.** This section consists of 48 general biology, microbiology, and anatomy and physiology questions. Thirty minutes are given to complete this section.
- **Reading Comprehension.** This section consists of six reading passages and 48 questions that test candidates' evaluation, comprehension, and analytical skills. Fifty minutes are given to complete this section.
- **Quantitative Ability.** This section consists of 48 basic math, algebra, pre-calculus, calculus, probability, and statistics questions. No calculators are allowed during the exam. Forty minutes are given to complete this section.

- **Chemistry.** This section consists of 48 general and organic chemistry questions. Some may involve calculations; remember, no calculators are allowed. Thirty minutes are given to complete this section.
- **Writing.** The candidate will be requested to compose two problem-solving essays. Thirty minutes will be given to write each essay.

Usually the PCAT exam includes multiple-choice experimental questions being tested for possible use in future exams. There is no way to know which items are experimental, so candidates will want to do their best to answer each question correctly.

The Exam

PCAT Sections	PCAT Section Subtests/% of Item Types 2011–2012 Cycle	PCAT Section Subtests/% of Item Types 2012–2013 Cycle	Number of Items in Section	Number of Minutes to Complete PCAT Section
1. Verbal Ability	Analogies—60% Sentence Completion—40%	Analogies—60% Sentence Completion—40%	48 Items	30 Minutes
2. Biology	General Biology—60% Microbiology—20% Anatomy & Physiology—20%	General Biology—50% Microbiology—20% Anatomy & Physiology—30%	48 Items	30 Minutes
3. Reading Comprehension	Comprehension—30% Evaluation—30% Analysis—40%	Comprehension—30% Evaluation—30% Analysis—40%	6 Reading Passages & 48 Items	50 Minutes
4. Quantitative Ability	Basic Math—15% Algebra—20% Probability & Statistics—20% Precalculus—22% Calculus—22%	Basic Math—15% Algebra—20% Probability & Statistics—20% Precalculus—22% Calculus—22%	48 Items	40 Minutes
5. Chemistry	General Chemistry—60% Organic Chemistry—40%	General Chemistry—50% Organic Chemistry—32% Basic Biochemistry Processes—18%	48 Items	30 Minutes
6. Writing	Problem Solving Conventions of Language	Problem Solving Conventions of Language	2 Topics	30 Minutes Each

Some slight modifications are being made to the PCAT sections following the 2011–2012 cycle. These differences may be demonstrated by examining the table on page 38 and comparing the Item Types for the 2011–2012 and 2012–2013 cycles. Please check the PCAT website, *www.pcatweb.info,* for the most up-to-date information.

PCAT Scoring

Your score report will include separate scaled scores and percentile scores for each of the five multiple-choice content areas. It will also include a composite scaled score and percentile score for the overall multiple-choice exam. Scaled scores are computed from raw scores for each individual test offering so that results can be compared from one test offering to the next. The scaled scores will range from 200 to 600.

Additionally, a percentile score is computed by distributing your performance in a norm group or pool of candidates. The percentile reported for individual sections and the composite score indicate the percentage of students who scored below you. For example, a 75th percentile score on the biology section indicates that you did better than 75% of the students in the norm group.

You will receive two scores for the writing section: one score for problem solving and one score for conventions of language. The scores for the writing section will be reported as raw scores on a scale of 1 to 5, with 5 representing the highest score possible. These scores will be reported on your individual score report and will be provided to the institutions to which you elected to submit your scores. The writing scores are not included in the composite score as detailed above; this will be discussed further in the Writing Exam section of this guide.

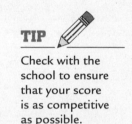

TIP

Check with the school to ensure that your score is as competitive as possible.

The scores used by numerous pharmacy programs in evaluating candidates vary. Some use scaled scores; others use percentiles. Some have minimum scores required in each of the PCAT sections; some use composite scores. Many will use a candidate's highest score on a single attempt if the candidate has taken the test more than once; however, this might not always be the case.

After a candidate has taken the PCAT five times, submission of a written request is required for a sixth test. Candidates registering for more than the fifth time still register online, but they must be prepared to provide documentation explaining the circumstances that require taking the PCAT again. If the requested documentation is not provided, a candidate's registration will be cancelled. Further details on this policy and the type of documentation that may be required can be found on the PCAT website.

When Is the PCAT Offered?

As of July 2011, the PCAT will be administered at Pearson VUE Test Centers on multiple dates. To obtain exact dates, visit the PCAT website at *www.pcatweb.info.* Accommodations may be made for individuals with disabilities. Deadlines for registration for the PCAT are generally approximately six weeks prior to the testing date—onsite, same-day registration is not available.

Fees

For the most current information visit the PCAT website at *www.pcatweb.info*. The following is the PCAT fee as of 2011.

Online Registration Fee $199.00

For more information concerning special fees, visit the PCAT website.

PCAT Information

For more information concerning the PCAT, contact Pearson at the address or phone number below:

Pearson
PSE Customer Relations—PCAT
19500 Bulverde Road
San Antonio, Texas 78259
1-800-622-3231
www.pcatweb.info

In the past, helpful instructional videos on procedures for taking the PCAT have been available at *www.pcatweb.info*. The authors of this guide recommend checking *www.pcatweb.info* to find out if instructional videos regarding computer-based versions of the PCAT have been made available. Additionally, the authors strongly recommend reviewing the PCAT candidate information booklet available at *www.pcatweb.info*.

When Should You Take the PCAT?

Many considerations are involved in the decision of when and how often to take the PCAT. Many colleges/schools of pharmacy do not penalize applicants for taking the test more than once and often use the highest scores. This practice differs from institution to institution, so you will need to check with the college/school that you are interested in attending. In addition, it is strongly recommended that you take the PCAT no later than the fall of the year prior to the semester that you want to begin pharmacy school. This strategy will allow you to retake the PCAT in the winter if desired or necessary.

The ultimate decision of when and how often to take the PCAT is an individualized one and depends on many circumstances, such as when you feel most comfortable taking the test (this may depend on the number of pre-pharmacy courses you have taken). Other factors that may affect your decision are the admissions policy of the pharmacy college or school you wish to attend and your previous PCAT scores.

CHAPTER 3

Strategies to Increase Your Score

PCAT STRATEGIES

When taking the PCAT, work at a comfortable pace but keep in mind that there is a time limit for each section. Be sure to answer every question. Your total PCAT score and the score you receive on each section of the test (excluding the PCAT essay) reflect the number of correct answers only. Some tests penalize for guessing by subtracting the number of wrong answers from the number of correct answers; with the PCAT, however, this is not the case. Although guesses are not likely to make much difference in your scores, you shouldn't ignore this chance to avoid the total loss of points from unanswered questions.

The PCAT is divided into six sections (please note, two essays are required to complete the writing section of the PCAT). Three sections are specifically related to coursework covered in the pre-pharmacy curriculum: chemistry, biology, and mathematics. Two sections are more comprehensive in nature and measure skills acquired through lifelong learning: verbal ability and reading comprehension. Because the verbal ability and reading comprehension sections assess skills acquired over a long period of time, they tend to be more difficult to study for in advance. The essays are a combination of comprehensive learning, life experiences, and skills potentially obtained during your pre-pharmacy work.

When you take the practice PCAT tests in this book and the actual PCAT test, make sure to keep track of the time allotted for each test section. Pace yourself and work quickly but calmly through all the questions. Although you may be forced to guess on some questions, there is a chance that some of your guesses will be correct.

FIFTEEN PRESCRIPTIONS TO INCREASE YOUR SCORE

The first section of this chapter discussed general PCAT strategies. In this section you are given fifteen "prescriptions" to improve your PCAT test scores. Students who have taken the PCAT and employed these test-taking tactics have found them quite useful:

- **Rx 1.** Get an adequate amount of sleep the night before the test.
- **Rx 2.** Allow yourself plenty of time to get to the testing site.
- **Rx 3.** Bring an accurate watch.

Remember

On the PCAT, your score is computed from the number of correct answers only. You are NOT penalized for guessing.

- **Rx 4.** Bring proper identification (e.g., driver's license).
- **Rx 5.** Wear comfortable clothes.
- **Rx 6.** Know what to expect. After studying this preparation manual, you will be familiar with the types of questions that may appear on the PCAT.
- **Rx 7.** Read and memorize the directions for each question type or section.
- **Rx 8.** Pace yourself. Work within the time restriction.
- **Rx 9.** Look at all the possible answers before making your final choice.
- **Rx 10.** Eliminate as many wrong answers as possible.
- **Rx 11.** Answer every question.
- **Rx 12.** In preparing for the verbal ability section, consider reviewing a vocabulary study manual.
- **Rx 13.** In the reading comprehension section, when asked to find the main idea, be sure to check the opening and summary sentences of the passage.
- **Rx 14.** You cannot use a calculator on the PCAT; therefore, rounding numbers to do the math problems accurately and quickly may be beneficial.
- **Rx 15.** Do not bring cell phones and other electronic devices to the PCAT as they are not allowed in the testing area. Your PCAT score will be cancelled if you break this rule.

CHAPTER 4

Verbal Ability Review and Practice

TIPS FOR THE VERBAL ABILITY SECTION

The verbal ability section of the PCAT is designed to test your knowledge of words (vocabulary) and the relationships between them by using sentence completion and analogy-type questions. This section consists of approximately 48 questions, with about 60% involving analogies and 40% involving sentence completion. You will have 30 minutes to complete the verbal ability section. To study for the verbal ability section, you can use texts designed to help you increase your "word power" or vocabulary. Studying material on the roots of words and on prefixes and suffixes may also help you prepare for this section of the PCAT.

Analogy questions test your understanding of how paired vocabulary words and ideas relate to each other. They are expressed as A : B :: C : D. In words, A is to B as C is to D; for example, meow is to cat as bark is to dog. The notion of a proportion should be familiar to you from mathematics. In an analogy, however, the proportion is a logical or verbal one.

There are a number of different kinds of analogy relationships, including cause and effect, part to whole, part to part, action to object, and analogies based on antonyms (words with the opposite meaning) or synonyms (words with the same or nearly the same meaning), purpose or use, place, association, sequence or time, characteristic, degree, and measurement; there are even grammatical analogies. It is not necessary for you to memorize all the types of analogies, but becoming familiar with some of the main types can help you identify them and answer the questions on the analogy section more quickly. You should first identify the part of speech represented by the words in the analogy; then look for that part of speech among the answer selections. The practice questions and answers in this chapter will demonstrate and explain the different types of analogies and provide insight into formulating a correct answer. For a complete survey of analogies, you may wish to consult *Barron's Miller Analogies Test.*

Once you have spent some time preparing yourself by studying vocabulary reviews and "word power" exercises and are ready to test your ability in this area, complete the verbal ability questions in this book. The explanatory answers for the analogy questions are designed to help you become familiar with the various types of analogies; therefore, you should read them carefully.

TIP

Be sure to familiarize yourself with the different kinds of analogy relationships.

Sentence completion questions are also included in the verbal section of the PCAT. You will be given a sentence in which either one word or two words will be omitted. You will be asked to choose which of the four answer choices provided best completes the sentence based on sentence context and reading comprehension. There will be only one correct response. The correct utilization of vocabulary skills, logic, grammar, and sentence tone and style will help you to eliminate the incorrect responses, allowing you to choose the answer that makes the most sense and best completes the sentence. In sentences that have two, or double, blanks, the correct answer will provide the best word choices for BOTH blanks. Even if you are unfamiliar with one or more of the words listed in the answer choices or the subject base of the sentence, by using clues embedded in the sentence you should still be able to choose the word or words that correctly complete the sentence. Thus, the sentence fragment may contain clues to help you eliminate unfamiliar words in the answers listed so that you may choose the correct answer.

Answer Sheet

VERBAL ABILITY

1 Ⓐ Ⓑ Ⓒ Ⓓ		26 Ⓐ Ⓑ Ⓒ Ⓓ
2 Ⓐ Ⓑ Ⓒ Ⓓ		27 Ⓐ Ⓑ Ⓒ Ⓓ
3 Ⓐ Ⓑ Ⓒ Ⓓ		28 Ⓐ Ⓑ Ⓒ Ⓓ
4 Ⓐ Ⓑ Ⓒ Ⓓ		29 Ⓐ Ⓑ Ⓒ Ⓓ
5 Ⓐ Ⓑ Ⓒ Ⓓ		30 Ⓐ Ⓑ Ⓒ Ⓓ
6 Ⓐ Ⓑ Ⓒ Ⓓ		31 Ⓐ Ⓑ Ⓒ Ⓓ
7 Ⓐ Ⓑ Ⓒ Ⓓ		32 Ⓐ Ⓑ Ⓒ Ⓓ
8 Ⓐ Ⓑ Ⓒ Ⓓ		33 Ⓐ Ⓑ Ⓒ Ⓓ
9 Ⓐ Ⓑ Ⓒ Ⓓ		34 Ⓐ Ⓑ Ⓒ Ⓓ
10 Ⓐ Ⓑ Ⓒ Ⓓ		35 Ⓐ Ⓑ Ⓒ Ⓓ
11 Ⓐ Ⓑ Ⓒ Ⓓ		36 Ⓐ Ⓑ Ⓒ Ⓓ
12 Ⓐ Ⓑ Ⓒ Ⓓ		37 Ⓐ Ⓑ Ⓒ Ⓓ
13 Ⓐ Ⓑ Ⓒ Ⓓ		38 Ⓐ Ⓑ Ⓒ Ⓓ
14 Ⓐ Ⓑ Ⓒ Ⓓ		39 Ⓐ Ⓑ Ⓒ Ⓓ
15 Ⓐ Ⓑ Ⓒ Ⓓ		40 Ⓐ Ⓑ Ⓒ Ⓓ
16 Ⓐ Ⓑ Ⓒ Ⓓ		41 Ⓐ Ⓑ Ⓒ Ⓓ
17 Ⓐ Ⓑ Ⓒ Ⓓ		42 Ⓐ Ⓑ Ⓒ Ⓓ
18 Ⓐ Ⓑ Ⓒ Ⓓ		43 Ⓐ Ⓑ Ⓒ Ⓓ
19 Ⓐ Ⓑ Ⓒ Ⓓ		44 Ⓐ Ⓑ Ⓒ Ⓓ
20 Ⓐ Ⓑ Ⓒ Ⓓ		45 Ⓐ Ⓑ Ⓒ Ⓓ
21 Ⓐ Ⓑ Ⓒ Ⓓ		46 Ⓐ Ⓑ Ⓒ Ⓓ
22 Ⓐ Ⓑ Ⓒ Ⓓ		47 Ⓐ Ⓑ Ⓒ Ⓓ
23 Ⓐ Ⓑ Ⓒ Ⓓ		48 Ⓐ Ⓑ Ⓒ Ⓓ
24 Ⓐ Ⓑ Ⓒ Ⓓ		49 Ⓐ Ⓑ Ⓒ Ⓓ
25 Ⓐ Ⓑ Ⓒ Ⓓ		50 Ⓐ Ⓑ Ⓒ Ⓓ

Practice Questions

50 Questions

ANALOGIES (25 QUESTIONS)

Directions: Choose the word that **best** completes the analogy.

1. SPIDER : WEB :: BIRD :

   (A) Deck
   (B) Wood
   (C) Nest ✓
   (D) Wing

2. PHARMACIST : PATIENT :: TEACHER :

   (A) Student ✓
   (B) Prescription
   (C) Education
   (D) Textbook

3. POLYPS : CORAL :: BEES :

   (A) Flowers
   (B) Colony
   (C) Hive
   (D) Honey ✓

4. HYPNOSIS : TRANCE :: STROKE :

   (A) Embolism
   (B) Paralysis ✓
   (C) Speech
   (D) Rehabilitation

5. HUMIDITY : SWAMP :: ARIDITY :

   (A) Ocean
   (B) Air conditioning
   (C) Sea level
   (D) Desert ✓

6. RIND : ORANGE :: BARK :

   (A) Tree ✓
   (B) Dog
   (C) Forest
   (D) Leaves

7. BIKINI : MARSHALL :: SAINT THOMAS :

   (A) Virgin ✓
   (B) Atlantic
   (C) Tourism
   (D) Haiti

8. DENTIST : DRILL :: ASTRONOMER :

   (A) Milky Way
   (B) Galaxies
   (C) Telescope ✓
   (D) Magnification

9. RED : RUDDY :: METAL :

   (A) Element
   (B) Metallic ✓
   (C) Strength
   (D) Gray

10. BOTANIST : PLANTS :: NEUROBIOLOGIST :

    (A) Neurotes
    (B) Experiment
    (C) Data
    (D) Neurotransmitter ✓

11. MILK : CASEIN :: WHEAT :

    (A) Bread
    (B) Carbohydrate
    (C) Gluten ✓
    (D) Grain

12. GANGES : INDIA :: MISSISSIPPI :

    (A) United States ✓
    (B) Continent
    (C) State
    (D) Delta

13. TRANSPARENT : CLEAR :: OPAQUE :

    (A) White
    (B) Heavy
    (C) Muddy ✓
    (D) Translucent

14. ABSTAIN : INDULGE :: LOOSEN :

    (A) Find
    (B) Tighten ✓
    (C) Yield
    (D) Corrupt

15. AIRPLANE : HANGAR :: AUTOMOBILE :

    (A) Garage ✓
    (B) Travel
    (C) Flight
    (D) Passenger

16. GRAIN : WOOD :: LUSTER :

    (A) Surface
    (B) Value
    (C) Diamond ✓
    (D) Shine

17. VIOLINS : ORCHESTRA :: PUPILS :

    (A) Symphony
    (B) Chorus
    (C) Conductor
    (D) Class ✓

18. ANACONDA : BOA :: TENNIS :

    (A) Racquet
    (B) Sport ✓
    (C) Court
    (D) Serve

19. LENS : MICROSCOPE :: HELMET :

    (A) Weapon
    (B) Battle
    (C) Armor ✓
    (D) Head

20. BERMUDA : WEST ATLANTIC :: MADAGASCAR :

    (A) Straits of Gibraltar
    (B) Outer Hebrides
    (C) Pacific
    (D) West Indian ✓

21. HAS FLOWN : WILL FLY :: HAS SHOWN :

    (A) Will show
    (B) Has been shown
    (C) Will be shown
    (D) Has fled

22. SINGER : MICROPHONE :: PHYSICIAN :

    (A) Hippocratic Oath
    (B) Stethoscope
    (C) Nurse
    (D) Surgery

23. BANYAN : TREE :: CHRYSANTHEMUM :

    (A) Stem
    (B) India
    (C) Japan
    (D) Flower

24. BOOLEAN : ALGEBRA :: EUCLIDEAN :

    (A) Smorgasbord
    (B) Geometry
    (C) Ghost
    (D) Gambling

25. MUZZLE : DOG :: CEREBELLUM :

    (A) Brain
    (B) Reticular activating system
    (C) Amygdala
    (D) Electrode

SENTENCE COMPLETIONS (25 QUESTIONS)

Directions: Select the word or set of words that makes the most sense when inserted into the sentence and that best fits the meaning of the sentence as a whole.

26. The teacher was _____ with the student, as the student was not honest or trustworthy.

    (A) impartial
    (B) understanding
    (C) disenchanted
    (D) elated

27. A _____ glance tends to overlook very important details.

    (A) versatile
    (B) cursory ✓
    (C) charitable
    (D) stable

28. Before giving an _____ solution, it is necessary to check the medication and dose against the patient's chart.

    (A) ambiguous
    (B) unlikely
    (C) eclectic
    (D) intravenous

29. _____ to an antibiotic means that a microorganism that was formerly _____ to the antibiotic is no longer affected by it.

    (A) Resistance; susceptible
    (B) Synergy; inhibited
    (C) Inhibition; nosocomial
    (D) Suicidal; caustic

30. Around strangers Karen may seem quiet and _____, but once she is around friends and family she is quite _____.

    (A) impartial; jaded
    (B) lurid; malleable
    (C) introverted; loquacious
    (D) impious; hostile

31. The next circus performer's act was very _____ because he had to juggle three balls while _____ balancing himself on a tightrope.

    (A) fickle; inadvertently
    (B) complicated; simultaneously
    (C) sufficient; hypothetically
    (D) germane; gradually

32. Her pride in her accomplishment was _____; she had just won a prestigious award.

    (A) justified
    (B) puzzling
    (C) cautious
    (D) damaged

33. We stood in _____ at how we were so easily dwarfed by the _____ sequoia trees.

    (A) bewilderment; versatile ✓
    (B) validation; execrable
    (C) remorse; elusive
    (D) veneration; gargantuan

34. The _____ left large sums of money in his will to be donated to many charitable foundations.

    (A) psychologist
    (B) connoisseur
    (C) philanthropist
    (D) sophisticate

35. While making the icing for the cake, we ran out of blue food coloring, so we had to _____ and use green instead.

    (A) implicate
    (B) substitute
    (C) effervesce
    (D) disseminate

36. Homeostasis is the maintenance of a _____ environment within the body.

    (A) different
    (B) sensitive
    (C) constant
    (D) disorganized

37. Don't be too _____ about the final results of the experiment; something _____ could happen and ruin the project like the test tube falling and shattering on the ground.

    (A) anxious; irreverent
    (B) predisposed; eclectic
    (C) dogmatic; ulterior
    (D) sanguine; unanticipated

38. As a sign of _____, one of the parties scheduled a peaceful conference where each party could negotiate and both reach an agreement.

    (A) hostility
    (B) indifference
    (C) prosperity
    (D) diplomacy

39. The wing of an eagle and the human arm are _____ structures.
    They differ in function but their anatomy is _____.

    (A) homologous; related
    (B) heterogeneous; stringent
    (C) benign; significant
    (D) simple; blatant

40. After reviewing the protocol from 20 years ago, we determined that it was
    _____ and that it needed to be revised and updated.

    (A) theoretical
    (B) intangible
    (C) beneficial
    (D) antiquated

41. The cerebrum, which is the largest portion of the brain, is divided into two
    _____.

    (A) hemispheres
    (B) communities
    (C) productions
    (D) concourses

42. When going from an area of bright sunlight into a dark room, the pupils
    of your eyes must dilate in order for you to _____ to your changed
    environment.

    (A) obscure
    (B) differentiate
    (C) adapt
    (D) stimulate

43. One way in which hormones may be _____ from the blood is by
    excretion into urine or bile.

    (A) celebrated
    (B) eliminated
    (C) replenished
    (D) ratified

44. Because he is so _____, he cannot play harmoniously with the other
    children in his class and does not have many friends.

    (A) pugnacious
    (B) dubious
    (C) suspicious
    (D) ingenious

45. The accusation of fraud that was printed in the newspaper was _____ and untrue; nonetheless, the organization's reputation was still _____.

    (A) intriguing; pragmatic
    (B) defamatory; besmirched
    (C) astute; commemorative
    (D) prevalent; exalted

46. After the demonstration, Sue realized that the actual product was not the same as what was advertised and she was very _____.

    (A) diversified
    (B) auspicious
    (C) exonerated
    (D) disillusioned

47. We are still _____ about our vacation plans for this year, unlike last year when we were _____ about where we wanted to go.

    (A) vehement; deceptive
    (B) amiss; repressed
    (C) amorphous; resolute
    (D) altruistic; dubious

48. When the doctor left the room, the patient became _____ and aggressive, but when the doctor returned she _____ her composure and became docile once again.

    (A) vicarious; sullied
    (B) supple; promoted
    (C) surly; fostered
    (D) belligerent; regained

49. A person with Type O blood is usually called a _____ donor, since he or she can give blood to a person with any blood type.

    (A) universal
    (B) ambivalent
    (C) confined
    (D) isolated

50. There are many _____ devices that can be used to help us _____ otherwise hard-to-remember concepts.

    (A) automatic; finesse
    (B) mnemonic; recollect
    (C) schematic; respire
    (D) pneumatic; inspire

Answer Key
VERBAL ABILITY

Analogies

1. **C**	6. **A**	11. **C**	16. **C**	21. **A**
2. **A**	7. **A**	12. **A**	17. **D**	22. **B**
3. **D**	8. **C**	13. **C**	18. **B**	23. **D**
4. **B**	9. **B**	14. **B**	19. **C**	24. **B**
5. **D**	10. **D**	15. **A**	20. **D**	25. **A**

Sentence Completion

26. **C**	31. **B**	36. **C**	41. **A**	46. **D**
27. **B**	32. **A**	37. **D**	42. **C**	47. **C**
28. **D**	33. **D**	38. **D**	43. **B**	48. **D**
29. **A**	34. **C**	39. **A**	44. **A**	49. **A**
30. **C**	35. **B**	40. **D**	45. **B**	50. **B**

EXPLANATORY ANSWERS

ANALOGIES

1. **(C)** This is an analogy of association. A spider is housed in its web just as a bird uses a nest for housing.

2. **(A)** A pharmacist cares for and instructs a patient just as a teacher instructs a student. This is an analogy of association.

3. **(D)** In this analogy of cause and effect, bees produce honey just as polyps cause or produce coral.

4. **(B)** This is an analogy of cause and effect. Just as hypnosis brings about a trance, a stroke may cause paralysis. (If you chose A by mistake, you identified a cause of stroke rather than its effect. Be careful to match the terms appropriately.)

5. **(D)** Humidity is associated with a swamp, and aridity with a desert. This may be considered an analogy of description or characteristic.

6. **(A)** In this "part to whole" analogy, the rind is the outer part of an orange, and the bark is the analogous (or corresponding) outer part of a tree. If you mistakenly chose B, you may have made a common error by assuming that bark was a verb rather than a noun.

7. **(A)** This is a geographical and also a "part to whole" analogy. Just as the island of Bikini is part of the Marshall Islands, so Saint Thomas is part of the Virgin Islands.

8. **(C)** The analogy is worker to tool. An astronomer uses a telescope just as a dentist uses a drill.

9. **(B)** In this grammatical analogy each noun is paired with an adjective derived from it. Ruddy means reddish in color, and metallic means "made from metal" or "metal-like."

10. **(D)** This analogy is one of association rather than worker to tool. Botanists are associated with the study of plants and neurobiologists with the study of neurotransmitters. (If you chose either C or B, your answer is too general to complete the analogy.)

11. **(C)** This is a "whole to part" analogy. Casein is a protein occurring in milk, and gluten is a protein occurring in wheat. In each case, the protein is part of the composition of the whole.

12. **(A)** This geographical analogy must be completed with the name of a country. The Ganges is a river in India, and the Mississippi is a river in the United States.

13. **(C)** This analogy is based on synonyms. Just as transparent and clear are synonymous, opaque and muddy also have the same or nearly the same meaning.

14. **(B)** This analogy is based on antonyms. Just as abstain and indulge have opposite meanings, loosen and tighten are also antonyms.

15. **(A)** In this analogy of association, an airplane is kept in a hangar and an automobile is kept in a garage.

16. **(C)** This is an analogy of characteristic or description. Grain is a characteristic of wood, and luster is a characteristic of a diamond.

17. **(D)** In this "part to whole" analogy, violins form part of an orchestra, and a pupil is part of a class.

18. **(B)** This is a "part to whole" analogy, since an anaconda is one type of boa, and tennis is one type of sport. To help clarify this kind of analogy, think of the group of all boas and the group of all sports as "wholes," of which the anaconda and tennis are merely respective parts.

19. **(C)** This is a "part to whole" analogy. Just as a lens is part of a microscope, a helmet is part of a suit of armor.

20. **(D)** In this geographical analogy, Bermuda is an island in the West Atlantic Ocean, and Madagascar is an island in the West Indian Ocean.

21. **(A)** In this grammatical analogy, will fly and will show are verbs in the future tense and the active voice. (When you are working with grammatical analogies, take care to be precise. If you chose C, the tense is correct, but the passive voice does not fit the analogy.)

22. **(B)** This is a "worker to tool" analogy. Just as a singer uses a microphone, a physician uses a stethoscope.

23. **(D)** Although the names of two countries are included in the answer selections, this is not a geographical analogy. In this analogy of part to whole, a banyan is one kind of tree; a chrysanthemum is one kind of flower.

24. **(B)** In this "part to whole" analogy, Boolean is a kind of algebra, and Euclidean is a kind of geometry.

25. **(A)** In this "part to whole" analogy, the muzzle is part of a dog, and the cerebellum is part of the brain. It is also necessary to be flexible enough to realize that "muzzle," as used here, means "the forward or projecting part of a dog's head," and not a device used to put over that part of the dog to keep it from barking, biting, or eating.

SENTENCE COMPLETIONS

26. **(C)** The blank indicates that the teacher's response to the student is affected by or related to something that the student did that is NOT honest or trustworthy. To be dishonest or untrustworthy has a negative connotation, so we can project that the correct word will have a negative connotation also. This eliminates Answer B (understanding) and Answer D (elated). Answer A (impartial), which means to be fair or without bias, doesn't make sense in this context, so Answer C (disenchanted) is the best answer.

27. **(B)** The placement of the blank indicates that the correct word will describe "glance," and that this type of glance is directly related to missing or ignoring very important details. Based on this, the projected word could mean "hasty," "superficial," or "short." The only word that matches this is Answer B (cursory).

28. **(D)** The words "medication," "dose," and "patient's chart" in this sentence indicate that the correct word will be related to health or medicine. This eliminates Answers A, B, and C, leaving Answer D (intravenous) as the correct response.

29. **(A)** The first blank in this sentence defines a microorganism's NEW reaction to an antibiotic's actions, in which it is "no longer affected." The word "formerly" preceding the second blank in the sentence provides a clue that there are two contrasting scenarios occurring; thus, the two correct words will most likely have opposite connotations. Accordingly, if the first blank means "impermeable" or "resistant," then the second blank must mean "susceptible" (unprotected or vulnerable). Based on this, Answer A is the best choice for this sentence.

30. **(C)** We are told that around strangers Karen is quiet, and the placement of the first blank indicates that the correct word will be synonymous with quiet. Because the word "but" comes before the second blank, we know that something contrasting or contradictory happens when she is around family and friends. From this, we can project that the two correct words will be opposites. This eliminates Answers A, B, and D, which leaves Answer C with the words "introverted" (meaning "shy" or "reclusive") and "loquacious" (meaning "talkative") as the correct answer.

31. **(B)** The word in the first blank most likely is an adjective that describes the circus performer's act of juggling three balls while balancing himself on a tightrope, which is not a simple task. Based on this we can project that the first correct word will mean "hard" or "difficult." Also, the word "very" in this sentence tells us that the performer's act is even more difficult due to some added element or component, indicated by the second blank. Based on these deductions, Answer B is the correct answer, with "complicated" and "simultaneous" as the best match for the sentence context.

32. **(A)** The placement of this blank indicates that the correct response will directly confirm, rationalize, or provide merit for her affirmative feelings and self-esteem in winning a distinguished or notable award. In reading each of the answers back into the sentence, Answer A makes sense and is therefore the best choice.

33. **(D)** Given the sentence context, the first blank indicates that an unexpected reaction, possibly amazement or astonishment, is elicited in response to being "so easily dwarfed." This eliminates Answer B. Sequoia trees, noted for their exceptional height as the tallest species of tree, would certainly dwarf a human. Among the remaining choices, Answer D ("veneration" and "gargantuan") provides the best fit for BOTH blanks in the sentence.

34. **(C)** The sentence describes someone or something who is very generous, altruistic, and who is freely giving in their monetary contributions. Philanthropy is a desire to help mankind by gifts and benevolent donations. Answer C, philanthropist, is the correct response that matches the sentence context.

35. **(B)** The word "instead" in association with the green food coloring in this sentence indicates that an improvised change or solution occurred directly related to the problem of running out of blue food coloring. This deviation from the blue icing preparation called for a replacement or alternate color to be used. Based on this, the only correct answer is B (substitute).

36. **(C)** The blank in this sentence describes the type of environment that is to be maintained within the body. The word "maintenance" denotes preservation, stability, or regularity. This eliminates Answers A, B, and D, leaving Answer C as the correct choice.

37. **(D)** The word to be placed in the first blank describes an action or reaction regarding the final results that should be avoided. In general, final results from a completed or finished experiment may bring some level of comfort or assuredness. Furthermore, a carefully organized and completed experiment could certainly be ruined by a shattered test tube. An event such as this one would be unexpected and unforeseen, and we can determine that the word in the second blank most likely will have a similar meaning. Based on this, we can eliminate Answers A, B, and C, leaving Answer D (sanguine and unanticipated).

38. **(D)** In this sentence, the correct word will be a symbol or gesture displayed by the scheduling of the peaceful conference—denoting "harmony" and "unity." Furthermore, all we know, based on the sentence, is that during the conference an agreement may be reached following the parties' negotiations. This denotes compromise and consideration. This eliminates Answers A, B, and C, leaving Answer D (diplomacy).

39. **(A)** The first sentence in this item tells us that the wing and the arm have alike or similar structure. However, the word "but" in the second sentence tells us that, although the structures are dissimilar when it comes to function, their anatomy somehow makes them equivalent—just as the first sentence implies. Therefore, the two correct answers should have parallel meanings. The only response that applies is Answer A.

40. **(D)** Based on the sentence context, the revisions and updates that need to be made are in direct response to the protocol being 20 years old, which is an extended time span. Based on this, our response should relate to time or something that results from a long duration of time. The only response that matches is Answer D, "antiquated," which means "outdated," "old-fashioned," or "obsolete."

41. **(A)** When something that is extensive and round is divided or separated into two, two "half spheres" are the result. Given the sentence's context, Answer A provides the best answer that makes sense.

42. **(C)** The clues in the sentence context suggest that pupil dilation, which occurs when "going from an area of bright sunlight into a dark room," will be associated with an adjustment or transition in the environment. The answer response that best fits the context is Answer C (adapt).

43. **(B)** The phrase "by excretion into urine or bile" tells us that the correct word will be closely related to the disposal or removal of the hormones from the blood. Thus, Answers A, C, and D can be ruled out, leaving Answer B (eliminated), meaning "to remove" or "to purge."

44. **(A)** To play "harmoniously" means to play peacefully or agreeably. The child in this sentence does not have many friends because he "cannot" play harmoniously. This is a clue that the correct word will mean the opposite of harmoniously— "argumentative," "antagonistic," or "combative." Answer A (pugnacious), meaning quarrelsome, is the correct response for this sentence.

45. **(B)** The context of the first blank tells us that the correct word will be closely associated with the word "untrue" or fraudulent. The second blank (describing

the organization's reputation resulting from the false fraud accusation) is preceded by the word "still." Since the accusation of fraud has a negative and unflattering connotation, we can assume that the correct word will also have an uncomplimentary tone. In addition, the word "nonetheless" (meaning "in spite of") tells us that this negative reputation will remain regardless of whether the accusation of fraud is untrue or not. Based on these deductions, the best match for the two blanks in this sentence is Answer B.

46. **(D)** Advertisements can often be misleading and exaggerated, which can result in false perceptions, and Sue's previous concept of the product was based on advertisement. However, after the demonstration, her new concept of the product was based on what she was able to see as real. Since the use of the phrase "not the same" tells us that the actual product and its advertisement are opposites, the correct word for the blank most likely describes Sue's disenchantment or disappointment when her previous perceptions or expectations of the product contradicted what was real. Of the words listed in the answer choices given, Answer D (disillusioned) makes the most sense.

47. **(C)** The word "unlike" gives us a clue that the correct words for the two blanks will probably be opposites; the vacation plans for this year are unlike or different compared to last year. Answer C provides the best match for the two blanks. "Amorphous" means vague or indefinite, and "resolute" means fixed, decided, or determined.

48. **(D)** We can tell by the placement of the first blank that the correct word will be synonymous with aggressive (meaning combative or hostile). Also, the patient's behavior described in the first blank is dependent upon the doctor leaving the room. When the doctor returns, however, something happens to the patient's composure, described by the second blank. From the sentence context we can project that a difference or change occurs, resulting in the patient's returning docility. Therefore, the answer choice that provides the best match based on these conclusions is Answer D, belligerent and regained.

49. **(A)** The word in the blank will be an adjective describing the type of donor who is associated with the ability to provide blood regardless of or unrestricted by the recipients' blood type. This type of donor will be able to be used in every instance, which can also be described as general, generic, or undifferentiated. Answer A (universal) best matches the sentence.

50. **(B)** Without the type of devices described in the first blank we might forget or have difficulty bringing back concepts to our mind. Thus, the second blank has to deal with recall, and the context of this sentence is related to memory. By reading each of the answer choices back into the sentence, Answer B (mnemonic and recollect) provides the best match for the sentence.

CHAPTER 5

Biology Review and Practice

TIPS FOR THE BIOLOGY SECTION

The biology section of the PCAT measures your knowledge and understanding of principles and concepts in basic biology (including general biology), microbiology, and human anatomy and physiology. Microbiology, human anatomy, and physiology may not be covered in general pre-pharmacy required biology courses. If you do not feel confident in these areas, you can probably improve your PCAT biology score by reviewing these subjects independently or by taking a course in these subjects.

The biology section of the real PCAT consists of approximately 48 questions (more have been included in this chapter for review purposes). You will have 30 minutes to complete the biology section. Be sure to answer all questions.

BIOLOGY REVIEW OUTLINE

I. **Molecular biology**
   A. Enzymes
   B. Energy
   C. Nucleic acids
   D. DNA
   E. RNA

II. **Cell biology**
   A. Structure
   B. Components
   C. Properties
   D. Energy (Krebs cycle)
   E. Cellular reproduction and division
      1. Mitosis
      2. Meiosis
   F. Membrane transport
   G. Cellular metabolism

III. **Health**

IV. Human anatomy and physiology
  A. Cells
  B. Tissues
  C. Organs
  D. Organ systems (anatomy and primary functions)
    1. Skeletal system
       a. Axial skeleton
       b. Appendicular skeleton
       c. Bones
       d. Joints
    2. Muscular system
    3. Circulatory system
       a. Blood
       b. Circulation
       c. Blood vessels
       d. Heart
    4. Respiratory system
       a. Ventilation
       b. Inspiration and expiration
       c. Gas exchange
    5. Urinary System
       a. Anatomy of kidney
       b. Role of kidney
    6. Liver
       a. Anatomy of liver
       b. Role of liver
    7. Integumentary system
       a. Skin
       b. Glands
       c. Hair
       d. Nails
       e. Role of integumentary system
    8. Digestive system
       a. Functions of digestive organs
       b. Digestive tract
       c. Digestive enzymes
       d. Digestive hormones
    9. Sensory organs
       a. Eye
       b. Ear
       c. Nose
       d. Tongue
    10. Nervous system
       a. Neuron
       b. Central nervous system
       c. Peripheral nervous system

11. Brain
    a. Parts
    b. Functions
12. Endocrine system
    a. Pancreas
    b. Thyroid gland
    c. Pituitary gland
    d. Parathyroid glands
    e. Adrenal glands
13. Reproductive system
    a. Reproductive organs (male and female)
    b. Hormones (hormonal regulation)
14. Immune system

V. **Nutrition**
    A. Protein
    B. Glucose—energy
    C. Vitamins
       1. Water soluble
       2. Fat soluble

VI. **Genetics**
    A. Chromosomes
    B. Genes
    C. Traits
    D. Genetic diseases

VII. **Microbiology**
    A. Microorganisms
    B. Infectious disease and prevention
    C. Medical microbiology
    D. Immunity

Answer Sheet
BIOLOGY

1 Ⓐ Ⓑ Ⓒ Ⓓ	26 Ⓐ Ⓑ Ⓒ Ⓓ	51 Ⓐ Ⓑ Ⓒ Ⓓ	76 Ⓐ Ⓑ Ⓒ Ⓓ
2 Ⓐ Ⓑ Ⓒ Ⓓ	27 Ⓐ Ⓑ Ⓒ Ⓓ	52 Ⓐ Ⓑ Ⓒ Ⓓ	77 Ⓐ Ⓑ Ⓒ Ⓓ
3 Ⓐ Ⓑ Ⓒ Ⓓ	28 Ⓐ Ⓑ Ⓒ Ⓓ	53 Ⓐ Ⓑ Ⓒ Ⓓ	78 Ⓐ Ⓑ Ⓒ Ⓓ
4 Ⓐ Ⓑ Ⓒ Ⓓ	29 Ⓐ Ⓑ Ⓒ Ⓓ	54 Ⓐ Ⓑ Ⓒ Ⓓ	79 Ⓐ Ⓑ Ⓒ Ⓓ
5 Ⓐ Ⓑ Ⓒ Ⓓ	30 Ⓐ Ⓑ Ⓒ Ⓓ	55 Ⓐ Ⓑ Ⓒ Ⓓ	80 Ⓐ Ⓑ Ⓒ Ⓓ
6 Ⓐ Ⓑ Ⓒ Ⓓ	31 Ⓐ Ⓑ Ⓒ Ⓓ	56 Ⓐ Ⓑ Ⓒ Ⓓ	81 Ⓐ Ⓑ Ⓒ Ⓓ
7 Ⓐ Ⓑ Ⓒ Ⓓ	32 Ⓐ Ⓑ Ⓒ Ⓓ	57 Ⓐ Ⓑ Ⓒ Ⓓ	82 Ⓐ Ⓑ Ⓒ Ⓓ
8 Ⓐ Ⓑ Ⓒ Ⓓ	33 Ⓐ Ⓑ Ⓒ Ⓓ	58 Ⓐ Ⓑ Ⓒ Ⓓ	83 Ⓐ Ⓑ Ⓒ Ⓓ
9 Ⓐ Ⓑ Ⓒ Ⓓ	34 Ⓐ Ⓑ Ⓒ Ⓓ	59 Ⓐ Ⓑ Ⓒ Ⓓ	84 Ⓐ Ⓑ Ⓒ Ⓓ
10 Ⓐ Ⓑ Ⓒ Ⓓ	35 Ⓐ Ⓑ Ⓒ Ⓓ	60 Ⓐ Ⓑ Ⓒ Ⓓ	85 Ⓐ Ⓑ Ⓒ Ⓓ
11 Ⓐ Ⓑ Ⓒ Ⓓ	36 Ⓐ Ⓑ Ⓒ Ⓓ	61 Ⓐ Ⓑ Ⓒ Ⓓ	86 Ⓐ Ⓑ Ⓒ Ⓓ
12 Ⓐ Ⓑ Ⓒ Ⓓ	37 Ⓐ Ⓑ Ⓒ Ⓓ	62 Ⓐ Ⓑ Ⓒ Ⓓ	87 Ⓐ Ⓑ Ⓒ Ⓓ
13 Ⓐ Ⓑ Ⓒ Ⓓ	38 Ⓐ Ⓑ Ⓒ Ⓓ	63 Ⓐ Ⓑ Ⓒ Ⓓ	88 Ⓐ Ⓑ Ⓒ Ⓓ
14 Ⓐ Ⓑ Ⓒ Ⓓ	39 Ⓐ Ⓑ Ⓒ Ⓓ	64 Ⓐ Ⓑ Ⓒ Ⓓ	89 Ⓐ Ⓑ Ⓒ Ⓓ
15 Ⓐ Ⓑ Ⓒ Ⓓ	40 Ⓐ Ⓑ Ⓒ Ⓓ	65 Ⓐ Ⓑ Ⓒ Ⓓ	90 Ⓐ Ⓑ Ⓒ Ⓓ
16 Ⓐ Ⓑ Ⓒ Ⓓ	41 Ⓐ Ⓑ Ⓒ Ⓓ	66 Ⓐ Ⓑ Ⓒ Ⓓ	91 Ⓐ Ⓑ Ⓒ Ⓓ
17 Ⓐ Ⓑ Ⓒ Ⓓ	42 Ⓐ Ⓑ Ⓒ Ⓓ	67 Ⓐ Ⓑ Ⓒ Ⓓ	92 Ⓐ Ⓑ Ⓒ Ⓓ
18 Ⓐ Ⓑ Ⓒ Ⓓ	43 Ⓐ Ⓑ Ⓒ Ⓓ	68 Ⓐ Ⓑ Ⓒ Ⓓ	93 Ⓐ Ⓑ Ⓒ Ⓓ
19 Ⓐ Ⓑ Ⓒ Ⓓ	44 Ⓐ Ⓑ Ⓒ Ⓓ	69 Ⓐ Ⓑ Ⓒ Ⓓ	94 Ⓐ Ⓑ Ⓒ Ⓓ
20 Ⓐ Ⓑ Ⓒ Ⓓ	45 Ⓐ Ⓑ Ⓒ Ⓓ	70 Ⓐ Ⓑ Ⓒ Ⓓ	95 Ⓐ Ⓑ Ⓒ Ⓓ
21 Ⓐ Ⓑ Ⓒ Ⓓ	46 Ⓐ Ⓑ Ⓒ Ⓓ	71 Ⓐ Ⓑ Ⓒ Ⓓ	96 Ⓐ Ⓑ Ⓒ Ⓓ
22 Ⓐ Ⓑ Ⓒ Ⓓ	47 Ⓐ Ⓑ Ⓒ Ⓓ	72 Ⓐ Ⓑ Ⓒ Ⓓ	97 Ⓐ Ⓑ Ⓒ Ⓓ
23 Ⓐ Ⓑ Ⓒ Ⓓ	48 Ⓐ Ⓑ Ⓒ Ⓓ	73 Ⓐ Ⓑ Ⓒ Ⓓ	98 Ⓐ Ⓑ Ⓒ Ⓓ
24 Ⓐ Ⓑ Ⓒ Ⓓ	49 Ⓐ Ⓑ Ⓒ Ⓓ	74 Ⓐ Ⓑ Ⓒ Ⓓ	99 Ⓐ Ⓑ Ⓒ Ⓓ
25 Ⓐ Ⓑ Ⓒ Ⓓ	50 Ⓐ Ⓑ Ⓒ Ⓓ	75 Ⓐ Ⓑ Ⓒ Ⓓ	100 Ⓐ Ⓑ Ⓒ Ⓓ

Practice Questions

100 Questions

Directions: Select the best answer to each of the following questions.

1. How much time is required for an adult human to produce detectable antibodies in the blood during a primary immune response?

   (A) 8 weeks
   (B) 6 weeks
   (C) 4 weeks
   (D) 1 week ✓

2. The relationship of microorganisms with one another and with their environment is called

   (A) micronology.
   (B) micrologies.
   (C) microbial ecologies. ✓
   (D) biologies.

3. In this organelle, sugar side chains are added to newly synthesized proteins.

   (A) Rough endoplasmic reticulum
   (B) Golgi complex ✓
   (C) Nuclear lamella
   (D) Smooth endoplasmic reticulum

4. A signal receptor that would respond to a steroid hormone

   (A) is located at the surface of a cell. ✓
   (B) binds to the hormone in the cytoplasm.
   (C) forms a hormone receptor complex and moves to the nucleus.
   (D) either B or C

5. The number and size of organelles in a cell correlates with that cell's function. A cell that has an extensive rough endoplasmic reticulum would be

   (A) undergoing rapid cell division.
   (B) actively moving about.
   (C) producing proteins that are secreted from the cell. ✓
   (D) producing fatty acids and other lipids.

6. Human sperm cells are mobile because of

   (A) mitochondria.
   (B) cilia.
   (C) flagella. ✓
   (D) the plasma membrane.

7. Different types of proteins are directed to different locations in a cell according to how they function. Their subcellular localization is determined by

   (A) entry into transport vesicles.
   (B) binding to receptor proteins.
   (C) binding to motor proteins.
   (D) localization signals in the proteins. ✓

8. Which of the following describes Stage 1 of sleep?

   (A) Characterized by drowsiness. The eyes may be closed, but the person is able to hear nearby activity. ✓
   (B) Characterized by alternating periods of muscle tension and relaxation. Heart rate slows and body temperature drops.
   (C) Little body movement, vivid dreaming.
   (D) Known as delta sleep. Breathing and heart rate slows.

9. In eukaryotes, glycolysis takes place in

   (A) cytoplasm. ✓
   (B) mitochondrial matrix.
   (C) inner membranes of the mitochondria.
   (D) Golgi complex.

10. Which of the following is the fluid medium of the nucleus?

    (A) Chloroplasm
    (B) Golgi complex
    (C) Nucleoplasm ✓
    (D) Nucleolus

11. Molecular biology is the study of _____ at a(n) _____ level.

    (A) biochemistry; molecular ✓
    (B) anatomy; gross
    (C) physics; quantum
    (D) health; individual

12. The pigment that is responsible for giving skin its color is called:

    (A) epidermis.
    (B) melanin. ✓
    (C) dermis.
    (D) subcutaneous layer.

13. Which statement is TRUE regarding enzymes?

    (A) An enzyme is a protein that acts as a catalyst.
    (B) An enzyme is temperature dependent.
    (C) An enzyme is pH dependent.
    (D) A, B, and C ✓

14. The sugar found in DNA has _____ carbons.

    (A) three
    (B) four
    (C) five ✓
    (D) six

15. Which part of the cell produces ribonucleoprotein?

    (A) Nuclear envelope
    (B) Chromosomes
    (C) Nucleoplasm
    (D) Nucleolus ✓

16. A clouding of the lens of the eye that causes blurred vision is known as

    (A) exetis.
    (B) dermatitis.
    (C) cataracts. ✓
    (D) pink eye.

17. The pineal gland produces which two hormones?

    (A) Melatonin and serotonin ✓
    (B) Adrenalin and nonadrenaline
    (C) Insulin and glucagon
    (D) None of the above

18. The theory of spontaneous generation states that:

    (A) microorganisms arise from lifeless matter. ✓
    (B) evolution has taken place in large animals.
    (C) humans have generated from apes.
    (D) viruses are degenerative forms of bacteria.

19. The affinity of hemoglobin for oxygen is affected by

    (A) pH level.
    (B) carbon dioxide.
    (C) neither A nor B.
    (D) A and B. ✓

20. Which vitamins are NOT lost in cooking?

    (A) Fat-soluble vitamins ✓
    (B) Water-soluble vitamins
    (C) None of the above
    (D) Both A and B

21. The spleen is involved with

    (A) blood cell formation.
    (B) blood cell storage.
    (C) blood filtration.
    (D) All of the above ✓

22. Fluoride deficiency problems include:

    (A) anemia.
    (B) muscle weakness.
    (C) osteoporosis. ✓
    (D) hair loss.

23. The primary transcription productions of most eukaryotic genes

    (A) are larger than the corresponding functional messenger RNA.
    (B) contain both introns and exons.
    (C) are processed by the spliceosome.
    (D) All of the above ✓

24. Diffusion is the
    (A) movement of molecules of one substance through the molecules of
        another substance from regions of lower concentration to regions
        of higher concentration by means of an outside energy source.
    (B) movement of molecules of one substance through the molecules of
        another substance from regions of higher concentration to regions
        of lower concentration by means of an outside energy source.
    (C) movement of molecules of one substance through the molecules of
        another substance from regions of lower concentration to regions
        of higher concentration by means of the molecules' own kinetic energy.
    (D) movement of molecules of one substance through the molecules of
        another substance from regions of higher concentration to regions
        of lower concentration by means of the molecules' own kinetic energy.

25. In eukaryotes, DNA is

    (A) naked.
    (B) bound by histone proteins to form chromatin.
    (C) transcribed into messenger RNA while in a condensed state.
    (D) may be a single-stranded molecule.

26. Which of the following statements about ultraviolet (UV) radiation is FALSE?

    (A) UV radiation is needed by our bodies to manufacture vitamin D.
    (B) UV radiation has no effects on plants and animals and is not mostly absorbed by the ozone layer.
    (C) Prolonged exposure to UV rays puts one at risk for a number of negative effects on the skin.
    (D) The strongest UV rays occur between 10 A.M. and 3 P.M.

27. In order for viruses to replicate in their host cells, all of the following must occur except:

    (A) the genome must be released in the host cell cytoplasm.
    (B) ATP must be synthesized within the virus.
    (C) the virus must unite with the correct host cell.
    (D) the host cell must contain ribosomes for the synthesis of proteins.

28. What are the health risks associated with tattooing?

    (A) Infection
    (B) Blood-borne diseases
    (C) There are no risks to tattooing
    (D) Both A and B

29. Microbial sterilization is used to

    (A) decrease the possibility of contaminants growing in a culture.
    (B) kill bacteria but not necessarily viruses or other microbes.
    (C) clean a work area.
    (D) kill all microbes.

30. Meiosis II is similar to which process?

    (A) Mitosis in a haploid cell
    (B) Meiosis I
    (C) Nondisjunction
    (D) Cytokinesis

31. Progression through the cell cycle is regulated by the oscillations in the concentrations of which types of molecules?

    (A) Suppressor proteins
    (B) Cyclin-dependent kinases
    (C) Cyclins
    (D) Tubulin

32. Which statement is FALSE?

    (A) Ribose is the sugar found in RNA.
    (B) DNA is double stranded.
    (C) RNA is mostly double stranded.
    (D) Deoxyribose is the sugar found in DNA.

33. During meiosis the number of chromosomes

    (A) remains the same.
    (B) decreases by 50 percent.
    (C) increases by 50 percent.
    (D) none of the above

34. The processing of glucose involves the process of

    (A) the Krebs cycle.
    (B) electron transport coupled with oxidative phosphorylation.
    (C) glycolysis.
    (D) All of the above

35. The stage in cell division marked by chromosome separation is

    (A) anaphase.
    (B) interphase.
    (C) prophase.
    (D) telophase.

36. The lac operon is usually in the _____ position and is activated by a(n) _____ molecule.

    (A) on; repressor
    (B) off; repressor
    (C) on; inducer
    (D) off; inducer

37. How many chromosomes are normally found in a human cell?

    (A) 23
    (B) 46
    (C) 92
    (D) None of the above

38. Which of the following describes Stage 3 of sleep?

    (A) Characterized by drowsiness. The eyes may be closed, but the person is able to hear nearby activity.
    (B) Characterized by alternating periods of muscle tension and relaxation. Heart rate slows and body temperature drops.
    (C) Little body movement, vivid dreaming.
    (D) Known as delta sleep. Breathing and heart rate slows.

39. Apoptosis plays a critical role in

    (A) pattern formation in normal development of complex organisms.
    (B) the replacement of cells in tissue at the end of their life span.
    (C) the prevention of tumor development.
    (D) All of the above

40. The amount of energy needed to carry out basic body functions when you are at rest is known as

    (A) resting metabolism.
    (B) complex metabolism.
    (C) catabolic metabolism.
    (D) basal metabolism.

41. Which of the following cells excavate bone cavities?

    (A) Osteoclasts
    (B) Osteoblasts
    (C) Osteomasts
    (D) Osteocytes

42. Which of the following hormones is involved in calcium homeostasis?

    (A) Parathyroid hormone
    (B) Calcitonin
    (C) Insulin
    (D) A and B

43. Which of the following cells form bone matrix?

    (A) Osteoclasts
    (B) Osteocytes
    (C) Osteoblasts
    (D) Osteomasts

44. The bones of the skeleton articulate with each other at

    (A) the appendicular skeleton.
    (B) the joints.
    (C) the axial skeleton.
    (D) cartilage.

45. Ball and socket, plane, gliding, hinge, and condylar are all types of

    (A) bones.
    (B) muscles.
    (C) cartilage.
    (D) joints.

46. Which of the following is (are) included in the function(s) of the circulatory system?

    (A) Supplies nutrients and oxygen to the tissues
    (B) Removes waste material
    (C) Initiates clotting
    (D) All of the above

47. Concerning nutrition, which statement is FALSE?

    (A) Being well nourished is not the same as being well fed.
    (B) Good nutrition is important so the body can best function.
    (C) Research indicates that teens are the most nutritious age group.
    (D) Long-term poor eating habits increase the risk for thin and brittle bones and high levels of blood fat.

48. What is the function of the middle ear?
    (A) It contains hair cells that detect specific frequencies of sound.
    (B) It transmits sound vibrations to the tympanic membrane.
    (C) It amplifies sound transmitted to the cochlea.
    (D) It vibrates in response to certain frequencies.

49. Blood is delivered to the heart from the lungs by the

    (A) renal veins.
    (B) pulmonary veins.
    (C) mitral arteries.
    (D) pulmonary arteries.

50. Which statement is FALSE?

    (A) Red blood cells transport oxygen.
    (B) Backflow of blood in the circulatory system is prevented by valves.
    (C) The liver returns blood via the hepatic veins to the inferior vena cava.
    (D) Plasma constitutes less than 23 percent of the blood volume.

51. What is another name for red blood cells?

    (A) Erythrocytes
    (B) Leukocytes
    (C) Lymphocytes
    (D) Basophils

52. Which of the following is found in gram-positive bacteria?

    (A) Pseudomurein
    (B) Sterol-rich membranes
    (C) Peptidoglycan
    (D) Amniotransports

53. Which are NOT leukocytes?

    (A) Neutrophils
    (B) Eosinophils
    (C) Basophils
    (D) Thrombophils

54. The primary function of platelets involves

    (A) blood formation.
    (B) blood clotting.
    (C) metabolism.
    (D) defense against infections.

55. What is (are) the primary function(s) of white blood cells?

    (A) Phagocytosis
    (B) Proteolysis
    (C) Antibody formation
    (D) All of the above

56. Albumin is a(n)

    (A) electrolyte.
    (B) trace element.
    (C) plasma protein.
    (D) mineral.

57. What is the functional unit of the nervous system?

    (A) Neuron
    (B) Nerve
    (C) Synapse
    (D) None of the above

58. Which of the following statements is(are) TRUE concerning the respiratory system?

    (A) Respiration refers to the gaseous exchanges that occur between the body and the environment.
    (B) During inspiration the thoracic cavity expands.
    (C) During inspiration air rushes into the respiratory tract because of the creation of negative pressure.
    (D) All of the above

59. Which of the following statements regarding cholesterol is FALSE?

    (A) Exercise tends to increase the level of high-density lipoprotein (HDL) cholesterol.
    (B) Smoking tends to increase HDL cholesterol.
    (C) Excessive sugar in the diet tends to lower HDL cholesterol.
    (D) None of the above

60. Which of the following statements is (are) TRUE concerning the urinary system?

    (A) The urinary system functions to help maintain homeostasis of the body by excreting waste and regulating the content of the blood.
    (B) The urinary system consists of two kidneys, two ureters, a urinary bladder, and a urethra.
    (C) The urinary system regulates the acid-base balance of the body.
    (D) All of the above

61. Which of the following is (are) NOT normally reabsorbed in the kidney?

    (A) Glucose
    (B) Creatinine
    (C) Sodium
    (D) A and C

62. How are carbohydrates digested?

    (A) By amylases in the mouth and small intestines
    (B) By pepsin and HCL acid in the stomach
    (C) By lipases in the small intestine
    (D) By nucleases in the stomach

63. What role do bile salts play in the digestion of complex fats?

    (A) They emulsify lipids by converting large masses of fat molecules into smaller masses.
    (B) They activate enzymes that digest fat.
    (C) They cleave the bonds releasing fatty acids and other small lipids.
    (D) The mechanism is unknown.

64. What is the name of the thin, mucus-secreting epithelial membrane that lines the interior surface of the eyelid?

    (A) Tarsal plate
    (B) Lacrimal gland
    (C) Conjunctiva
    (D) Sclera

65. Cholesterol

    (A) is responsible for blockage of arteries leading to heart attacks and strokes.
    (B) is used in the synthesis of bile salts.
    (C) is transported in the blood in two distinct forms.
    (D) All of the above

66. The term "oral cavity" refers to the

    (A) stomach.
    (B) intestine.
    (C) mouth.
    (D) liver.

67. The fat-soluble vitamins include all of the following EXCEPT

    (A) vitamin D.
    (B) vitamin K.
    (C) vitamin A.
    (D) vitamin B_1.

68. Which statement is FALSE concerning the digestive system?

    (A) The small intestine has three major regions—the duodenum, jejunum, and ileum.
    (B) Most nutrients are absorbed by the large intestine.
    (C) The pancreas synthesizes and secretes a number of digestive enzymes.
    (D) Water is reabsorbed from the residue of the food mass as it passes through the large intestine.

69. Animal viruses are classified into taxonomic groups based on

    (A) their type of genetic material.
    (B) the kind of cells they infected.
    (C) their replication strategy.
    (D) whether they are naked or enveloped.

70. The water-soluble vitamins include all of the following EXCEPT

    (A) thiamine.
    (B) niacin.
    (C) folic acid.
    (D) vitamin E.

71. What is the primary function of the gallbladder?

    (A) To store gastrin
    (B) To store bile
    (C) To synthesize insulin
    (D) To store amylase

72. Which of the following statements is FALSE?

    (A) Excess weight increases risk for heart disease and stroke.
    (B) The Centers for Disease Control and Prevention (CDC) estimates that excess weight and physical inactivity combined account for approximately 10,000 premature deaths in the United States per year.
    (C) The more overweight a person is, the greater his or her chances for developing weight-related health problems.
    (D) Excess weight increases the risk for diabetes and cancer.

73. Which of the following enhance(s) the intestinal absorption of fatty acids?

    (A) Bile salts
    (B) Amylase
    (C) Hydrochloric acid
    (D) Pepsin

74. If the blood pH of a subject is measured immediately before and after hyperventilation, which of the following results is expected?

    (A) There is no difference between the pH measurements.
    (B) The pH will be lower after hyperventilating.
    (C) The pH will be higher after hyperventilating.
    (D) The pH will be higher before hyperventilating but will rapidly fall.

75. Which is NOT a function of the medulla oblongata?

    (A) Arteriole wall contraction
    (B) Respirations
    (C) Heartbeat
    (D) Verbal communication

76. Which of the following is (are) included among the function(s) of the thyroid gland?

    (A) Controlling the rate of metabolism
    (B) Controlling the growth of the organism
    (C) Influencing nervous system activity
    (D) All of the above

77. Antibiotics are molecules that kill bacteria and

    (A) are frequently produced naturally by soil-dwelling fungi.
    (B) may act by preventing bacterial cell wall synthesis.
    (C) may disrupt bacterial translation.
    (D) All of the above

78. Which statement is TRUE concerning the parathyroid glands and/or the hormone they produce?

    (A) There are usually four parathyroid glands, which are embedded in the thyroid gland.
    (B) The parathyroid glands produce parathyroid hormone.
    (C) Parathyroid hormone regulates calcium levels.
    (D) All of the above

79. Koch's postulate defines the criterion used to demonstrate that

    (A) an organism is a heterotrophy.
    (B) an organism causes a specific disease.
    (C) a disease-causing organism also has harmless variants.
    (D) organisms that lack cell walls undergo lyses in hypotonic solutions.

71

67

Water soluble:
thiamine
niacin
folic acid

Not:
Vitamin E

Fat Soluble Vitamins:
Vitamin D, K, A

Not: Vitamin B₁

Figure 1 is needed to answer question 80.

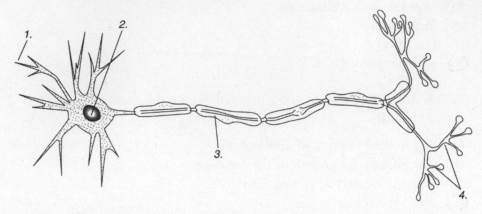

Figure 1.

80. Figure 1 illustrates a typical neuron. Which number on the figure indicates where impulses from other neurons are picked up?

(A) 1
(B) 2
(C) 3
(D) 4

81. Which of the following is NOT a neurotransmitter?

(A) Albuterol
(B) Serotonin
(C) Acetylcholine
(D) Norepinephrine

82. Which of the following is(are) responsible for the removal and destruction of erythrocytes?

(A) Liver
(B) Gallbladder
(C) Kidneys
(D) Pancreas

83. In humans, which of the following is(are) NOT vestigial in nature?

(A) Appendix
(B) Stomach
(C) Wisdom teeth
(D) A and C

84. Which of the following nutrients has(have) the highest caloric value per gram?

    (A) Protein
    (B) Glucose
    (C) Fat
    (D) Carbohydrates

85. _____ is a condition where a person eats a great deal of food and then vomits or uses other purging methods.

    (A) Binge-eating disorder
    (B) Bulimia nervosa
    (C) Anorexia nervosa
    (D) Disordered-eating pattern

86. Many animal viruses contain a membrane-like envelope structure that includes viral proteins protruding from a lipid bilayer. When do viruses acquire an envelope?

    (A) During the assembly in the cytoplasm of the cell
    (B) During the budding from the host cell
    (C) During the entry of the virus into the host cell
    (D) All of the above

87. Viruses are obligate intracellular parasites. Which statement below is NOT correct?

    (A) Virus particles are self-assembled.
    (B) Viruses must degrade host DNA and RNA to obtain nucleotides for their replication.
    (C) Energy for virus replication is provided by the host cell.
    (D) Enveloped viruses acquire a cellular membrane during particle release.

88. What do host cells NOT provide viruses?

    (A) Enzymes to assemble virus particles
    (B) Nucleotides and amino acids
    (C) ATP
    (D) Ribosomes

89. The Rh factor in blood is a

    (A) protein.
    (B) carbohydrate.
    (C) blood cell.
    (D) nuclear acid.

90. In _____ drug dependence, the user's body needs the drug to avoid the discomfort of withdrawal.

    (A) physical
    (B) psychological
    (C) sociological
    (D) None of the above

91. If Y represents yellow (dominant color) and y represents green (recessive color), which of the following crosses would be expected to result in 75 percent yellow offspring?

    (A) Yy × yy
    (B) YY × yy
    (C) Yy × Yy
    (D) Yy × YY

92. _____ is the process in which energy is released as electrons pass through a series of electron acceptors to either oxygen or another inorganic compound.

    (A) Oxidative phosphorylation
    (B) Phosphorylation
    (C) Photosynthetic phosphorlyation
    (D) Substrate-level phosphorylation

93. Blue (B) is the dominant color for the Figbird, whereas white (w) is the alternative recessive color. When a homozygous blue bird is crossed with a homozygous white bird, what percentage of the offspring is expected to be white?

    (A) 0
    (B) 25
    (C) 50
    (D) 100

94. Blue (B) is the dominant color for the Figbird, whereas white (w) is the alternative recessive color. When a homozygous blue bird is crossed with a homozygous white bird, what percentage of the offspring is expected to be blue heterozygous?

    (A) 0
    (B) 25
    (C) 50
    (D) 100

95. Which of the following provide(s) daylight color vision and is (are) responsible for visual acuity?

    (A) Rods
    (B) Cones
    (C) Optic disc
    (D) Retina

96. Which of the following events is NOT involved in the inflammatory response?

    (A) Mast cells secrete chemical messengers that increase blood flow.
    (B) Cytotoxic T-cells kill infected host cells.
    (C) Macrophages release chemical messengers that increase body temperature.
    (D) Neutrophils phagocytize pathogens.

97. A person who is heterozygous at the gene locus of a disorder, but shows no signs of the disorder, is called a(n) _____ of the disorder.

    (A) infector
    (B) carrier
    (C) infection
    (D) holder

98. Cystic fibrosis develops in individuals who inherit two copies of a recessive gene (c). If a man with cystic fibrosis marries a woman who does not have the disease but is a carrier of it, what percentage of their offspring is expected to have the disease?

    (A) 0
    (B) 25
    (C) 50
    (D) 75

99. Sickle-cell anemia develops in individuals who inherit two copies of a recessive gene(s). If a man with sickle-cell anemia marries a woman who does not have the disease but is a carrier of it, what percentage of their offspring is expected to have the disease or to be a carrier of it?

    (A) 25
    (B) 50
    (C) 75
    (D) 100

100. If green eyes are dominant and blue eyes are recessive, what percentage of the offspring can be expected to have blue eyes if one parent has green eyes and one parent has blue eyes?

(A) 0
(B) 25
(C) 50
(D) Cannot be determined from the information given

Answer Key
BIOLOGY

1.	D	26.	B	51.	A	76.	D
2.	C	27.	B	52.	C	77.	D
3.	B	28.	D	53.	D	78.	D
4.	A	29.	D	54.	B	79.	B
5.	C	30.	A	55.	D	80.	A
6.	C	31.	B	56.	C	81.	A
7.	D	32.	C	57.	A	82.	A
8.	A	33.	B	58.	D	83.	B
9.	A	34.	D	59.	B	84.	C
10.	C	35.	A	60.	D	85.	B
11.	A	36.	D	61.	B	86.	B
12.	B	37.	B	62.	A	87.	B
13.	D	38.	D	63.	A	88.	A
14.	C	39.	D	64.	C	89.	A
15.	D	40.	D	65.	D	90.	A
16.	C	41.	A	66.	C	91.	C
17.	A	42.	D	67.	D	92.	A
18.	A	43.	C	68.	B	93.	A
19.	D	44.	B	69.	C	94.	D
20.	A	45.	D	70.	D	95.	B
21.	D	46.	D	71.	B	96.	B
22.	C	47.	C	72.	B	97.	B
23.	D	48.	C	73.	A	98.	C
24.	D	49.	B	74.	C	99.	D
25.	B	50.	D	75.	D	100.	D

EXPLANATORY ANSWERS

1. **(D)** In general, it takes approximately one week (or within one week), for an adult human to produce detectable antibodies in the blood during a primary immune response.

2. **(C)** No explanation needed.

3. **(B)** The Golgi complex adds carbohydrate side chains to create glycosylated proteins.

4. **(A)** The signal receptors that respond to steroid hormones are located inside the cell. Steroid hormones are lipid soluble and readily diffuse through the plasma membrane. The hormones then bind to a receptor in the cytoplasm and are transported to the nucleus.

5. **(C)** A cell with an extensive rough endoplasmic reticulum would be producing proteins that are secreted from the cell. Ribosomes that translate messenger RNAs that encode secretory proteins bind to the rough endoplasmic reticulum and the protein being synthesized enters the lumen of the rough endoplasmic reticulum. The proteins destined for secretion move to the Golgi vesicles that, ultimately, fuse with the cell membrane releasing the protein from the cell.

6. **(C)** Both flagella (C) and cilia (B) provide cell locomotion. However, human sperm cells move by means of flagella.

7. **(D)** Inside cells proteins are transported to their destination with the help of "zip codes." Zip codes are localization sequences in the protein itself that allow the protein to be transported to its appropriate location in the cell.

8. **(A)** Stage 1 of sleep is characterized by drowsiness and the eyes may be closed, but the person is able to hear nearby activity. Stage 2 of sleep is characterized by light sleep and alternating periods of muscle tension and relaxation; the heart rate slows and body temperature drops. Stage 3 of sleep is known as delta sleep; breathing and heart rate slows. Stage 4 of sleep is the deepest stage of delta sleep and is the stage during which it is the most difficult to rouse the sleeper; the stage when the body produces growth hormone and repairs itself from injuries. During the final stage, REM sleep, there is little body movement and vivid dreaming.

9. **(A)** Glycolysis takes place in the cytoplasm of the cell.

10. **(C)** Nucleoplasm, meaning protoplasm of the nucleus, is the fluid medium of the nucleus.

11. **(A)** No explanation needed.

12. **(B)** There are specialized cells in the deepest level of the epidermis, or outer layer of the skin, that produce a pigment called melanin. Melanin is responsible for giving color to skin.

13. **(D)** An enzyme is a protein that acts as a catalyst (a catalyst regulates the rate of a reaction). The rate of enzyme activity is temperature and pH dependent.

14. **(C)** The sugar found in DNA is deoxyribose, and it is a 5-carbon sugar.

15. **(D)** The nucleolus, a small, rounded mass in the cell nucleus, is where ribonucleoprotein is produced.

16. **(C)** No explanation needed.

17. **(A)** The pineal gland produces melatonin and serotonin. The adrenal glands produce adrenaline and noradrenaline. The pancreas produces insulin and glucagon.

18. **(A)** The theory of spontaneous generation states that certain living things arose from vital forces present in living or nonliving decomposers.

19. **(D)** Since hemoglobin in red blood cells transports oxygen and carbon dioxide to provide oxygen to the body's tissues, it should come as no surprise that factors affecting the affinity of hemoglobin for oxygen include the body's pH (acid-base level) and level of carbon dioxide present.

20. **(A)** No explanation needed.

21. **(D)** No explanation needed.

22. **(C)** No explanation needed.

23. **(D)** Most eukaryotic genes contain noncoding sequences called introns that interrupt the coding sequences. During primary transcription, all of the sequences in a gene are transcribed into a single RNA molecule and the introns are subsequently removed to produce the function messenger RNA.

24. **(D)** No explanation needed.

25. **(B)** Eukaryotic DNA is bound by histones and condensed to form chromatin. The regions of the DNA that are transcribed into RNA are not condensed.

26. **(B)** UV radiation *does* have effects on plants and animals and *is* mostly absorbed by the ozone layer.

27. **(B)** In order for viruses to replicate in their host cells all of the listed choices must occur except for ATP synthesizing within the virus.

28. **(D)** Infection is a risk because tattoos create open wounds that bleed after the procedure. It is very important that the wound be kept clean and protected from infection. Blood-borne diseases are also a risk of tattooing as transmission of HIV or hepatitis C is possible if equipment is not properly sterilized.

29. **(D)** Microbial sterilization kills all microbes that are present.

30. **(A)** After chromosomes are replicated in somatic cells, mitosis distributes one chromosome copy to each daughter cell. Sister chromatids are separated during Meiosis II to produce four haploid gametes in sexually reproducing animals. Both processes involve chromosome segregation.

31. **(B)** The cyclin concentrations of a cell cycle in dividing cells. Cyclin concentrations are greatest in the M phase. Protein kinases and cyclins blend to form

a mitosis-promoting complex that activates other proteins leading to initiation of the M phase.

32. **(C)** While DNA consists of a double strand, RNA is mostly single stranded (certain viruses are exceptions).

33. **(B)** Meiosis is a process of cell division comprising two nuclear divisions in succession. It results in four gametocytes, each containing half the number of chromosomes (B) as the parent cell.

34. **(D)** The processing of glucose involves glycolysis, the Krebs cycle, and electron transport coupled with oxidative phosphorylation.

35. **(A)** The stages of cellular division include prophase, metaphase, anaphase, and telophase. During prophase (C) the chromosomes condense, the nuclear membrane deteriorates, and the spindle microtubules attach to the chromosomes. During metaphase the chromosomes move to the center of the cell. During anaphase (A) each kinetochore divides, and the chromosomes separate. During telophase (D) the nuclear membrane reforms around each new daughter cell's nucleus.

36. **(D)** The lac operon is usually in the off position and is activated by an inducer molecule.

37. **(B)** No explanation needed.

38. **(D)** Stage 3 of sleep is known as delta sleep; breathing and heart rate slows. Stage 1 of sleep is characterized by drowsiness and the eyes may be closed, but the person is able to hear nearby activity. Stage 2 of sleep is characterized by light sleep and alternating periods of muscle tension and relaxation; the heart rate slows and body temperature drops. Stage 4 of sleep is the deepest stage of delta sleep and is the stage during which is it most difficult to rouse the sleeper; the stage when the body produces growth hormone and repairs itself from injuries. During the final stage, REM sleep, there is little body movement and vivid dreaming.

39. **(D)** Apoptosis plays an important role in development and regeneration. Programmed cell death also is used to destroy tumor cells. In order for tumor cells to survive, they activate genes to suppress apoptosis.

40. **(D)** No explanation needed.

41. **(A)** In the bone remolding cycle, osteoclasts (A) are cells that remove bone, and osteoblasts (B) are cells that form bone. Choices C and D are irrelevant.

42. **(D)** Both parathyroid hormone (A) and calcitonin (B) are involved in calcium homeostasis. Parathyroid hormone, secreted by the parathyroid glands, causes (1) bones to release calcium into the bloodstream, (2) the kidneys to conserve calcium lost through the urine, and (3) intestinal absorption of calcium. Calcitonin promotes a decrease in blood calcium, thereby antagonizing the effects of parathyroid hormone. Insulin (C) promotes glucose utilization and glycogen storage.

43. **(C)** See explanatory answer for question 41.

44. **(B)** Joints (B) are the place of union between two or more bones whereas cartilage (D) is a type of connective tissue with a solid elastic matrix. Choices A and C are irrelevant.

45. **(D)** No explanation needed.

46. **(D)** Blood in the circulatory system supplies nutrients and oxygen to tissues, removes waste material, and initiates clotting. Oxygen is supplied to the tissues primarily by the lungs and red blood cells. Erythrocytes (red blood cells) carry oxygen to the tissues' cells. In the lungs, oxygen from the inhaled air attaches to hemoglobin molecules within the erythrocytes and is transported to the cells for aerobic respiration. The lungs also eliminate carbon dioxide produced by cell respiration. Metabolic waste is filtered through the capillaries of the kidneys and excreted in urine. Platelets (thrombocytes) in the blood play a major role in blood clotting.

47. **(C)** Teens are the most poorly nourished age group in the United States.

48. **(C)** The middle ear amplifies the sound energy transmitted to the cochlea.

49. **(B)** To answer this question correctly, it is important to remember two principles: (1) arteries carry blood away from the heart, while veins carry blood to the heart; and (2) the pulmonary circulation consists of blood vessels that transport blood to the lungs and then to the heart. Therefore, the correct choice is pulmonary veins (B), not pulmonary arteries (D). Choices A and C are irrelevant.

50. **(D)** All of the statements are true (A, B, and C) except D. Approximately 55 percent, not 23 percent, of the blood is plasma.

51. **(A)** No explanation needed.

52. **(C)** In gram-positive bacteria, peptidoglycan is found within the cell wall.

53. **(D)** White blood cells are called leukocytes. Neutrophils (A), eosinophils (B), basophils (C), lymphocytes, and monocytes are types of white blood cells.

54. **(B)** No explanation needed.

55. **(D)** No explanation needed.

56. **(C)** Protein in the blood is composed of albumin and globulin, with albumin being the most abundant serum protein. The total quantity of albumin is two to three times the level of globulin. Choices A, B, and D are irrelevant.

57. **(A)** No explanation needed.

58. **(D)** No explanation needed.

59. **(B)** Smoking tends to lower high-density lipoprotein (HDL) cholesterol (or "good" cholesterol). It is considered beneficial to *increase* HDL cholesterol through exercise and reducing sugar intake.

60. **(D)** No explanation needed.

61. **(B)** Glucose (A) and sodium (C) are reabsorbed in the kidney. However, creatinine is not absorbed by the kidneys, thereby making it a good indicator of renal function.

62. **(A)** Carbohydrates are digested by amylases in the mouth and small intestines. Pepsin digests proteins, lipase lipids, and nucleases nucleic acids.

63. **(A)** Before lipases can act on the fat that enters the small intestine, they must first be broken down into smaller fat globules. This emulsification process is carried out by bile salts.

64. **(C)** The tarsal plates (A) are made of dense fibrous connective tissue and are important in maintaining the shape of the eyelids. The lacrimal gland (B) secretes lacrimal fluid through the ducts into the conjunctival sac of the upper eye. The answer is (C), the conjunctiva is the thin, mucus-secreting epithelial membrane that lines the interior surface of the eyelid.

65. **(D)** Cholesterol, when deposited in the body's large arteries, causes atherosclerosis that can lead to heart attacks and strokes. Cholesterol is used in the synthesis of cellular membranes and bile salts. It is transferred in the blood in two different forms: low-density lipoprotein (LDL) and high-density lipoprotein (HDL) particles.

66. **(C)** No explanation needed.

67. **(D)** Fat-soluble vitamins include vitamins A, D, E, and K. B_1 is a water-soluble vitamin, not a fat-soluble vitamin.

68. **(B)** All of the statements are true except B. Most nutrients are absorbed by the small intestines rather than the large intestines.

69. **(C)** Animal viruses are classified on the basis of their replication strategy.

70. **(D)** Vitamin E is a fat-soluble vitamin. Fat-soluble vitamins include vitamins A, D, E, and K. Thiamine (B_1), riboflavin (B_2), and folic acid (B_9) are water-soluble vitamins. +Vitamin C, Niacin (B_3), Pyridoxine (B_6), Inositol (B_8)

71. **(B)** The gallbladder serves as a reservoir for bile (B). Bile aids in the emulsification of fats. The beta cells of the pancreas produce insulin (C), not the gallbladder. Choices A and D are irrelevant.

72. **(B)** The Centers for Disease Control and Prevention (CDC) estimates that excess weight and physical inactivity combine to account for more than 300,000 premature deaths in the United States annually.

73. **(A)** Bile salts enhance the intestinal absorption of fatty acids. The other three choices are involved in the digestion of food.

74. **(C)** If an individual hyperventilates, a change in blood pH is likely to occur, thus ruling out choice A. To reason the correct solution, one must know that hyperventilation (rapid breathing) results in a loss of CO_2—thereby increasing blood pH. Therefore, choices B and D are incorrect.

75. **(D)** The medulla oblongata controls autonomic respirations and functions of the cardiac centers (e.g., heartbeat) and the vasomotor center (e.g., arteriole wall constriction). Verbal communication is a function of the frontal lobe of the brain, not the medulla oblongata.

76. **(D)** No explanation needed.

77. **(D)** Most of the antibiotics used today are natural products produced by fungi. Many antibiotics act by either preventing bacterial cell wall synthesis or interfering with ribosome function.

78. **(D)** No explanation needed.

79. **(B)** Koch's postulate defines the criterion used to demonstrate that an organism is responsible for causing a specific disease.

80. **(A)** Impulses from other neurons are picked up by dendrites (A).

81. **(A)** A neurotransmitter is a specific chemical agent in the body released by presynaptic cells, upon excitation, that crosses the synapse to stimulate or inhibit the postsynaptic cells. Serotonin (B), acetylcholine (C), and norepinephrine (D) are neurotransmitters. On the other hand, albuterol (D) is not. Albuterol is a medication used to bronchodilate.

82. **(A)** No explanation needed.

83. **(B)** Although the stomach (B) is not vestigial (remnants of organs that do not serve a true function, but are believed to have served a function in the past), the appendix (A) and the wisdom teeth (C) are vestigial in nature.

84. **(C)** No explanation needed.

85. **(B)** Bulimia nervosa is an eating disorder in which a person eats a great deal of food and then vomits or uses other purging methods. Anorexia nervosa is an eating disorder in which individuals do not eat enough to maintain body function at a normal level. Individuals with binge-eating disorder eat large amounts of food frequently and repeatedly. Disordered-eating patterns occur when concerns about dieting, food restriction, fear of becoming overweight, and dissatisfaction with body image interfere with normal daily life.

86. **(B)** Viruses obtain their envelope by budding through host cell membranes at sites where viral proteins have been inserted.

87. **(B)** Viruses do not degrade host cell nucleic acids to obtain nucleotides for replication.

88. **(A)** Virus particles self-assemble. Neither enzymes nor ATP are required to assemble virus particles.

89. **(A)** No explanation needed.

90. **(A)** Physical drug dependence results when an individual's body needs a drug to avoid withdrawal. Psychological drug dependence occurs when the drug is constantly on the user's mind and he or she feels an overwhelming need to use the drug often. Answer C is a nonsense answer.

91. **(C)** The best way to solve this problem is to find the cross that will most likely result in 75 percent yellow offspring given that yellow is dominant over green. After making your selection from the four possible choices, you should perform the cross by using a Punnett square. For example, let's cross choice C (Yy and Yy):

	Y	y
Y	YY	Yy
y	Yy	yy

YY = homozygous yellow;
Yy = heterozygous yellow;
yy = green

This cross will result in 75 percent yellow offspring.
To check the other choices, set up each of them in a Punnett square. Choice A will result in 50 percent yellow and 50 percent green. Choice B will result in 100 percent yellow offspring. Choice D will result in 100 percent yellow.

92. **(A)** Oxidative phosphorylation is the process in which energy is released as electrons pass through a series of electron acceptors to either oxygen or another inorganic compound.

93. **(A)** A homozygous (having the same pair) blue bird is represented by BB, and a homozygous white bird is represented by ww. Cross the two in the following Punnett square:

	w	w
B	Bw	Bw
B	Bw	Bw

Bw = blue

A cross between a homozygous blue bird (BB) and a homozygous white bird (ww) will result in 0 percent white birds.

94. **(D)** Follow the same procedure as in question 93:

	w	w
B	Bw	Bw
B	Bw	Bw

Bw = blue

A cross between a homozygous blue bird and a homozygous white bird will result in 100 percent blue heterozygous (Bw) birds.

95. **(B)** Cones (B) provide daylight color vision and are responsible for visual acuity. Rods (A) respond to dim light for black-and-white vision. The optic disc (C) is a small region of the retina where the fibers of the ganglion neurons exit from the eyeball. The retina (D) is the inner layer of eyeball, and it contains the rods and cones.

96. **(B)** The immune system employs two major responses to inhibit an invading organism: an innate and an acquired response. The innate response includes the inflammatory response and is not directed against a specific disease agent. The acquired immune response, involving either T or B cells, is directed against a specific agent.

97. **(B)** No explanation needed.

98. **(C)** Set up the cross between the individual carrying the disease (represented by Cc) and the individual with the disease (represented by cc = two recessive genes):

	C	c
c	Cc	cc
c	Cc	cc

Cc = do not have disease but are carriers;
cc = have the disease

Therefore, 50 percent are expected to have the disease.

99. **(D)** Similar to question 98, set up the cross between the individual carrying the disease (Ss) and the individual with the disease (ss):

	S	s
s	Ss	ss
s	Ss	ss

Ss = carrier of disease;
ss = have the disease

Therefore, 100 percent are expected to either be a carrier or have the disease.

100. **(D)** The percentage cannot be determined from the information given. You need to know if the parent is heterozygous green or homozygous green.

CHAPTER 6

Chemistry Review and Practice

TIPS FOR THE CHEMISTRY SECTION

The chemistry section of the PCAT consists of approximately 48 questions. You will have 30 minutes to complete the chemistry section. General chemistry, organic chemistry, and biochemistry questions are asked.

GENERAL CHEMISTRY REVIEW OUTLINE

I. Matter and the Periodic Table
 A. Three states of matter
  1. Solid
  2. Liquid
  3. Gas
 B. Chemical and physical properties
 C. Elements, compounds, and mixtures
 D. Metals and nonmetals
 E. Electrolytes and nonelectrolytes
 F. Sizes of atoms
 G. Electronegativity
 H. Phase changes

II. Simple mathematics
 A. Density
 B. Percent composition
 C. Average atomic weight
 D. Conversions (e.g., English and metric systems; see Appendix)

III. Atomic structure
 A. Atomic particles
  1. Protons
  2. Neutrons
  3. Electrons
 B. Atomic number

C. Atomic mass (atomic weight)
D. Molecular weight
E. Formula weight
F. Isotopes
G. Allotropes
H. Moles and Avogadro's number

IV. **Oxidation and reduction**
A. Oxidation number
B. Formal charge
C. Oxidizing agents
D. Reducing agents

V. **Balancing equations**
A. Simple equations
B. Redox equations

VI. **Solutions**
A. Concentration
  1. Molarity
  2. Molality
  3. Percent composition
  4. Mole fraction
B. Dilution of solutions
C. Colligative properties
  1. Depression of vapor pressure
  2. Elevation of boiling point
  3. Depression of freezing point
  4. Osmosis
D. Solubility rules

VII. **Gas laws**
A. Boyle's law
B. Charles's law
C. Ideal gas law
D. Dalton's law of partial pressure
E. Real gases
F. Effusion and diffusion

VIII. **Bonding**
A. Ionic
B. Covalent
C. Polar covalent
D. Intermolecular forces
  1. Hydrogen bonding
  2. Van der Waals forces

IX. Stoichiometry and equations
   A. Molar relationships
   B. Volume relationships
   C. Limiting reagent
   D. Percent yield

X. Nomenclature and writing formulas

XI. Molecular geometry
   A. Hybridization
   B. Bond angles
   C. Dipole moment

XII. Resonance

XIII. Electromagnetic spectrum
   A. Quantum theory and quantum numbers
   B. Electron configuration
   C. Lewis dot structures

XIV. Calorimetry
   A. Specific heat
   B. Heat capacity

XV. Acids and bases
   A. Definitions–Arrhenius, Brönsted-Lowry (conjugate pairs), Lewis
   B. Strengths of acids and bases
   C. pH
   D. Neutralization
   E. Buffers
   F. Acidic, basic, and amphoteric oxides

XVI. Kinetics
   A. First-order reactions
   B. Second-order reactions
   C. Half-life
   D. Determination of reaction orders
   E. Graphs

XVII. Equilibrium
   A. Equilibrium constants
      1. Acid
      2. Base
      3. Solubility product
      4. Complex ion formation
   B. Le Châtelier's principle

XVIII. **Electrochemistry**
- A. Electrolytic and galvanic cells
- B. Oxidation and reduction
- C. Anode and cathode

XIX. **Radioactivity**
- A. Nuclear particles
- B. Balancing equations
- C. Fission
- D. Fusion

ORGANIC CHEMISTRY REVIEW OUTLINE

I. **Formulas for families**
- A. RCOOH, carboxylic acid, etc.
- B. General formulas for families (e.g., alkanes are C_nH_{2n+2})
- C. Empirical, molecular, and structural formulas
- D. Hybridation states of carbon

II. **Physical properties of various organic families**

III. **Nomenclature**

IV. **Isomerism**
- A. Geometric
- B. Optical
  1. Enantiomer
  2. Diastereomer
  3. Stereocenter
  4. Racemic mixture

V. **Examples of simple reactions**
- A. Addition
  1. Electrophilic addition to alkenes/alkynes
  2. Nucleophilic addition to carbonyl compounds
- B. Substitution
  1. Electrophilic substitution of benzene compounds
  2. Nucleophilic substitution of alkyl halides, acid derivatives
  3. Alpha substitution of carbonyl compounds
- C. Oxidation
  1. Cleavage of alkenes/alkynes
  2. Alcohols
- D. Reduction
  1. Alkenes/alkynes
  2. Carbonyl compounds

    E. Elimination
    F. Free-radical substitution
    G. Condensations of carbonyl compounds
        1. Aldol condensation
        2. Claisen condensation

VI. Resonance
    A. Benzene
    B. Cations, anions
    C. Radicals

VII. Spectroscopy
    A. Infrared (IR)
    B. Nuclear magnetic resonance (NMR)

BIOCHEMISTRY REVIEW OUTLINE

I. DNA, RNA
    A. Structures
    B. Processes
        1. Transcription
        2. Translation
        3. Replication

II. Lipids
    A. Structures
    B. Processes
        1. Storage, triglycerides
        2. Energy production, beta oxidation
        3. Membrane formation
        4. Steroid hormones

III. Proteins
    A. Levels of structure
        1. Primary
        2. Secondary
        3. Tertiary
        4. Quaternary
    B. Processes
        1. Synthesis, translation
        2. Degradation, digestion

Answer Sheet
CHEMISTRY

1 Ⓐ Ⓑ Ⓒ Ⓓ	26 Ⓐ Ⓑ Ⓒ Ⓓ	51 Ⓐ Ⓑ Ⓒ Ⓓ	76 Ⓐ Ⓑ Ⓒ Ⓓ
2 Ⓐ Ⓑ Ⓒ Ⓓ	27 Ⓐ Ⓑ Ⓒ Ⓓ	52 Ⓐ Ⓑ Ⓒ Ⓓ	77 Ⓐ Ⓑ Ⓒ Ⓓ
3 Ⓐ Ⓑ Ⓒ Ⓓ	28 Ⓐ Ⓑ Ⓒ Ⓓ	53 Ⓐ Ⓑ Ⓒ Ⓓ	78 Ⓐ Ⓑ Ⓒ Ⓓ
4 Ⓐ Ⓑ Ⓒ Ⓓ	29 Ⓐ Ⓑ Ⓒ Ⓓ	54 Ⓐ Ⓑ Ⓒ Ⓓ	79 Ⓐ Ⓑ Ⓒ Ⓓ
5 Ⓐ Ⓑ Ⓒ Ⓓ	30 Ⓐ Ⓑ Ⓒ Ⓓ	55 Ⓐ Ⓑ Ⓒ Ⓓ	80 Ⓐ Ⓑ Ⓒ Ⓓ
6 Ⓐ Ⓑ Ⓒ Ⓓ	31 Ⓐ Ⓑ Ⓒ Ⓓ	56 Ⓐ Ⓑ Ⓒ Ⓓ	81 Ⓐ Ⓑ Ⓒ Ⓓ
7 Ⓐ Ⓑ Ⓒ Ⓓ	32 Ⓐ Ⓑ Ⓒ Ⓓ	57 Ⓐ Ⓑ Ⓒ Ⓓ	82 Ⓐ Ⓑ Ⓒ Ⓓ
8 Ⓐ Ⓑ Ⓒ Ⓓ	33 Ⓐ Ⓑ Ⓒ Ⓓ	58 Ⓐ Ⓑ Ⓒ Ⓓ	83 Ⓐ Ⓑ Ⓒ Ⓓ
9 Ⓐ Ⓑ Ⓒ Ⓓ	34 Ⓐ Ⓑ Ⓒ Ⓓ	59 Ⓐ Ⓑ Ⓒ Ⓓ	84 Ⓐ Ⓑ Ⓒ Ⓓ
10 Ⓐ Ⓑ Ⓒ Ⓓ	35 Ⓐ Ⓑ Ⓒ Ⓓ	60 Ⓐ Ⓑ Ⓒ Ⓓ	85 Ⓐ Ⓑ Ⓒ Ⓓ
11 Ⓐ Ⓑ Ⓒ Ⓓ	36 Ⓐ Ⓑ Ⓒ Ⓓ	61 Ⓐ Ⓑ Ⓒ Ⓓ	86 Ⓐ Ⓑ Ⓒ Ⓓ
12 Ⓐ Ⓑ Ⓒ Ⓓ	37 Ⓐ Ⓑ Ⓒ Ⓓ	62 Ⓐ Ⓑ Ⓒ Ⓓ	87 Ⓐ Ⓑ Ⓒ Ⓓ
13 Ⓐ Ⓑ Ⓒ Ⓓ	38 Ⓐ Ⓑ Ⓒ Ⓓ	63 Ⓐ Ⓑ Ⓒ Ⓓ	88 Ⓐ Ⓑ Ⓒ Ⓓ
14 Ⓐ Ⓑ Ⓒ Ⓓ	39 Ⓐ Ⓑ Ⓒ Ⓓ	64 Ⓐ Ⓑ Ⓒ Ⓓ	89 Ⓐ Ⓑ Ⓒ Ⓓ
15 Ⓐ Ⓑ Ⓒ Ⓓ	40 Ⓐ Ⓑ Ⓒ Ⓓ	65 Ⓐ Ⓑ Ⓒ Ⓓ	90 Ⓐ Ⓑ Ⓒ Ⓓ
16 Ⓐ Ⓑ Ⓒ Ⓓ	41 Ⓐ Ⓑ Ⓒ Ⓓ	66 Ⓐ Ⓑ Ⓒ Ⓓ	91 Ⓐ Ⓑ Ⓒ Ⓓ
17 Ⓐ Ⓑ Ⓒ Ⓓ	42 Ⓐ Ⓑ Ⓒ Ⓓ	67 Ⓐ Ⓑ Ⓒ Ⓓ	92 Ⓐ Ⓑ Ⓒ Ⓓ
18 Ⓐ Ⓑ Ⓒ Ⓓ	43 Ⓐ Ⓑ Ⓒ Ⓓ	68 Ⓐ Ⓑ Ⓒ Ⓓ	93 Ⓐ Ⓑ Ⓒ Ⓓ
19 Ⓐ Ⓑ Ⓒ Ⓓ	44 Ⓐ Ⓑ Ⓒ Ⓓ	69 Ⓐ Ⓑ Ⓒ Ⓓ	94 Ⓐ Ⓑ Ⓒ Ⓓ
20 Ⓐ Ⓑ Ⓒ Ⓓ	45 Ⓐ Ⓑ Ⓒ Ⓓ	70 Ⓐ Ⓑ Ⓒ Ⓓ	95 Ⓐ Ⓑ Ⓒ Ⓓ
21 Ⓐ Ⓑ Ⓒ Ⓓ	46 Ⓐ Ⓑ Ⓒ Ⓓ	71 Ⓐ Ⓑ Ⓒ Ⓓ	96 Ⓐ Ⓑ Ⓒ Ⓓ
22 Ⓐ Ⓑ Ⓒ Ⓓ	47 Ⓐ Ⓑ Ⓒ Ⓓ	72 Ⓐ Ⓑ Ⓒ Ⓓ	97 Ⓐ Ⓑ Ⓒ Ⓓ
23 Ⓐ Ⓑ Ⓒ Ⓓ	48 Ⓐ Ⓑ Ⓒ Ⓓ	73 Ⓐ Ⓑ Ⓒ Ⓓ	98 Ⓐ Ⓑ Ⓒ Ⓓ
24 Ⓐ Ⓑ Ⓒ Ⓓ	49 Ⓐ Ⓑ Ⓒ Ⓓ	74 Ⓐ Ⓑ Ⓒ Ⓓ	99 Ⓐ Ⓑ Ⓒ Ⓓ
25 Ⓐ Ⓑ Ⓒ Ⓓ	50 Ⓐ Ⓑ Ⓒ Ⓓ	75 Ⓐ Ⓑ Ⓒ Ⓓ	100 Ⓐ Ⓑ Ⓒ Ⓓ

Practice Questions

100 Questions

Directions: Select the best answer to each of the following questions.

1. Which of the following statements describes a chemical property?

   (A) Liquid water is converted to water vapor by application of heat.
   (B) Salt, NaCl, dissolves in water.
   (C) A stone displaces its volume in a liquid.
   (D) Milk sours more readily at room temperature than in the refrigerator.

2. Which of the following theories would describe the covalent bond in water as the overlap of a half-filled 1s orbital with a half-filled sp^3 orbital?

   (A) Molecular Orbital Theory
   (B) Valence Shell Electron Pair Repulsion Theory (VSEPR)
   (C) Valence Bond Theory
   (D) Kinetic Molecular Theory

3. If the volume of a sample of gas at 1 atm and 25°C is reduced, what will be TRUE if the temperature remains constant?

   (A) pressure will decrease
   (B) gas particles will slow down
   (C) Boyle's law will be demonstrated
   (D) Charles's law will be demonstrated

4. Which of the following is NOT a nuclear reaction?

   (A) A sodium atom becomes a sodium ion.
   (B) A uranium atom becomes a barium atom and a krypton atom.
   (C) A thorium atom releases a gamma particle.
   (D) An iodine atom becomes a different isotope of iodine.

5. Which of the following statements is NOT true concerning DNA?

   (A) It contains deoxyribonucleotides.
   (B) It contains adenine, guanine, cytosine, and thymine.
   (C) It exists as a double helix in the cell.
   (D) It is commonly found in the cytoplasm of animal cells.

6. How many neutrons are contained in the following atom of the element scandium: $^{45}_{21}Sc$?

   (A) 21
   (B) 66
   (C) 45
   (D) 24

   45 − 21 = 24   *protons*

   neutrons   *e⁻*

7. The classification of macromolecules as lipids is primarily based on the

   (A) cellular function of the molecule.
   (B) nonpolarity of the molecule.
   (C) absence of phosphate groups.
   (D) presence of peptide bonds.

8. The mass of 1 mole of copper (Cu) atoms equals 63.55 grams. What is the weight, in grams, of one atom of Cu?

   [Avogadro's number = 6×10^{23}]

   (A) 1.06×10^{-24}
   (B) 9.47×10^{-23}
   (C) 9.47×10^{-21}
   (D) 1.06×10^{-22}

   molcu
   mo

   $$\frac{63.55 grams}{1 mol} \times \frac{1 mol}{6 \times 10^{23}}$$

9. Calculate the formula weight, in atomic mass units (amu), of the salt ammonium sulfate, $(NH_4)_2SO_4$. (S = 32 amu, O = 16 amu, N = 14 amu, H = 1 amu)

   (A) 72
   (B) 132
   (C) 128
   (D) 114

   14 + 4

   $\times \frac{16}{4}{64}$

   28 + 8 + 32 + 16(4) =

   28 + 40 = 68 ≠ 64 = 132

10. What is the percentage of hydrogen, H, present in dimethyl ether, C_2H_6O?
    (C = 12 amu, H = 1 amu, O = 16 amu)

    (A) 2
    (B) 13
    (C) 52
    (D) 35

    24 + 6 = 30 + 16 = 46

    $\frac{6}{46} =$

11. The primary structure of proteins is

    (A) the order of the amino acids in the polymer.
    (B) the result of hydrogen bonding between amino acids.
    (C) irrelevant to the protein's function.
    (D) destroyed by denaturation.

12. When the following equation is balanced with the smallest set of whole numbers, what is the coefficient of H_2SO_4?

    $\underline{1}\,Na_2CO_3 + \underline{2}\,H_2SO_4 \rightarrow \underline{2}\,NaHSO_4 + \underline{1}\,H_2O + \underline{1}\,CO_2$

    $11=0 \qquad\qquad 8+$

    (A) 1
    (B) 2
    (C) 3
    (D) 5

13. What is the oxidation number of sulfur, S, in H_2SO_3?

    (A) 2
    (B) 4
    (C) 5
    (D) 6

    $$H$$
    $$(+2) + x + (-6) = 0$$

14. What is the reducing agent in the following equation?

    $$Zn + CuSO_4 \rightarrow ZnSO_4 + Cu$$
    $$\;0\quad\; +\qquad\quad +\qquad -$$

    (A) Zn
    (B) $CuSO_4$
    (C) $ZnSO_4$
    (D) Cu

15. RNA differs from DNA in that it

    RNA =

    DNA =

    (A) cannot base-pair.
    (B) doesn't contain phosphate groups.
    (C) is not used to synthesize new molecules of itself.
    (D) contains uracil rather than thymine found in DNA.

16. In the following reaction, how many moles of O_2 are necessary to react with 5 moles of NH_3? (O = 16 amu, N = 14 amu, H = 1 amu)

    $$4NH_3 + 5O_2 \rightarrow 4NO + 6H_2O$$

    $\dfrac{25}{4} =$

    (A) 4.0
    (B) 5.0
    (C) 5.5
    (D) 6.3

    $\dfrac{4NH_3}{5O_2}$

    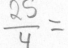 $5\,mol\,NH_3 \times \dfrac{5\,mol\,O_2}{4\,mol\,NH_3} =$

17. How many liters of oxygen gas, O_2, will react completely with 3.5 liters of carbon disulfide gas, CS_2, in the following reaction?

$$CS_2 + 2O_2 \rightarrow CO_2 + 2SO_2$$

(A) 14.0
(B) 3.5
(C) 7.0
(D) 1.8

$$3.5 \text{ Liters } CS_2 \times \frac{2 \text{ mol } O_2}{1 \text{ mol } CS_2}$$

18. In the following reaction, how many grams of H_2O are produced from 17.0 g of NH_3? (O = 16 amu, N = 14 amu, H = 1 amu)

$$4 NH_3 + 5 O_2 \rightarrow 4 NO + 6 H_2O$$

(A) 1.5
(B) 18
(C) 27
(D) 2.4

$$17g\ NH_3 \times \frac{1\,mol}{17g} \times \frac{6\ H_2O\ mol}{4\ NH_3} \times \frac{18}{1\,mol}$$

19. In the following reaction, how many liters of NO are produced from 1.70 g of NH_3 at standard temperature and pressure conditions? (O = 16 amu, N = 14 amu, H = 1 amu)

$$4 NH_3 + 5 O_2 \rightarrow 4 NO + 6 H_2O$$

(A) 2.24
(B) 1.70
(C) 8.96
(D) 0.026

$$1.7g\ NH_3 \times \frac{1\,mol}{17g} \times \frac{4\,mol}{4\,mol} \times \frac{22.4\,L}{1\,mol} =$$

$$1\,mol = 22.4\ Liters$$

20. In the following reaction, how many molecules of NO are produced from 0.17 g of NH_3? (O = 16 amu, N = 14 amu, H = 1 amu)

$$4 NH_3 + 5 O_2 \rightarrow 4 NO + 6 H_2O$$

(A) 6.0×10^{21}
(B) 1.4×10^{22}
(C) 4.0×10^{23}
(D) 2.9×10^{23}

$$.17g\ NH_3 \times \frac{1\,mol}{17g} \times \frac{4\,mol}{4} \times \frac{6 \times 10^{23}}{1\,mol}$$

$$=$$

21. A 100-milliliter sample of oxygen, O_2, is collected over water at 25°C and 750 mm Hg pressure. The pressure of water vapor at 25°C is 23.76 mm Hg. Which of the following equations is correct to calculate the number of grams of oxygen collected? (R = 0.082 L-atm/K-mole)

(A) $750\,\text{mm}(100\,\text{ml}) = \dfrac{x}{16\,\text{g/mole}}\left(\dfrac{0.082\ \text{L-atm}}{\text{K-mole}}\right)(25°C)$

(B) $\dfrac{726.24\,\text{mm}(0.100\ \text{liter})}{760\,\text{mm/atm}} = \dfrac{16\,\text{g/mole}}{x}\left(\dfrac{0.082\ \text{L-atm}}{\text{K-mole}}\right)(25°C)$

(C) $\dfrac{750\,\text{mm}(100\,\text{ml})}{760\,\text{mm/atm}} = \dfrac{x}{32\,\text{g/mole}}\left(\dfrac{0.082\ \text{L-atm}}{\text{K-mole}}\right)(298K)$

(D) $\dfrac{726.24\,\text{mm}(0.100\,\text{liter})}{760\,\text{mm/atm}} = \dfrac{x}{32\,\text{g/mole}}\left(\dfrac{0.082\ \text{L-atm}}{\text{K-mole}}\right)(298K)$

[handwritten: $PV = nRT$; $\dfrac{PV}{RT}$; $n = \dfrac{PV}{RT}$]

22. What is the molarity (M) of a solution prepared by dissolving 1.8 grams of sugar, $C_6H_{12}O_6$, in 1000 milliliters of solution? (O = 16 amu, C = 12 amu, H = 1 amu)

(A) 0.01
(B) 1.80
(C) 0.0018
(D) 0.10

[handwritten: $\dfrac{1.8\,g}{1L} = \dfrac{g/mol}{L}$]

23. How many grams of nitrogen gas, N_2, are present in a bulb of volume 1.0 liter, at 27°C and 1 atmosphere? (R = 0.082 liter-atm/K-mole, N = 14 amu)

(A) 7.9×10^{-2}
(B) 1.0×10^5
(C) 1.1
(D) 8.4×10^{-3}

[handwritten: $PV = nRT$; $\dfrac{}{RT}$; 298; $\dfrac{g}{mol\,wt.} = x = \dfrac{(1\,atm)(1)}{(0.082)(300)} = \dfrac{1}{24.6} = 0.04065\,mol \times \dfrac{28}{1\,mol}$]

24. How many milliliters of 5.0 M, sodium hydroxide, NaOH, solution must be used to prepare 200 milliliters of 2.5 M solution?

(A) 440
(B) 36
(C) 500
(D) 100

[handwritten: $\dfrac{g/mol}{L}$; $\dfrac{2.5M}{0.2} = 12.5$; $200(2.5) = 5(x)$; $\dfrac{5\,g/mol}{1L}$]

25. Which of the following compounds would be expected to have the highest boiling point?

(A)

(B)

(C)

(D)

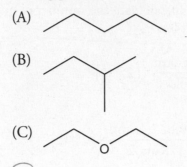

26. How many milliliters of 2.0 M lithium hydroxide, LiOH, solution are necessary to neutralize 10 milliliters of 3.0 M sulfuric acid, H_2SO_4, according to the following equation?

$$2\ LiOH + H_2SO_4 \rightarrow Li_2SO_4 + 2H_2O$$

(A) 60
(B) 30
(C) 15
(D) 12

$2x = 10 \times 3$

$2 = 30$

$15\,mL\ x$

$\dfrac{2\ LiOH}{1\ H_2SO_4}$

27. A bubble of gas (1.4 mL) is at the bottom of a lake where the temperature and pressure are 7°C and 2.0 atmospheres, respectively. The temperature and pressure at the surface of the lake are 27°C and 1.0 atmosphere. What is the volume, in milliliters, of a gas bubble at the surface of the lake?

(A) 2.6
(B) 3.0
(C) 0.75
(D) 0.65

$1.4\,mL(7)(2) - (27)(1)$ ✗

$\dfrac{19.6}{27}$

$\dfrac{PV}{T} = \dfrac{P_2 V_2}{T_2}$ ✓

28. Ammonia, NH_3, and oxygen, O_2, are gases at standard temperature and pressure. They are combined to produce nitrous oxide gas, NO, and water vapor. How many liters of NO can be produced at 27°C and 2.0 atmospheres from 1.7 g of NH_3? (O = 16 amu, N = 14 amu, H = 1 amu, R = 0.082 liter-atm/K-mole).

$$4NH_3 + 5O_2 \rightarrow 4NO + 6H_2O$$

(A) 2.2
(B) 1.2
(C) 4.0
(D) 0.8

$1.7g\ NH_3 \times \dfrac{1\,mol}{17g} \times \dfrac{4\,mol}{4\,mol} \times \dfrac{30g}{1\,mol} = 0.1\,\cancel{4}mol$

$PV = nRT$

$\dfrac{}{P}$

$V = \dfrac{\overset{0.1}{0.14}\ (0.082)\ 300}{2}$

29. Two gases—oxygen, O_2, and hydrogen, H_2—effuse (escape from one part of a container to another part by passing through a small hole). What is the rate of effusion of hydrogen as compared to that of oxygen at the same temperature and pressure? (O = 16 amu, H = 1 amu)

    (A) 16.0
    (B) 0.25
    (C) 4.00
    (D) 0.06

    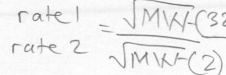

    $$\frac{rate\ 1}{rate\ 2} = \frac{\sqrt{MW\ (32)}}{\sqrt{MW\ (2)}}$$

30. Specify the absolute configuration of each chiral center in:

    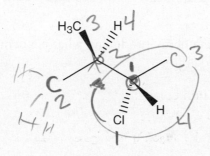

    (A) 2R
    (B) 2S
    (C) 2R, 3R
    (D) 2S, 3S

31. The specific heat of copper, Cu, is 0.385 joule per gram °C. What is the heat capacity, in joules per °C, of 10.0 grams of copper?

    (A) 0.03
    (B) 15.4
    (C) 3.85
    (D) 38.9

    $C = M\ S$

    $mas \times sph$

32. All of the following are uses of lipids EXCEPT

    (A) hormones.
    (B) energy production.
    (C) cell membrane construction.
    (D) gene composition.

33. Name the following molecule.

    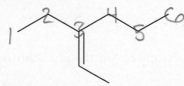

    (A) 3-ethylenehexane
    (B) (E)-3-propyl-2-pentene
    (C) (Z)-3-ethyl-2-hexene
    (D) (E)-3-ethyl-2-hexene

Use the periodic table to answer questions 34, 35, 37–43.

H																	He
Li	Be											B	C	N	O	F	Ne
Na	Mg											Al	Si	P.	S	Cl.	Ar
K	Ca	Sc	Ti	V	Cr	Mn	Fe	Co	Ni	Cu	Zn	Ga	Ge	As	Se	Br	Kr
Rb	Sr	Y	Zr	Nb	Mo	Tc	Ru	Rh	Pd	Ag	Cd	In	Sn	Sb	Te	I	Xe
Cs	Ba	La	Hf	Ta	W	Re	Os	Ir	Pt	Au	Hg	Tl	Pb	Bi	Po	At	Rn
Fr	Ra	Ac	Rf	Ha	Sg	Ns	Hs	Mt									

Ce	Pr	Nd	Pm	Sm	Eu	Gd	Tb	Dy	Ho	Er	Tm	Yb	Lu
Th	Pa	U	Np	Pu	Am	Cm	Bk	Cf	Es	Fm	Md	No	Lr

34. Radium undergoes beta decay producing what element?

$$^{228}_{88}Ra \rightarrow ^{0}_{-1}e + ?$$

(A) Fr
(B) Rn
(C) Ac
(D) Ra

35. The electron configuration for the sulfide ion, S^{2-}, is

(A) $1s^2 2s^2 2p^6 3s^2 3p^6$.
(B) $1s^2 2s^2 2p^6 3s^2 3p^4$.
(C) $1s^2 2s^2 2p^6 3s^2 3p^2$.
(D) $1s^2 2s^2 2p^6 3s^2 3p^6 4s^2$.

36. An example of secondary structure in proteins includes a

(A) tetramer.
(B) peptide bond.
(C) beta sheet.
(D) double helix.

37. What is the maximum number of electrons possible in the p orbitals of an atom?

(A) 6
(B) 10
(C) 5
(D) 3

38. How many unshared electrons are on the phosphorus atom in the Lewis dot structure for PCl_5?

(A) 5
(B) 2
(C) 0
(D) 8

39. What is the formal charge on the carbon atom in the carbonate ion, CO_3^{2-}?

    (A) 0
    (B) +1
    (C) −1
    (D) +4

    $x + (-6) = -2$ no!

    #valance e^- − #bonding e^- − $\frac{1}{2}$bond = 0

40. The compound with the greatest amount of ionic bonding character is

    (A) CO_2
    (B) Li_2O
    (C) CH_4
    (D) NH_3

41. What is the molecular geometry of the silicon hydride, SiH_4, molecule?

    (A) Linear
    (B) Bent
    (C) Tetrahedral
    (D) Trigonal pyramid

    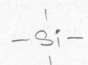

42. What is the approximate value of the bond angle for the H-S-H bond in hydrogen sulfide, H_2S?

    (A) 105°
    (B) 120°
    (C) 180°
    (D) 90°

    H − S̈ − H

43. What is the hybridization state of the aluminum (Al) atom in $AlCl_3$?

    (A) sp
    (B) sp^2
    (C) sp^3
    (D) sp^3d^2

    Cl − Al − Cl

44. The synthesis of protein directly involves all of the following EXCEPT

    (A) amino acids.
    (B) DNA.
    (C) ribosomes.
    (D) RNA.

45. Name the following molecule.

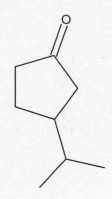

    (A) 3-isopropylcyclopentanone
    (B) 1-isopropyl-2-cyclopentanone
    (C) 2-oxo-1-isopropylcyclopentane
    (D) 2-isopropyl-3-oxocyclopentane

46. What is the product of the following reaction?

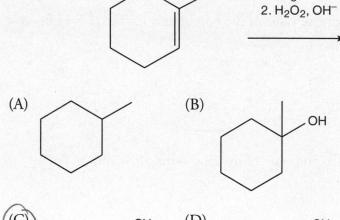

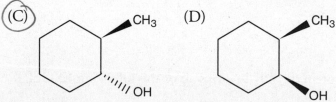

47. Which of the following molecules has a dipole moment of zero?

    (A) CO_2
    (B) H_2O
    (C) HF
    (D) NH_3

48. In the process of replication

    (A) the DNA duplex does not melt (unwind).
    (B) the two resulting DNA molecules are identical.
    (C) both new DNA molecules are synthesized discontinuously.
    (D) the raw material nucleotides are carried by tRNA.

49. How many resonance structures are possible for the carbonate ion, CO_3^{2-}?

    (A) 1
    (B) 2
    (C) 3
    (D) 4

50. What reagent would accomplish the following conversion?

    $$CH_3CH_2CHO \rightarrow CH_3CH_2CH_2OH$$

    (A) PCC (pyridinium chlorochromate)
    (B) $NaBH_4$
    (C) H_2
    (D) $KMnO_4$

51. What is a product of the following reaction?

    (A)   (B)

    (C)   (D)

52. The process by which an RNA molecule is synthesized based on the nucleotide sequence in DNA is called

    (A) transcription.
    (B) translation.
    (C) replication.
    (D) respiration.

53. The major kind of lipid found in cell membranes is

    (A) triglycerides.
    (B) phospholipids.
    (C) waxes.
    (D) starch.

54. Which of the following types of RNA carries amino acids to the ribosome for protein synthesis?

    (A) mRNA messanger
    (B) rRNA ribosomal
    (C) tRNA
    (D) aRNA

55. What is the half life, in seconds, for a first-order reaction having a rate constant of 6.93×10^2 per second?

    (A) $1.0 \times 10^{+1}$
    (B) 1.0×10^{-3}
    (C) 1.0×10^{-1}
    (D) $1.0 \times 10^{+5}$

$$t_{1/2} = \frac{0.693}{6.93 \times 10^2} = 1.0 \times 10^{-3}$$

56. What functional group is formed by the following reaction?

$$CH_3OH + (CH_3)_2CHCOBr \rightarrow$$

    (A) Ester
    (B) Acid
    (C) Acid anhydride
    (D) Ketone

57. What is the structure of the starting material if, after the addition of potassium permanganate, the products are carbon dioxide and acetone?

(A)   (B)

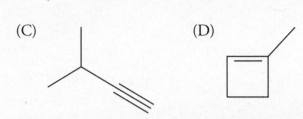

PMg

(C)   (D)

58. What is the equilibrium constant for the following reaction when [H₂] = 0.25 M, [I₂] = 0.25 M and [HI] = 0.50 M?

$$H_2 + I_2 \leftrightarrow 2HI$$

(A) 4.0
(B) 0.25
(C) 8.0
(D) 0.13

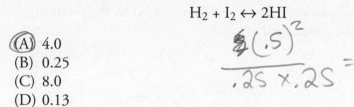

$$\frac{(.5)^2}{.25 \times .25} =$$

59. Which of the following changes will NOT cause the reaction equilibrium shown below to shift toward the products on the right?

$$Heat + N_2O_4(g) \leftrightarrow 2NO_2\ (g)$$

(A) A decrease in temperature
(B) Addition of more N_2O_4 right
(C) Removal of some NO_2 shift right (products)
(D) An increase in temperature

60. What reagent is needed for the following conversion?

$$CH_3CH_2CH(CH_3)CO_2H \rightarrow CH_3CH_2CH(CH_3)CH_2OH$$

(A) $NaBH_4$
(B) H_2
(C) $LiAlH_4$
(D) $KMnO_4$

61. What is the major product of the following elimination?

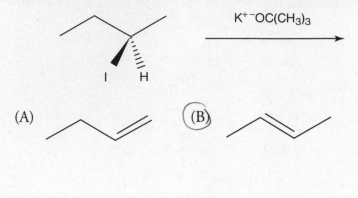

(A)

(B)

(C)

(D)

OC(CH₃)₃

62. What kind of condensation reaction is demonstrated by the following reaction under basic conditions?

(A) Claisen
(B) Williamson
(C) Michael
(D) Aldol

63. What are the monomeric units of peptides and proteins?

(A) Amino acids
(B) Aminoalcohols
(C) Aminals
(D) β–hydroxyacids

64. Which of the following is a resonance structure of

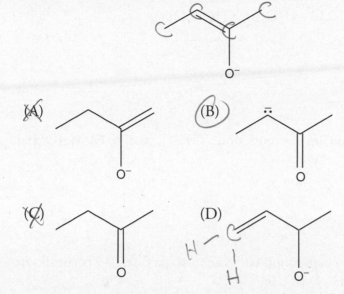

65. What is the pH of a solution having a hydroxide ion concentration, $[OH^-]$, equal to 0.01 M?

(A) 2
(B) 10
(C) 12
(D) 14

$$pOH = -\log (10^{-2})$$

$$14 - 2 = 12 \; pH$$

66. The intermolecular force that holds the two strands of DNA in a helical form is called

(A) base-pairing.
(B) covalent bonding.
(C) hydrogen bonding.
(D) both (A) and (C).

67. The infrared spectrum of a substance has a strong absorption at 3300 cm^{-1} and at 1700 cm^{-1}. What functional group is present in the substance?

(A) Ester
(B) Alcohol
(C) Acid
(D) Aldehyde

68. Which statement is TRUE concerning triglycerides?

(A) They are stored in smooth muscle.
(B) Basic hydrolysis yields soap.
(B) They are triesters of glucose.
(B) Their long carbon chains are used to generate ATP via gluconeogenesis.

69. What is the conjugate base of NH_4^+ in the following reaction?

$$NH_3 + H_2O \leftrightarrow NH_4^+ + OH^{-1}$$

(A) NH_3
(B) H_2O
(C) OH^{-1}
(D) None of the above

70. What is the hydroxide ion concentration, $[OH^{-1}]$, in 2.50 M $Mg(OH)_2$?

(A) 2.50 M
(B) 1.25 M
(C) 5.00 M
(D) 7.25 M

$POH = -\log[OH]$

71. Which structure for a compound with the formula $C_9H_{10}O$ is consistent with the following ^1H NMR data?

δ 1.4 ppm, triplet, 3H
δ 4.1 ppm, quartet, 2H
δ 7.0 ppm, doublet, 2H
δ 7.8 ppm, doublet, 2H
δ 9.8 ppm, singlet, 1H

(A)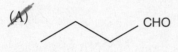

(B)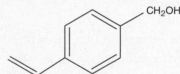

(C)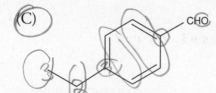

(D)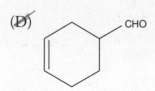

72. Beta oxidation is a metabolic pathway involving the oxidation of

(A) polysaccharides.
(B) nucleic acids.
(C) fatty acids.
(D) polypeptides.

73. If the value of K_A for an acid, HY, is 5×10^{-5}, what is the value of K_B for the conjugate ion, Y^{-1}?

(A) 2.0×10^{-10}
(B) 2.0×10^{-8}
(C) 2.0×10^{-18}
(D) 2.0×10^{-20}

1×10^{-14}

$K_a \times 5 \times 10^{-5} = 1 \times 10^{-14}$

74. Which of the following weak acids is the strongest acid? (The ionization constants are given.)

	K_A
(A) Benzoic acid	6.5×10^{-5}
(B) Nitrous acid	4.5×10^{-4}
(C) Formic acid	1.7×10^{-4}
(D) Acetic acid	1.8×10^{-5}

75. Which is a product of the following reaction?

(A)

(B)

(C)

(D)

76. Which of the following compounds is insoluble in water?

(A) NaOH
(B) NH_4Cl
(C) $LiNO_3$
(D) $CaCO_3$

77. Amino acids used in translation come from

(A) biosynthesis reactions.
(B) digestion of dietary fats.
(C) degradation of cellular nucleic acids.
(D) the citric acid cycle.

78. Which of the following slightly soluble salts is the most soluble? (The solubility product constants are given.)

		Ksp
(A)	Copper (II) sulfide	6.0×10^{-37}
(B)	Nickel (II) sulfide	1.4×10^{-24}
(C)	Silver chloride	1.6×10^{-10}
(D)	Lead (II) chromate	2.0×10^{-14}

79. Which of the following complex ions is the most stable? (The formation constants, K_f, are given.)

		K_f
(A)	$Ag(NH_3)_2^{+1}$	1.5×10^7
(B)	$Zn(NH_3)_4^{2+}$	2.0×10^9
(C)	HgI_4^{2-}	2.0×10^{30}
(D)	$Cd(CN)_4^{2-}$	7.1×10^{16}

80. Proteins are composed of twenty amino acids that

(A) are joined by glycosidic bonds.
(B) differ in the identity of a group at the alpha carbon.
(C) are all essential.
(D) are not water soluble.

81. In which of the following solutions will aluminum hydroxide, $Al(OH)_3$, be the LEAST soluble?

(A) H_2O
(B) 0.5 M $Al(NO_3)_3$
(C) 1.6 M NaOH
(D) 0.3 M HCl

82. Which of the following molecules is a lipid?

(A)

(B)

(C)

(D)

Use the following table of standard reduction potentials to answer questions 83–84.

			emf°
Li^+ (aq) + e^-	$\rightarrow$	Li (s)	−3.05
Ca^{2+} (aq) + $2e^-$	$\rightarrow$	Ca (s)	−2.87
Zn^{2+} (aq) + $2e^-$	$\rightarrow$	Zn (s)	−0.76
Sn^{+2} (aq) + $2e^-$	$\rightarrow$	Sn (s)	−0.14
$2 H^+$ (aq) + $2e^-$	$\rightarrow$	H_2 (g)	0.00
Cu^{2+} (aq) + $2e^-$	$\rightarrow$	Cu (s)	+0.34
Fe^{3+} (aq) + e^-	$\rightarrow$	Fe^{2+}	+0.77
Br_2 (ℓ) + $2e^-$	$\rightarrow$	$2 Br^{-1}$	+1.07

83. In the following overall reaction:

$$Zn\ (s) + Cu^{+2} \rightarrow Zn^{2+} + Cu\ (s)$$

which partial reaction shows the reagent that is oxidized?

(A) Zn^{2+} (aq) + $2e^-$ $\rightarrow$ Zn (s)   oxidized = 0 → 2

(B) Cu^{2+} (aq) + $2e^-$ $\rightarrow$ Cu (s) reduced

(C) Zn (s) $\rightarrow$ Zn^{2+} (aq) + $2e^-$ reduced = 2 → 0

(D) Cu (s) $\rightarrow$ Cu^{2+} (aq) + $2e^-$

84. Which of the following species is the strongest reducing agent?

(A) Li^+

(B) Br_2

(C) Br^{-1}

(D) Li

85. Which of the following statements describes the reaction which occurs at the cathode in an electrochemical cell?

(A) The cathode is the electrode at which electrons are lost and oxidation occurs.

(B) The cathode is the electrode at which electrons are lost and reduction occurs.

(C) The cathode is the electrode at which electrons are gained and oxidation occurs.

(D) The cathode is the electrode at which electrons are gained and reduction occurs.

86. The general formula RCOOH is the formula for

(A) an aldehyde.

(B) a ketone.

(C) an ester.

(D) a carboxylic acid.

87. What is the general formula for a cycloalkane?

(A) C_nH_{2n+2}
(B) C_nH_{2n}
(C) C_nH_n
(D) C_nH_{2n-2}

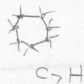

C_7H

88. Which of the following formulas represents an unsaturated compound?

(A) C_2H_6
(B) C_3H_6
(C) C_2H_6O
(D) CH_3Cl

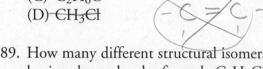

double "c" bond .

89. How many different structural isomers can be formed by the compound having the molecular formula C_4H_9Cl?

(A) 1
(B) 2
(C) 3
(D) 4

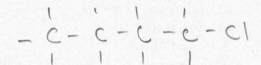

90. How many different compounds (ignoring stereoisomers) can be formed by the monochlorination of pentane?

(A) 1
(B) 2
(C) 3
(D) 4

91. What is the name of the following compound?

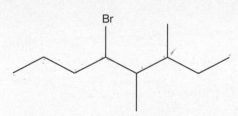

(A) 5-Bromo-3,4-dimethyloctane
(B) 4-Bromo-2-ethyl-3-methylheptane
(C) 4-Bromo-6-ethyl-5-methylheptane
(D) 4-Bromo-5,6-dimethyloctane

92. A stereocenter is one to which are attached

    (A) four groups that are the same.
    (B) three groups that are the same, one group that is different.
    (C) four groups that are different.
    (D) two groups that are the same, and another two groups which are the same yet different from the first two groups.

93. The two formulas shown below represent

$$CH_3 \quad CH_3 \qquad\qquad CH_3 \quad Cl$$
$$\diagdown\quad\diagup \qquad\qquad\qquad \diagdown\quad\diagup$$
$$C = C \qquad\qquad\qquad C = C$$
$$\diagup\quad\diagdown \qquad\qquad\qquad \diagup\quad\diagdown$$
$$Cl \quad Cl \qquad\qquad\qquad Cl \quad CH_3$$

    (A) geometric isomers.
    (B) a racemic mixture.
    (C) enantiomers.
    (D) diastereomers.

94. The carbon atom in methane, CH_4, has the hybridization

    (A) sp.
    (B) sp^2.
    (C) sp^3.
    (D) sp^3d^2.

95. The carbon atom in ethylene, $H_2C = CH_2$, has the hybridization

    (A) sp.
    (B) sp^2.
    (C) sp^3.
    (D) sp^3d^2.

96. Oxidation of the secondary alcohol 2-propanol

$$CH_3-CH-CH_3$$
$$|$$
$$OH$$

    yields:

    (A) ethanol.
    (B) propanone.
    (C) propanal.
    (D) dimethyl ether.

97. Which of the following compounds is the most water soluble?

(A) Ethyl ether, $CH_3CH_2OCH_2CH_3$
(B) Ethyl chloride, CH_3CH_2Cl
(C) Ethane, CH_3CH_3
(D) Benzene, C_6H_6

98. After reaction workup, the reaction of the Grignard reagent, methyl magnesium bromide, CH_3MgBr, with the aldehyde, acetaldehyde, CH_3CHO, produces as a product

(A) methyl ethyl ether.
(B) 2-propanol.
(C) 1-propanol.
(D) dimethyl ketone.

99. Dehydration of an alcohol produces

(A) a ketone.
(B) an alkene.
(C) an aldehyde.
(D) an alkyl halide.

OH leaves O

100. A mixture of equal amounts of a pair of enantiomers is called a

(A) pair of diastereomers.
(B) conformational mixture.
(C) meso compound.
(D) racemic mixture.

Answer Key
CHEMISTRY

1. **D**	26. **B**	51. **C**	76. **D**
2. **C**	27. **B**	52. **A**	77. **A**
3. **C**	28. **B**	53. **B**	78. **C**
4. **A**	29. **C**	54. **C**	79. **C**
5. **D**	30. **B**	55. **B**	80. **B**
6. **D**	31. **C**	56. **A**	81. **C**
7. **B**	32. **D**	57. **B**	82. **A**
8. **D**	33. **C**	58. **A**	83. **C**
9. **B**	34. **C**	59. **A**	84. **D**
10. **B**	35. **A**	60. **C**	85. **D**
11. **A**	36. **C**	61. **B**	86. **D**
12. **B**	37. **A**	62. **D**	87. **B**
13. **B**	38. **C**	63. **A**	88. **B**
14. **A**	39. **A**	64. **B**	89. **D**
15. **C**	40. **B**	65. **C**	90. **C**
16. **D**	41. **C**	66. **D**	91. **A**
17. **C**	42. **A**	67. **C**	92. **C**
18. **C**	43. **B**	68. **B**	93. **A**
19. **A**	44. **B**	69. **A**	94. **C**
20. **A**	45. **A**	70. **C**	95. **B**
21. **D**	46. **C**	71. **C**	96. **B**
22. **A**	47. **A**	72. **C**	97. **A**
23. **C**	48. **B**	73. **A**	98. **B**
24. **D**	49. **C**	74. **B**	99. **B**
25. **D**	50. **B**	75. **A**	100. **D**

EXPLANATORY ANSWERS

1. **(D)** Physical changes are illustrated by answers A, B, and C. Most physical changes are reversible. For example, water vapor can be converted back to liquid water by cooling, salt can be separated from water by evaporating the water, and the volume of the liquid returns to its original volume when the stone is removed. Answer D, however, represents a chemical change. Once milk sours, the original chemicals present in the milk are converted to new compounds and the change is not reversible. Some chemical changes are reversible, but most are not.

2. **(C)** The Valence Bond Theory is a theory concerning how atoms share electrons in covalent bonds. It views covalent bonds as being the overlap of an atomic orbital from each of the involved atoms. The Molecular Orbital Theory is also a theory of covalent bonding but it views the covalent bonding in molecules as being the addition of the individual atoms' atomic orbitals creating new orbitals that encompass the molecule (called molecular orbitals) that replace the atomic orbitals. The Valence Shell Electron Pair Repulsion Theory is used to predict the geometry of molecules and says that the electron pairs around a central atom in a molecule will spread out as far as possible. The Kinetic Molecular Theory is the theory that brings together the observed properties of gases.

3. **(C)** If the volume of a gas is reduced (and the temperature remains constant), then the pressure must increase. This is stated formally in Boyle's law ($P_1V_1 = P_2V_2$). The movement of the gas particles is dependent on the temperature so (B) is not correct. Charles's law has to do with changes in volume and temperature ($V_1/T_1 = V_2/T_2$).

4. **(A)** Nuclear reactions are reactions involving the nucleus. When a sodium atom becomes a sodium ion, an electron is lost from the valence shell of sodium (not from the nucleus). All of the other reactions are nuclear reactions. Option (B) is an example of fission (two nuclei are produced from one). Emission of gamma particles and conversion of one isotope of an element into another are both nuclear processes.

5. **(D)** DNA is contained in the nucleus of animal cells (eucaryotes).

6. **(D)** In the symbol, 45 is the mass number, or atomic weight (number of protons plus number of neutrons), and 21 is the atomic number (number of protons) of scandium, Sc. Subtracting 21 from 45 gives the number of neutrons, 24.

7. **(B)** The feature that all lipids share is that they are poorly water soluble (hydrophobic or nonpolar) due to extensive numbers of carbon-hydrogen bonds. The functions of lipids are varied and include incorporation into cell membranes, energy storage in adipose tissue, and the steroid hormones.

8. **(D)** Use the factor-label method to calculate the weight of one atom of Cu.

Avogadro's number $\cong 6 \times 10^{23}$ atoms = 1 mole

63.55 g Cu = 1 mole

$$\frac{63.55 \text{ g}}{1 \text{ mole}} \times \frac{1 \text{ mole}}{6 \times 10^{23} \text{ atoms}} = 10.59 \times 10^{-23} = 1.06 \times 10^{-22} \text{ g}$$

9. **(B)** A formula weight (or molecular weight) is calculated by adding the number of atoms of each element multiplied by its atomic mass, or weight; a total weight in atomic mass units for $(NH_4)_2SO_4$.

$$\begin{array}{rcl}
2N = 2(14) & = & 28 \\
8H = 8(1) & = & 8 \\
1S = 1(32) & = & 32 \\
4O = 4(16) & = & \underline{64} \\
& & 132 \text{ amu}
\end{array}$$

10. **(B)** Percentage equals part divided by whole times 100.

$$\frac{\text{Part}}{\text{Whole}} \times 100 = \%$$

$$\frac{6 \text{ H}}{C_2H_6O} \times 100 = \frac{6}{46} \times 100 = 13\%$$

11. **(A)** With respect to proteins, primary structure is the sequence of amino acids in the protein, secondary structure is localized patterns that arise due to hydrogen bonding between peptide bonds in the protein, tertiary structure is the overall folding pattern of the protein, and quaternary structure is the association of multiple proteins (not all proteins exhibit quaternary structure). All of the levels of structure are important in the protein's function. Denaturation disrupts the noncovalent interactions in the protein (secondary through quaternary structure), but the primary structure (which involves covalent bonds) is not affected.

12. **(B)** The coefficient of H_2SO_4 is 2 as shown in the balanced equation below:

$$Na_2CO_3 + 2H_2SO_4 \rightarrow 2 \text{ NaHSO}_4 + H_2O + CO_2$$

13. **(B)** The oxidation number of hydrogen, H, in a compound is +1, except when that element is present as a hydride [eg., LiH (–1)], and the oxidation number of oxygen, O, in a compound is –2, except when that element is present as a peroxide [eg., Na_2O_2 (–1)].

$$\overset{+2}{\underset{2(+1)}{}} \quad \overset{-6}{\underset{3(-2)}{}}$$
$$H_2SO_3$$

Since sulfurous acid, H_2SO_3, is a neutral compound, the sum of the oxidation numbers for hydrogen, sulfur, and oxygen must equal zero; +2 (for H) plus +4 (for S) combine with –6 (for O) to equal zero.

14. **(A)** Oxidation is the loss of electrons; the substance oxidized is the reducing agent. Reduction is the gain of electrons; the substance reduced is the oxidizing agent. In the given equation, Zn loses electrons while Cu^{2+} gains electrons. Thus, Zn^0 (which is oxidized to Zn^{2+}) is the reducing agent; Cu^{2+} (which is reduced to Cu^0) is the oxidizing agent.

$$Zn + CuSO_4 \rightarrow ZnSO_4 + Cu$$
$$Zn^0 \rightarrow Zn^{2+} + 2\ e^-$$
$$Cu^{2+} + 2\ e^- \rightarrow Cu$$

15. **(C)** RNA (ribonucleic acid) and DNA (deoxyribonucleic acid) are both polymers of nucleotides (nucleotides are composed of a purine or pyrimidine base, a ribose or deoxyribose sugar, and a phosphate). The purines in both RNA and DNA are named guanine and adenine. Both RNA and DNA contain the pyrimidine cytosine but only RNA contains the pyrimidine uracil and only DNA contains the pyrimidine thymine. Base-pairing refers to hydrogen bonding between nucleotides so both RNA and DNA are capable of base-pairing. The synthesis of RNA molecules is called transcription and uses the nucleotide sequence in DNA as a template for synthesis. The synthesis of DNA is called replication and uses the nucleotide sequence in DNA as a template for synthesis.

16. **(D)** The coefficients of the reactants and products in a balanced equation represent *volume* for gases, as well as *molecules* and *moles*. These are the only direct relationships involving coefficients that exist in a balanced equation. Use the factor-label method to calculate the number of moles of oxygen formed when the reaction begins with 4 moles of ammonia.

$$4NH_3(g) + 5O_2(g) \rightarrow 4NO(g) + 6H_2O(g)$$

Two fractions are possible from the relationship that 4 moles NH_3 require 5 moles O_2:

$$\frac{4 \text{ moles } NH_3}{5 \text{ moles } O_2} \qquad \frac{5 \text{ moles } O_2}{4 \text{ moles } NH_3}$$

Having 5 moles of NH_3, multiply by the appropriate fraction so that only moles of O_2 remain.

$$5 \text{ moles } NH_3 \ \times \frac{5 \text{ moles } O_2}{4 \text{ moles } NH_3} = 6.3 \text{ moles } O_2$$

17. **(C)** Refer to the explanation for question 16.

18. **(C)** Convert 17.0 g of NH_3 to moles NH_3:

$$17.0 \text{ g} \times \frac{1 \text{ mol } NH_3}{17.0 \text{ g } NH_3} = 1 \text{ mol } NH_3$$

Use the coefficients in the equation to find moles of H_2O:

$$1 \text{ mol NH}_3 \times \frac{6 \text{ mol H}_2\text{O}}{4 \text{ mol NH}_3} = 1.5 \text{ mol H}_2\text{O}$$

Convert mol H_2O to grams H_2O:

$$1.5 \text{ mol H}_2\text{O} \times \frac{18 \text{ g H}_2\text{O}}{1 \text{ mol H}_2\text{O}} = 27 \text{ g H}_2\text{O}$$

19. **(A)** Follow the same method as shown in the explanation to problem 18, except convert from moles NO to liters NO. Remember, 1 mole of any gas at standard temperature and pressure, STP, 0°C and 1 atm, occupies 22.4 liters.

$$\underline{\text{g NH}_3} \;\rightarrow\; \underline{\text{moles NH}_3} \;\rightarrow\; \underline{\text{moles NO}} \;\rightarrow\; \underline{\text{liters NO}}$$

$\underline{\text{g NH}_3}$

17.0 g NH_3

$\underline{\text{moles NH}_3}$

$$\frac{1.70 \text{ g}}{17 \text{ g/mole}} = 0.10 \text{ mole NH}_3$$

$\underline{\text{moles NO}}$

$$0.10 \text{ mole NH}_3 \times \frac{4 \text{ moles NO}}{4 \text{ moles NH}_3} = 0.10 \text{ mole NO}$$

$\underline{\text{liters NO}}$

$$0.10 \text{ mole NO} \times \frac{22.4 \text{ liters NO}}{1 \text{ mole NO}} = 2.24 \text{ liters NO}$$

20. **(A)** Follow the same method as shown in the explanations to problems 18 and 19, except convert from moles NO to molecules NO. Remember, 1 mole of any substance contains 6×10^{23} particles.

$$\underline{\text{g NH}_3} \;\rightarrow\; \underline{\text{moles NH}_3} \;\rightarrow\; \underline{\text{moles NO}} \;\rightarrow\; \underline{\text{molecules NO}}$$

$\underline{\text{g NH}_3}$

0.17 g NH_3

$\underline{\text{moles NH}_3}$

$$\frac{0.17 \text{ g NH}_3}{17 \text{ g/mole}} = 0.01 \text{ mole NH}_3$$

$\underline{\text{moles NO}}$

$$0.01 \text{ mole NH}_3 \times \frac{4 \text{ moles NO}}{4 \text{ moles NH}_3} = 0.01 \text{ mole NO}$$

$\underline{\text{molecules NO}}$

$$0.01 \text{ mole NO} \times \frac{6 \times 10^{23} \text{ molecules NO}}{1 \text{ mole NO}} = 6 \times 10^{21} \text{ molecules NO}$$

21. **(D)** The equation used to solve the problem is

$$PV = nRT$$

The symbol P is pressure in atmospheres, V is volume in liters, n is number of moles, which equals grams/molar mass, R is the gas constant, and T is temperature in Kelvin. Because the oxygen is collected over water, both water and oxygen contribute to the pressure of the gas. The contribution of water, 23.76 mm, must be subtracted from the total pressure, 750 mm, in order to determine the pressure contributed by the oxygen, 726.24 mm. Pressure must be converted to atmospheres, volume converted to liters, and temperature converted to Kelvin. In addition, oxygen is a diatomic gas and, consequently, its molar mass is 32 amu.

22. **(A)** Molarity is defined as moles of solute divided by liters of solution.

$$M = \frac{\text{moles of solute}}{\text{liters of solution}} = \frac{\text{g/mol. wt.}}{\text{liters of solution}}$$

Sugar, $C_6H_{12}O_6$, has a molecular weight of 180 g/mole. Substitute 1.8 g, 180 g/mole, and 1.0 L into the above equation to obtain the molarity of the solution.

$$M = \frac{1.8\ g / 180\ g / mole}{1.0\ L} = 0.01\ \frac{\text{mole}}{\text{liter}} = 0.01M$$

23. **(C)** The ideal gas law, PV = nRT, or

$$PV = \left(\frac{\# g}{\text{mol. wt.}}\right)(RT)$$

is used to solve this problem. Pressure is used in atmospheres, volume in liters, and temperature in Kelvin. Moles of gas is represented by n, which equals grams divided by molecular weight. The molar mass of nitrogen is 28 grams/mole since nitrogen is a diatomic molecule, N_2. Substituting the given data into the above formula gives:

$$1\ atm\ (1.0\ liter) = \frac{x}{28\ \text{grams/mole}}\left(0.082\frac{\text{L-atm}}{\text{K-mole}}\right)(273+27)\ K$$

$$x = 1.1\ g$$

24. **(D)** In a dilution problem, # moles of solute before dilution = # moles of solute after dilution. Therefore

Molarity × volume (before dilution) = Molarity × volume (after dilution)

$$2.5\ \frac{\text{moles}}{L} \times 0.2\ L = 5.0\ \frac{\text{moles}}{L} \times \text{volume}$$

$$0.100\ L = \text{volume}$$

To prepare the 2.5 M solution of NaOH, dilute 100 mL of the 5.0 M solution to 200 mL.

25. **(D)** Boiling point is based on molecular weight (how heavy the molecule is) and the strength of the intermolecular forces of attraction that occur between

molecules. The heavier the molecule, the more energy will be required to get it into the gaseous state and the boiling point will increase. The stronger the intermolecular forces of attraction between molecules, the more energy it will take to break these forces and liberate the molecules in the gas form so the higher the boiling point. All of the selections have about the same molecular weight so the determining factor will be the strength of the intermolecular forces possible in a sample of each. Since the molecule in choice (D) has an alcohol functional group that can hydrogen bond (the strongest of all the available intermolecular forces) with other alcohol functional groups on nearby molecules, it will have the highest boiling point. Remember that in order for a molecule to be capable of hydrogen bonding, it must have a hydrogen atom covalently attached to a small electronegative element (N, O, halogen)—so the molecule in choice (D) is the only one capable of hydrogen bonding.

26. **(B)** Neutralization is the reaction of acid plus base to produce salt plus water.

$$2LiOH + H_2SO_4 \rightarrow Li_2SO_4 + 2H_2O$$

The balanced equation shows that twice as many moles of LiOH are needed to completely react with H_2SO_4. Given the volume and molarity of the sulfuric acid, 10 mL of 3 M H_2SO_4, calculate the number of moles of sulfuric acid.

$$M = \frac{\# \text{ moles}}{\# \text{ liters}} \qquad 3M = \frac{\# \text{moles}}{0.01 \text{ L}} \qquad \# \text{ moles } H_2SO_4 = 0.03$$

Multiply the moles of acid by 2 (factor-label method from balanced equation) to determine the number of moles of lithium hydroxide.

$$0.03 \text{ mole } H_2SO_4 \times \frac{2 \text{ moles LiOH}}{1 \text{ mole } H_2SO_4} = 0.06 \text{ mole LiOH}$$

Finally, determine the volume of lithium hydroxide necessary to contain that number of moles of 2 M lithium hydroxide.

$$M = \frac{\# \text{moles}}{\# \text{liters}} \qquad 2M = \frac{0.06 \text{ mole}}{\# \text{liters}} \qquad \# \text{liters LiOH} = 0.03 \text{ (30 mL)}$$

27. **(B)** The bubble at the bottom of the lake has a volume of 1.4 mL at $(7 + 273)$K and 2.0 atm pressure. To determine the volume of the bubble at the surface of the lake at $(27 + 273)$K and 1.0 atm pressure, use the equation shown below.

$$\frac{P_1 V_1}{T_1} = \frac{P_2 V_2}{T_2} = \frac{2.0 \text{ atm } (1.4 \text{ mL})}{280 \text{ K}} = \frac{1 \text{ atm } V_2}{300 \text{ K}} \qquad V_2 = 3.0 \text{ mL}$$

Since pressure and volume are present on both sides of the equation, any pressure or volume term (atm, psi, mL, liters, etc.) can be used as long as the term is the same on both sides of the equation. The pressure units cancel, and the volume term is part of the answer.

Also, one can predict that the volume of the gas bubble will increase since, as temperature rises, volume increases, and as pressure decreases, volume increases.

28. **(B)** This problem involves calculating the number of liters of NO produced at STP, 0°C, and 1.0 atm, and converting that volume to the new volume at 27°C and 2.0 atm.

$$4\ NH_3\ (g) + 5\ O_2\ (g) \rightarrow 4\ NO\ (g) + 6\ H_2O\ (g)$$

$$\underline{g\ NH_3} \rightarrow \underline{moles\ NH_3} \rightarrow \underline{moles\ NO} \rightarrow \underline{liters\ NO\ at\ STP}$$

$$1.7 \qquad \frac{1.7}{17} = 0.10 \qquad \frac{0.10(4)}{4} = 0.10 \qquad 0.10(22.4) = 2.2\ L$$

After finding the volume at STP, convert this volume to the volume at 2.0 atm and (27 + 273)K.

$$\frac{P_1V_1}{T_1} = \frac{P_2V_2}{T_2} = \frac{1.0\ atm\ (2.2\ L)}{(0+273)\ K} = \frac{2.0\ atm\ V_2}{(27+273)\ K}$$

$$V_2 = 1.2\ L\ at\ 27°C\ and\ 2.0\ atm$$

An alternative solution involves use of the ideal gas law equation, $PV = nRT$.

$$(2.0\ atm)V = \frac{1.7\ g}{17\ g/mole}\left(0.082\frac{L\text{-}atm}{K\text{-}mole}\right)(27+273)\ K$$

$$V = 1.2\ liters\ at\ 27°C\ and\ 2.0\ atm$$

29. **(C)** The rate of effusion or diffusion (mixing of gases) of a gas is inversely proportional to the square root of its molecular weight. The rates of effusion can be compared by using the following equation:

$$\frac{Rate\ 1}{Rate\ 2} = \sqrt{\frac{molecular\ weight\ 2}{molecular\ weight\ 1}}$$

Let the rate of hydrogen be rate 1, and the rate of oxygen be rate 2. The molecular weight 1 is the molecular weight of hydrogen gas and molecular weight 2 is the molecular weight of oxygen gas.

$$\frac{Rate\ 1}{Rate\ 2} = \sqrt{\frac{32}{2}} = \sqrt{16} = 4$$

Therefore the rate of effusion of hydrogen is 4 times faster than that of oxygen. Lighter gases move faster than heavier ones.

30. **(B)** To determine absolute configuration of a chiral center (a carbon with four different groups attached to it), prioritize the four groups according to atomic number. Place the fourth priority group pointed away from you and look at the priorities of the other three groups. If their priority of 1, 2, 3 is arranged clockwise, the chiral center is designated as R and if counterclockwise, S. In this molecule, there is only one chiral center and the chlorine will be priority 1, the isopropyl group will be priority 2, the methyl will be priority 3, and the hydrogen will be priority 4. Directing the hydrogen away from you places the other three groups in a counterclockwise priority order. Note: Since the isopropyl and the methyl groups begin with a carbon, determining their priorities requires a look at the atoms the first carbon of each group is attached to.

In the case of the isopropyl group, the first carbon of that group is attached to a hydrogen and two carbons, whereas the first carbon in the methyl group is attached to three hydrogens. Because the isopropyl carbon is attached to carbons that have a higher atomic number than the hydrogens of the methyl group, the isopropyl group has a higher priority than the methyl group.

31. **(C)** The heat capacity, *C*, of a substance equals the specific heat, *s*, times the mass of the material, *m*.

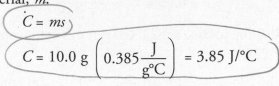

$$C = ms$$

$$C = 10.0 \text{ g} \left(0.385 \frac{J}{g°C} \right) = 3.85 \text{ J/°C}$$

32. **(D)** See the answer to question 7 above. Genes are composed of DNA.

33. **(C)** When naming alkenes, find the longest carbon chain that includes the double bond. In this case, it's 6 carbons with the double bond at carbon 2, so immediately you know that either (C) or (D) is correct. To assign E or Z to the double bond, prioritize the two groups at each end of the double bond according to atomic number (as described in question 30). If the alkene has both its priority 1 groups on the same side of the double bond, it is designated as a Z alkene as is the case with this molecule. If the two priority 1 groups are on opposite sides of the double bond, it is designated E.

34. **(C)** To balance nuclear equations, the mass numbers on each side of the equation must be equal and the atomic numbers on each side of the equation must be equal. For the given equation, the atomic number of the element produced would have to be 89, meaning the element's symbol would be the one right of Ra in the periodic table.

35. **(A)** The correct electron configuration for the sulfide ion, S^{2-}, is $1s^2 2s^2 2p^6 3s^2 3p^6$. The letters *s*, *p*, *d*, and *f* indicate the type of orbital. The number in front of the symbols, as in 1s, indicates the number of the orbital, in this case 1. The superscript, as in $1s^2$, indicates the number of electrons present in the orbital, in this case 2. The electron configuration for the sulfur atom, S, which is $1s^2 2s^2 2p^6 3s^2 3p^4$, shows the 16 electrons present in the atom. The sulfur ion, S^{2-}, has two more electrons in the p orbital: $1s^2 2s^2 2p^6 3s^2 3p^6$.

36. **(C)** See question 11 above. The two most common examples of secondary structure are alpha helices and beta (pleated) sheets. A tetramer would be an example of quaternary structure, and peptide bonds are what connect amino acids so they are involved in the primary structure. A double helix refers to the arrangement of DNA molecules (which aren't proteins).

37. **(A)** In the first shell around the nucleus of the atom, there is one *s* orbital. In the second shell, there are one *s* orbital and three *p* orbitals. In the third shell, there are one *s* orbital, three *p* orbitals and five *d* orbitals. In the fourth shell, there are one *s* orbital, three *p* orbitals, five *d* orbitals, and seven *f* orbitals. Each orbital is capable of containing a maximum of two electrons. Therefore, there are six electrons possible in the three *p* orbitals.

38. **(C)** Draw the Lewis structure of the molecule by adding up the valence electrons for the atoms in the formula. Phosphorus has 5 and each chlorine has 7. That's a total of 40 valence electrons to distribute. Place the phosphorus in the center and arrange the chlorines symmetrically around it using a pair of electrons to attach each chlorine atom to the central phosphorus. Now, complete the octet for each chlorine by adding 6 unshared electrons on each. That uses up all of the valence electrons so there are no unshared electrons on the phosphorus atom.

39. **(A)** The formal charge on a bonded atom equals the number of valence electrons in the nonbonded atom minus the number of nonbonded electrons in the bonded atom minus one-half the number of bonding electrons in the bonded atom.

The number of valence electrons in the nonbonded atom (Lewis dot formula)	$\cdot C \cdot = 4$
The number of nonbonded electrons in the bonded atom (Lewis dot structure)	$=C-$ $= 0$
One-half the number of bonding electrons in the bonded atom	$=C-$ $\frac{1}{2}(8) = 4$

The formal charge on a bonded atom $\qquad 4 - 0 - 4 = 0$

40. **(B)** The farther two elements are from each other in the periodic table, one being a metal and the other a nonmetal, the more ionic the bond between them. Consequently, of the compounds listed, Li_2O has the most ionic bond.

For the other compounds, CO_2, CH_4, and NH_3, the bonding is covalent because the atoms are close to each other and the compounds are nonmetals. Although hydrogen, H, may be located a distance from carbon, C, and from nitrogen, N, this element is an anomaly and has unique properties.

41. **(C)** The molecular geometry of SiH_4, like that of CH_4, is tetrahedral. Carbon is above silicon in the periodic table; consequently, if the same number of bonds is formed by the 4 hydrogen atoms to the central atom, Si or C, the geometry of the molecule is the same. If there are 2 bonding electron pairs around the central atom, as in BeF_2, the molecule is linear. If there are 3 bonding electron pairs around the central atom, as in BF_3, the molecule is trigonal planar. With 4 bonding electron pairs, as in SiH_4 or CH_4, the molecule is tetrahedral. In the molecule NH_3, there are 4 electron pairs but 1 is a nonbonding pair (only 3 hydrogen atoms), and the molecule is described as being a trigonal pyramid. In H_2O, there are 4 electron pairs but only 2 pairs participate in bonding to the 2 hydrogen atoms, and the molecule is bent.

42. **(A)** The molecule H_2S has the same geometry as does H_2O, which is bent. Sulfur, S, is under oxygen, O, in the periodic table and has the same number of atoms bonded to it, two hydrogens in each case. A bent molecule has a bond angle of about 105°, a trigonal pyramid an angle of 107°, a tetrahedron an angle of 109°, a trigonal planar molecule an angle of 120°, and a linear molecule an angle of 180°.

43. **(B)** The molecule $AlCl_3$, a trigonal planar molecule, has sp^2 hybridization. The linear molecule BeF_2 is sp hybridized. The tetrahedral CH_4, as well as the trigonal pyramid, NH_3, and the bent molecule, H_2O, are all sp^3 hybridized.

44. **(B)** Protein synthesis (translation) involves the covalent connection of amino acids associated with the cellular structure called the ribosome. Several types of RNA are involved in the process: mRNA (messenger RNA) provides the "instructions" for the amino acid sequence, rRNA (ribosomal RNA) is part of the ribosome structure, and tRNA (transfer RNA) brings the appropriate amino acids to the ribosome for incorporation into the growing protein.

45. **(A)** When a molecule contains a ring, the ring is the parent unless there is a functional group in a side chain. In this case, the ring has the functional group on it so the ring is the parent and named cyclopentanone. The numbering of the carbons of the ring would begin at the ketone carbon making the isopropyl branch at carbon 3.

46. **(C)** These reagents represent hydroboration-oxidation, which is a method of hydrating an alkene (adding the components of water across the double bond). It occurs with anti-Markovnikov regiochemistry (meaning the H goes on the more highly substituted carbon of the alkene and the OH goes on the less highly substituted carbon of the alkene) and with syn stereochemistry (meaning the new H and OH add to the ring from the same side and will therefore be cis to each other). The other method of hydration of alkenes, oxymercuration-demercuration, occurs with Markovnikov regiochemistry and anti-stereochemistry.

47. **(A)** The dipole moment is a measure of the polarity of a molecule, that is, one part of the molecule is partially positive and one part partially negative. The greater the dipole moment, the more polar a molecule is. Carbon dioxide, CO_2, has a dipole moment of zero because the molecule is linear with carbon in the middle and one oxygen atom on either side of the carbon. Although each individual $C - O$ bond is polar, the two bonds balance each other to produce a nonpolar molecule.

    H_2O, HF, and NH_3 are all polar molecules. The water molecule is bent with the electrons being drawn toward the oxygen. The hydrogen fluoride molecule is linear, but the $H - F$ bond is polar with the electrons drawn toward the fluorine. The ammonia molecule is trigonal pyramidal with the electrons drawn toward the nitrogen.

48. **(B)** Replication is the process whereby DNA is duplicated. The DNA duplex unwinds to expose its nucleotide sequence and new DNA molecules are synthesized complementary to each of the exposed DNA molecules resulting in two molecules of DNA having identical nucleotide sequences. Since the involved synthetic enzymes (DNA polymerases) can synthesize new DNA in only one direction and since the two DNA molecules composing the original duplex are antiparallel to each other, only one of the new DNA molecules can be synthesized continuously (without interruption). The other new DNA molecule is synthesized in pieces (called Okazaki fragments) or discontinuously.

49. **(C)** Three structures may be drawn for the carbonate ion, CO_3^{-2}.

$$\overset{\displaystyle O}{\underset{\displaystyle \overset{-1}{O} - \overset{\parallel}{C} - \overset{-1}{O}}{}} \qquad \overset{\displaystyle \overset{-1}{O}}{\underset{\displaystyle O = C - \overset{-1}{O}}{|}} \qquad \overset{\displaystyle \overset{-1}{O}}{\underset{\displaystyle \overset{-1}{O} - C = O}{|}}$$

The double bond between the carbon atom and one of the oxygen atoms may be in any one of three possible positions.

50. **(B)** The conversion of an aldehyde to an alcohol is a reduction. Hydride donors like $NaBH_4$ and $LiAlH_4$ are used to perform this reduction. H_2 is used to reduce alkenes and alkynes. PCC and $KMnO_4$ are both oxidizing agents and would oxidize the aldehyde to the carboxylic acid.

51. **(C)** Bromine with $FeBr_3$ is used to accomplish electrophilic aromatic substitution on arene rings. A bromine atom will substitute for a hydrogen on the ring. The ring already has an amino group on it and an amino group is an ortho,para director (and also an activator by electron donation through resonance) so choice (C) is correct.

52. **(A)** Transcription is the synthesis of RNA, translation is the synthesis of protein, replication is the synthesis of DNA, and respiration is the oxidation of molecules for energy production.

53. **(B)** The first three options are lipids. Triglycerides are the lipids found in adipose tissue and waxes are used to coat fruits or animal hair. Starch is not a lipid; it is a carbohydrate.

54. **(C)** See question 44.

55. **(B)** In a first-order reaction, the half-life, that is, the length of time for one-half of the concentration to be reacted, is dependent only on the rate constant, not on the original concentration. If the rate constant, k, is 6.93×10^2 / sec, the length of time needed for one-half of the starting material to be reacted is

$$4t_{1/2} = \frac{0.693}{k}$$

$$t_{1/2} = \frac{0.693}{6.93 \times 10^2 \text{ / sec}} = 1.0 \times 10^{-3} \text{ sec}$$

56. **(A)** When an alcohol reacts with an acid halide, an ester results through nucleophilic acyl substitution. All acid derivatives (acid halides, anhydrides, esters, and amides) undergo this type of reaction. In questions like this using condensed formulas, it is always a good idea to draw the line-bond structure before selecting an answer so that you can see clearly what types of functional groups are present (they are sometimes hard to see in a condensed structure).

57. **(B)** When potassium permanganate is added to an alkene or an alkyne, oxidative cleavage occurs. In the case of alkenes, the double bond is cut and each carbon of the double bond becomes doubly bonded to an oxygen atom. If any products are aldehydes, then they are further oxidized to carboxylic acids and if any resulting carboxylic acids are one-carbon acids, they are further oxidized to carbon dioxide. For alkynes, oxidative cleavage cuts the triple bond and both carbons of the triple bond become carboxylic acid groups. Again, if any one-carbon acids are formed, they are further oxidized to carbon dioxide.

58. **(A)** An equilibrium constant may be written for the following reaction. An equilibrium constant is equal to the product of the products divided by the product of the reactants, each raised to the power as indicated in the balanced equation.

$$H_2 + I_2 \leftrightarrow 2\,HI \qquad K = \frac{[HI]^2}{[I_2][H_2]} \qquad K = \frac{(0.5)^2}{(0.25)(0.25)} = 4$$

59. **(A)** According to Le Châtelier's principle, any stress applied to a system in equilibrium will cause the equilibrium to shift so as to relieve the stress. For example, in the given system:

$$\text{Heat} + N_2O_4\,(g) \leftrightarrow 2NO_2\,(g)$$

think of heat as one of the reactants. An increase in any reactant concentration on the left will cause the equilibrium to shift to the right, to the products. An increase in the product concentration on the right will cause the equilibrium to shift left, to the reactants. A decrease in any reactant concentration will cause the equilibrium to shift to the left. A decrease in any product concentration will cause the equilibrium to shift to the right. Therefore, a decrease in temperature or heat will cause the reaction to shift to the left, NOT to the right.

An increase in the concentration of N_2O_4, a decrease in the concentration of NO_2, and an increase in temperature will all cause the equilibrium to shift to the right.

60. **(C)** The conversion of a carboxylic acid to an alcohol is a reduction. Hydride-reducing agents are used to reduce carboxylic acids but $NaBH_4$ (a hydride reducing agent) is a mild hydride donor and is not powerful enough to reduce an acid. See question 50.

61. **(B)** Potassium t-butoxide is a strong base and is used to perform an E2 elimination by causing the removal of HI on this alkyl halide, creating an alkene. The most stable alkene will predominate. Remember, trans alkenes are more stable than cis alkenes, and more highly substituted alkenes are more stable than less highly substituted ones.

62. **(D)** When aldehydes and ketones condense in the presence of a base and either a beta-hydroxy carbonyl compound or an alpha beta-unsaturated carbonyl compound (as in this case) results, an aldol condensation has occurred. A Claisen condensation involves an ester, a Williamson is used to make an

ether, and a Michael is the reaction between an enolate and an alpha beta-unsaturated carbonyl compound.

63. **(A)** Proteins and peptides are polymers of amino acids joined by amide bonds (called peptide bonds).

64. **(B)** Resonance structures have the same atom connections but different placements of pi and unshared electrons. Only choice (B) has all of the atoms in the same place.

65. **(C)** The acidity of a solution can be measured by determining the pH or the pOH.

$$pH = - \log [H^+] \qquad pOH = - \log [OH^-]$$

The pH and pOH values are related by the following equations:

$$pH + pOH = 14 \text{ and } [H^+][OH^-] = 10^{-14}$$

Calculating the pH when the $[OH^-] = 0.01$ M gives

$$pOH = -\log [OH^-] = -\log (10^{-2}) = - (-2) = 2$$
$$pH + 2 = 14$$
$$pH = 12$$

66. **(D)** The DNA helix is composed of two molecules of DNA (strands) that are intertwined and held together by hydrogen bonding between the purine and pyrimidine bases of each strand. This type of hydrogen bonding is called base-pairing.

67. **(C)** The most important infrared (IR) absorptions are around 3000 cm^{-1} for O-H or N-H, around 2100 cm^{-1} for triple bonds, and around 1600–1700 cm^{-1} for double bonds. The only functional group that would have bands at both 3300 and 1700 is the acid.

68. **(B)** Triglycerides are lipids stored in adipose tissue. They are triesters of glycerol with three fatty acids (long-chain carboxylic acids). Basic hydrolysis of triglycerides (i.e., reaction with water and base, also called saponification) yields glycerol and three molecules of deprotonated fatty acid (also called soap). These fatty acids can be liberated from adipose tissue for beta-oxidation that results in the production of ATP.

69. **(A)** In the equilibrium reaction between ammonia, NH_3, and water, H_2O, ammonium ion, NH_4^{+1}, and hydroxide ion, OH^{-1}, are formed as products.

$$NH_3 + H_2O \rightarrow NH_4^{+1} + OH^{-1}$$

Using the Brönsted-Lowry definitions of acid and base, NH_3 is the base accepting an H^{+1} ion from the acid H_2O to form the NH_4^{+1} ion. The NH_4^{+1} ion is the acid donating the H^{+1} ion to the base, OH^{-1} ion, to form H_2O.

$$NH_3 + H_2O \rightarrow NH_4^{+1} + OH^{-1}$$
$$\text{base} \quad \text{acid} \quad \text{acid} \quad \text{base}$$

The NH_4^{+1} and the NH_3 are a conjugate acid-base pair and the H_2O and the OH^{-1} are a conjugate acid-base pair.

70. **(C)** Magnesium hydroxide, $Mg(OH)_2$, is a strong base. Strong bases ionize completely.

$$Mg(OH)_2 \rightarrow Mg^{2+} + 2OH^-$$

From the balanced equation above, we see that, for every 1 mole of magnesium hydroxide, 2 moles of hydroxide ion are formed. If the concentration of magnesium hydroxide is 2.5 M, or 2.5 moles/L, then the concentration of the hydroxide ion, $[OH^-]$, is 2×2.5 M = 5.0 M, that is, 5.0 moles/L.

Strong acids also ionize completely and their concentrations are calculated in the same manner as shown above for NaOH. A balanced equation for hydrochloric acid, HCl, is shown below.

$$HCl \rightarrow H^+ + Cl^-$$

71. **(C)** ^1H NMR gives information about the hydrogens in a molecule. Since there are five signals, there are five kinds of hydrogen in the molecule. Choice (A) can be excluded since the molecule has only four kinds of hydrogen and choice (D) can be excluded since the molecule has seven kinds of hydrogen. After comparing the number of signals in the spectrum to the number of different kinds of hydrogen in the molecule, look at the splitting pattern and integration information. Simple splitting patterns follow the n + 1 rule meaning that the splitting pattern for a group of hydrogens will be equal to the number of neighboring hydrogens (those on an adjacent carbon) plus one. For example, a triplet indicates that the hydrogens represented by that signal have two neighboring hydrogens, and a quartet indicates that the hydrogens represented by that signal have three neighboring hydrogens. Since the data include a triplet that integrates for 3H and a quartet that integrates for 2H, there must be an ethyl group, meaning choice (C) is the answer.

72. **(C)** Beta oxidation refers to the series of reactions that results in the oxidation of the carbons of fatty acids resulting in ATP synthesis (through oxidative phosphorylation). Polysaccharides (after conversion to monosaccharides) are oxidized through glycolysis followed by the citric acid cycle resulting in ATP synthesis.

73. **(A)** The constant K_B may be defined for the Y^{-1} ion, a base. The base, Y^{-1}, reacts with water, which is the acid, and an equilibrium expression for a base can be written.

$$Y^{-1} + H_2O \leftrightarrow HY + OH^{-1} \qquad K_B = \frac{[HY][OH^{-1}]}{[Y^{-1}]}$$

Since water is present in large excess in a dilute solution, its concentration does not change significantly, and therefore its concentration is included in the constant K_B.

The relationship that exists between K_A and K_B is as follows:

$$(K_A)(K_B) = K_w = 1 \times 10^{-14}$$

where K_w is the ionization constant for water.

Substituting the given K_A value for HY, 5×10^{-5}, into the above equation gives a value of 2×10^{-10} for K_B.

74. **(B)** The larger the value of the equilibrium constant, K_A, the greater the amount of products, the greater the amount of ionization of the acid (or base), or the stronger the acid (or base). See the equation below for acetic acid, a weak acid.

$$HAc \leftrightarrow H^+ + Ac^- \qquad K_A = \frac{[H^+][Ac^-]}{[HAc]}$$

Of the acids listed, nitrous acid (HNO_2) has the largest ionization constant and is the strongest acid. Conversely, the smaller the equilibrium constant, the weaker the acid (or base).

75. **(A)** When a Grignard reagent reacts with an ester, a tertiary alcohol results. The Grignard reagent first attacks the ester converting it into a ketone by nucleophilic acyl substitution (see question 56) but a second Grignard reagent attacks the ketone carbonyl resulting in an alcohol after protonation.

76. **(D)** Calcium carbonate, $CaCO_3$ (marble), is insoluble in water. The other compounds—NaOH, NH_4Cl, and $LiNO_3$—are all water soluble. The solubility rules include the following:

All salts formed with the alkali metals, for example, any member of the lithium family, are soluble.

All ammonium salts (NH_4^+) and all nitrate salts (NO_3^-) are soluble.

Many chlorides (Cl^-), bromides (Br^-), and iodides (I^-) are soluble.

Many sulfates (SO_4^{2-}) are soluble.

77. **(A)** One source of amino acids for protein synthesis is cellular biosynthesis (the other source is dietary protein).

78. **(C)** The larger the value of K_{sp}, the more silver and chloride ions are present in solution and hence the more soluble the salt. Of the salts listed, silver chloride is the most soluble.

79. **(C)** The formation constant for the formation of a complex ion, K_f, may be defined for the silver ammonia complex, $Ag(NH_3)_2^{+1}$, as shown below.

$$Ag^{+1} + 2NH_3 \leftrightarrow Ag(NH_3)_2^{+1} \qquad K_f = \frac{\left[Ag(NH_3)_2^{+1}\right]}{\left[Ag^{+1}\right]\left[NH_3\right]^2}$$

The concentration of each of the species in the equation is raised to the power shown in the balanced equation. As can be seen from the equation above, K_f will have a large value when the concentration of the complex ion, $[Ag(NH_3)_2^{+1}]$, is high. When much complex ion is formed the ion must be stable. Hence the largest value for the formation complex, 2.0×10^{30} for HgI_4^{-2}, gives the most stable ion.

80. **(B)** Proteins are polymers of amino acids joined by peptide bonds, a kind of amide bond. The different amino acids differ in a group attached to the alpha carbon (the carbon to which the amine and acid groups are attached)—this group is often called the side chain. The term "essential," when used in reference to amino acids, specifically means amino acids that cannot be biosynthesized and are therefore essential in the diet.

81. **(C)** Aluminum hydroxide, $Al(OH)_3$, dissolves in water to produce aluminum ions, Al^{+3}, and hydroxide ions, OH^{-1}.

$$Al(OH)_3 \text{ (s)} \leftrightarrow Al^{+3} \text{ (aq)} + 3OH^{-1} \text{ (aq)}$$

An equilibrium exists in solution between undissolved aluminum hydroxide, $Al(OH)_3$ (s), and dissolved aluminum hydroxide, Al^{+3} (aq) + $3OH^{-1}$ (aq).

Dissolving aluminum hydroxide in either **B**, 0.5 M $Al(NO_3)$, or **C**, 1.6 M NaOH, will decrease its solubility relative to its solubility in water. Since aluminum nitrate, $Al(NO_3)$, is a soluble salt, the concentration of the aluminum ion, Al^{+3}, will be 0.5 M (0.5 mole/ liter) in a solution of 0.5 M $Al(NO_3)_3$.

$$Al(NO_3)_3 \text{ (s)} \quad \rightarrow \quad Al^{+3} \text{ (aq)} \quad + \quad 3NO_3^{-1} \text{ (aq)}$$

$$\frac{0.5 \text{ mole}}{\text{liter}} \qquad \frac{0.5 \text{ mole}}{\text{liter}} \qquad \frac{3(0.5 \text{ mole})}{\text{liter}}$$

In the same way, the concentration of the hydroxide ion, OH^{-1}, in a solution of 1.6 M sodium hydroxide, NaOH (s), a soluble base, will be 1.6 M.

$$NaOH \text{ (s)} \quad \rightarrow \quad Na^{+1} \text{ (aq)} \quad + \quad OH^{-1} \text{ (aq)}$$

$$\frac{1.6 \text{ moles}}{\text{liter}} \qquad \frac{1.6 \text{ moles}}{\text{liter}} \qquad \frac{1.6 \text{ moles}}{\text{liter}}$$

Both the aluminum and hydroxide ions result in solution from dissolving solid aluminum hydroxide in water. According to LeChâtelier's Principle, increasing the concentration of either ion on the right side of the equation will shift the equilibrium to the left and decrease the solubility of $Al(OH)_3$ (s). Therefore, the presence of aluminum ions in the aluminum nitrate solution and the presence of hydroxide ions in the sodium hydroxide solution decrease the solubility of aluminum hydroxide in either of these solutions. The concentration of hydroxide in the sodium hydroxide solution is 1.6 M which is larger than the concentration of the aluminum ion, 0.5 M, in the aluminum nitrate solution. The 1.6 M sodium hydroxide solution will decrease the solubility of aluminum hydroxide more than the 0.5 M aluminum nitrate solution will.

Adding solid aluminum hydroxide to the 0.3 M hydrochloric acid, HCl, will increase the solubility of the aluminum hydroxide relative to its solubility in water, since the hydroxide ion concentration would be reduced by reacting with the hydrogen ion, H^{+1}, of the hydrochloric acid, HCl, and the equilibrium would shift to the right. More aluminum hydroxide would dissolve.

82. **(A)** Lipids are nonpolar molecules meaning they have lots of carbon-hydrogen bonds (which are nonpolar) and very few, if any, polar bonds (like carbon-oxygen, nitrogen-hydrogen, or oxygen-hydrogen bonds).

83. **(C)** Oxidation is the loss of electrons; reduction is the gain of electrons. The oxidizing agent is the material reduced, and the reducing agent is the material oxidized.

In the given reaction between zinc and the ion Cu^{2+}:

$$Zn + Cu^{2+} \rightarrow Zn^{2+} + Cu$$

Zn is oxidized because it has lost electrons to form Zn^{2+} as in answer C, and consequently is the reducing agent. The ion Cu^{2+} has gained electrons to form copper, Cu, and is the oxidizing agent.

84. **(D)** Refer to the answer given to question 83. The reducing agent is the species that loses electrons, Li or Br^{-1}. The equation with the more negative value for emf^0 indicates the species with the greater tendency to lose electrons, Li. The equation with the more positive value indicates the species with the greater tendency to gain the electrons, Br_2.

85. **(D)** An electrochemical cell is made up of two electrodes connected in solution and by wires. One of the chemical species in solution loses electrons, the process of oxidation, to an electrode, the anode. Oxidation occurs at the anode. The electrons travel from the anode, through the wire, to the cathode where another species in solution gains the electrons, the process of reduction, supplied by the cathode. Reduction occurs at the cathode.

86. **(D)** RCOOH is the general formula for a carboxylic acid.

$CH_3 - CH_3$	an alkane, specifically ethane
$CH_2 = CH_2$	an alkene, specifically ethene
$HC \equiv CH$	an alkyne, specifically ethyne
C_6H_6	benzene
CH_3CHO	an aldehyde, specifically ethanal, acetaldehyde
CH_3COCH_3	a ketone, specifically propanone, acetone
CH_3CH_2Cl	an alkyl halide, specifically chloroethane, ethyl chloride
CH_3COOH	a carboxylic acid, specifically ethanoic acid, acetic acid
CH_3COOCH_3	an ester, specifically methyl ethanoate, methyl acetate
CH_3CH_2OH	an alcohol, specifically ethanol, ethyl alcohol
CH_3CONH_2	an amide, specifically ethanamide, acetamide
$CH_3CH_2NH_2$	an amine, specifically aminoethane, ethyl amine
CH_3OCH_3	an ether, specifically dimethyl ether

87. **(B)** The following general formulas represent the following general types of compounds:

C_nH_{2n+2}	an alkane
C_nH_{2n}	an alkene or a cycloalkane
C_nH_{2n-2}	an alkyne or a cycloalkene
C_nH_n	benzene when n = 6

88. **(B)** The formula, C_3H_6, is one for either an alkene or a cycloalkane, both of which are unsaturated. The formula C_2H_6 represents an alkane; the formula

C_2H_6O represents a fully saturated compound and could be dimethyl ether or ethyl alcohol; the formula CH_3Cl represents an alkyl halide, methyl chloride.

89. **(D)** Four different structural isomers can be formed by C_4H_9Cl.

$CH_3 - CH_2 - CH_2 - CH_2 - Cl$	1-chlorobutane
$CH_3 - CH_2 - CHCl - CH_3$	2-chlorobutane
$(CH_3)_2 - CH - CH_2Cl$	1-chloro-2-methylpropane
$(CH_3)_3 - C - Cl$	2-chloro-2-methylpropane

90. **(C)** Draw pentane and then draw it again substituting a chlorine atom for one of the hydrogens. Now draw it again substituting a different hydrogen with a chlorine atom. See how many different compounds can be drawn by this method. If in doubt about whether a structure you've drawn is different from a previous one, name your structures. If they have the same name, they are the same compound. The three compounds that can be formed from this monochlorination are 1-chloropentane, 2-chloropentane, and 3-chloropentane (4-chloropentane is actually 2-chloropentane, and 5-chloropentane is actually 1-chloropentane).

91. **(A)** Pick the longest straight chain for the base name of the alkane, in this case octane. Next, name each of the substituents, two methyl groups and one bromo group. Give each substituent the lowest possible number and arrange the substituents in alphabetical order. The name is 5-bromo-3,4-dimethyloctane.

    The base names are listed below for the straight-chain alkanes with the general formula C_nH_{2n+2}. The names of compounds in other families can be derived from these names by using the proper suffix.

1 Carbon	methane
2 Carbons	ethane
3 Carbons	propane
4 Carbons	butane
5 Carbons	pentane
6 Carbons	hexane
7 Carbons	heptane
8 Carbons	octane
9 Carbons	nonane
10 Carbons	decane

92. **(C)** A stereocenter is an atom to which four different groups are attached. The different groups may be atoms such as the chlorine atom, Cl, or the bromine atom, Br, or they may be groups of atoms such as the methyl group, CH_3, or the ethyl group, CH_3CH_2. The underlined C in the following molecule, 2-bromo-2-chlorobutane, is a stereocenter.

$$CH_3$$
$$|$$
$$Cl - \underline{C} - CH_2 - CH_3$$
$$|$$
$$Br$$

93. **(A)** The two molecules pictured in question 93 have carbon-carbon double bonds. It is not possible to freely rotate around a carbon-carbon double bond as it is around a carbon-carbon single bond. Therefore, when a carbon-carbon double bond is present in a compound, two different compounds, geometric isomers, exist. In the example shown in question 93, the two chlorine atoms are on the same side of the double bond in one compound and on opposite sides of the double bond in the other compound. One could just as easily compare the positions of the two methyl groups relative to the carbon-carbon double bond and arrive at the same conclusion.

Racemic mixture – Refer to the explanation for question 100.

Enantiomers are a form of stereoisomers, i.e. compounds which have the same groups within the molecules but differ from each other because of the arrangement of groups in the molecules. Enantiomers are two compounds having the same four different groups bonded to the stereocenter in each compound, but because of the different positions in which these groups are placed relative to each other, i.e. because of different configurations, they are nonsuperimposable mirror images. Enantiomers are identical in almost all their physical and chemical properties. The Fischer projections of enantiomers of 1-chloro-1-iodoethane are shown below.

$$
\begin{array}{ccc}
& CH_3 & \\
& | & \\
H- & C & -Cl \\
& | & \\
& I &
\end{array}
\qquad\qquad
\begin{array}{ccc}
& CH_3 & \\
& | & \\
Cl- & C & -H \\
& | & \\
& I &
\end{array}
$$

Diastereomers are also a form of stereoisomers. Diastereomers are two compounds, each having at least two different stereocenters. The diastereomers have the arrangement of the four different groups at one of the stereocenters identical in both molecules but the arrangement of another four different groups at the other stereocenter different in both compounds. In other words, diastereomers with two stereocenters have the same configuration at one of the stereocenters but opposite configurations at the other stereocenter. Diastereomers are nonsuperimposable and have different physical and chemical properties. The Fischer projections of one pair of diastereoisomers of 2-bromo-3-chlorobutane are shown below.

$$
\begin{array}{ccc}
& CH_3 & \\
& | & \\
H- & C & -Cl \\
& | & \\
H- & C & -Br \\
& | & \\
& CH_3 &
\end{array}
\qquad\qquad
\begin{array}{ccc}
& CH_3 & \\
& | & \\
H- & C & -Cl \\
& | & \\
Br- & C & -H \\
& | & \\
& CH_3 &
\end{array}
$$

94. **(C)** Refer to the explanation for question 43.

95. **(B)** The carbon atom in ethylene has four pairs of electrons around it.

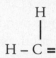

Based upon the explanation given to questions 41, 42, and 43, one might expect the hybridization to be sp^3. However, when a multiple bond such as the carbon-carbon double bond in ethylene is present, the multiple bond is considered as one pair of electrons for the purpose of determining hybridization. The carbon atom is considered to have three pairs of electrons around it and consequently has sp^2 hybridization.

96. **(B)** Oxidation may be defined as the loss of hydrogen. Oxidation of the secondary alcohol results in the loss of the two underlined hydrogen atoms, one bonded to the carbon atom and one bonded to the oxygen atom. A double bond forms between the two atoms which lost the hydrogen atoms. The product is a ketone.

$$CH_3 — \underset{\underset{O\underline{H}}{|}}{C\underline{H}} — CH_3 \quad \rightarrow \quad CH_3 — \underset{\underset{O}{\|}}{C} — CH_3$$

2-propanol   Propanone or acetone

97. **(A)** Water-soluble compounds are substances whose structures are most like the structure of water. An ether, alkyl chloride, alkane, and benzene are given as possible answers. Ethyl ether or diethyl ether contains an oxygen atom, as does water. The hydrogen atoms in water are capable of hydrogen bonding to the oxygen atom in the ether, just as they can hydrogen bond to other water molecules.

Of the compounds listed, ether is not only the most soluble in water; it is the only one that is slightly soluble. The other functional groups are totally water insoluble.

98. **(B)** A Grignard Reagent reacts with an aldehyde to produce, upon subsequent workup with water, a secondary alcohol. The reaction consists of addition across the carbon-oxygen double bond, with the alkyl group from the Grignard Reagent adding to the carbon atom and hydrogen adding to the oxygen atom. The methyl of the Grignard Reagent adds to the carbon atom of the double bond and the hydrogen adds to the oxygen to produce 2-propanol.

$$CH_3 - \underset{\underset{}{\overset{O}{\|}}}{C} - H \xrightarrow[\text{2. }H_2O]{\text{1. }CH_3MgBr} CH_3 - \underset{\underset{CH_3}{|}}{\overset{\overset{OH}{|}}{C}} - H$$

acetaldehyde   2-propanol
or ethanol

99. **(B)** The term dehydration means loss of water. When the elements of water are lost from an alcohol, the OH of the alcohol and the hydrogen atom on a carbon atom adjacent to the carbon atom bonded to the OH group are lost. The underlined atoms shown in the formula below are the ones most likely to be lost. An alkene is produced.

$$
\begin{array}{c}
CH_3 \\
|\\
CH_3 - CH - C - \underline{H} \qquad\qquad CH_3 - CH = C(CH_3)_2 \\
|\quad\quad| \\
\underline{OH}\quad CH_3
\end{array}
$$

  3-methyl-2-butanol   2-methyl-2-butene

100. **(D)** Each member of a pair of enantiomers rotates plane polarized light to an equal extent but in opposite directions. If one enantiomer rotates plane polarized light +42°, the other enantiomer of the pair rotates the light −42°. When the two enantiomers are mixed together in equal amounts, the mixture does not rotate plane polarized light and is called a racemic mixture (Answer D). A conformational mixture is a mixture of conformers, i.e. structures that differ from each other only in orientation of groups but that can be converted into each other by rotation around a carbon-carbon single bond. A meso compound is one in which the molecule can be visualized as two parts which are nonsuperimposable mirror images of each other, i.e. a pair of enantiomers in one molecule. Refer to the answer to question 93 for an explanation of diastereomers.

CHAPTER 7

Quantitative Ability Review and Practice

TIPS FOR THE QUANTITATIVE ABILITY SECTION

The quantitative ability section of the PCAT consists of approximately 48 math problems. You will have 40 minutes to complete the quantitative ability section. This section is the one that most students say they are unable to finish. Therefore, it is important that you pace yourself and answer all questions. There are 100 questions in this section to give you sufficient practice.

Currently, the use of calculators during the PCAT is prohibited. Therefore, it is important to brush up on your math skills!

QUANTITATIVE ABILITY REVIEW OUTLINE

I. **Basic mathematic calculations**

II. **Whole numbers and their operations**
   A. Addition of negative and positive integers
   B. Subtraction of negative and positive integers
   C. Multiplication of negative and positive integers
   D. Division of negative and positive integers
   E. Absolute value
   F. Factorial
   G. Order of operations

III. **Fractions**
   A. Adding fractions
   B. Subtracting fractions
   C. Multiplying fractions
   D. Dividing fractions
   E. Comparing fractions: Which is larger or smaller?

IV. **Decimals**
  A. Adding decimals
  B. Subtracting decimals
  C. Multiplying decimals
  D. Dividing decimals

V. **Percentages**
  A. Calculating percents
  B. Adding percentages
  C. Subtracting percentages
  D. Multiplying percentages
  E. Dividing percentages
  F. Percent increase and decrease (percent change)
  G. Simple and compound interest

VI. **Converting percents, fractions, and decimals**
  A. Converting fractions to percents
  B. Converting percents to fractions
  C. Converting fractions to decimals
  D. Converting decimals to fractions
  E. Converting percents to decimals
  F. Converting decimals to percents

VII. **Ratios and proportions**

VIII. **Powers and exponents**

IX. **Logarithms**
  A. Base 10 and natural logarithm
  B. Solving equations with logarithms or exponents
  C. Laws of logarithms
    1. Addition
    2. Subtraction
    3. Multiplication
    4. Division

X. **Roots and radicals**
  A. Square root
  B. Cube root
  C. Addition of radicals
  D. Subtraction of radicals
  E. Multiplying radicals

XI. Statistics
    A. Mean
    B. Median
    C. Mode
    D. Probability

XII. Basic Algebra
    A. Simplifying variable expressions
    B. Factoring
    C. Slope of a line
    D. Linear equations
    E. Quadratic equations and the discriminant
    F. Rational equations
    G. Logarithmic equations

XIII. Precalculus
    A. Functions and graphs
    B. Domain, range, symmetry
    C. Inverse functions
    D. Linear functions
    E. Quadratic functions
    F. Rational functions and asymptotes
    G. Function composition
    H. Distance formula, Midpoint formula
    I. Circle equations, completing the square
    J. Average rate of change
    K. Graphing via transformations (shifting, stretching, compressing, reflecting)
    I. Piecewise functions

XIV. Calculus
    A. Derivatives of functions
    B. Product Rule, Quotient Rule
    C. Limits
    D. Slope of a tangent line to a curve
    E. Instantaneous rate of change
    F. Integrals of functions
    G. Area under a curve
    H. Inflection points and concavity

XV. Operations concerning the conversion of basic units of measure
(see Appendix)

XVI. **Word-problem solving—analytical reasoning**

XVII. **Interpretation of graphs and figures**

XVIII. **Probabilities**
A. Venn diagrams and set operations
B. Counting combinations
C. Counting permutations
D. Calculating probabilities of indepedent events

Answer Sheet

QUANTITATIVE ABILITY

1 Ⓐ Ⓑ Ⓒ Ⓓ	26 Ⓐ Ⓑ Ⓒ Ⓓ	51 Ⓐ Ⓑ Ⓒ Ⓓ	76 Ⓐ Ⓑ Ⓒ Ⓓ
2 Ⓐ Ⓑ Ⓒ Ⓓ	27 Ⓐ Ⓑ Ⓒ Ⓓ	52 Ⓐ Ⓑ Ⓒ Ⓓ	77 Ⓐ Ⓑ Ⓒ Ⓓ
3 Ⓐ Ⓑ Ⓒ Ⓓ	28 Ⓐ Ⓑ Ⓒ Ⓓ	53 Ⓐ Ⓑ Ⓒ Ⓓ	78 Ⓐ Ⓑ Ⓒ Ⓓ
4 Ⓐ Ⓑ Ⓒ Ⓓ	29 Ⓐ Ⓑ Ⓒ Ⓓ	54 Ⓐ Ⓑ Ⓒ Ⓓ	79 Ⓐ Ⓑ Ⓒ Ⓓ
5 Ⓐ Ⓑ Ⓒ Ⓓ	30 Ⓐ Ⓑ Ⓒ Ⓓ	55 Ⓐ Ⓑ Ⓒ Ⓓ	80 Ⓐ Ⓑ Ⓒ Ⓓ
6 Ⓐ Ⓑ Ⓒ Ⓓ	31 Ⓐ Ⓑ Ⓒ Ⓓ	56 Ⓐ Ⓑ Ⓒ Ⓓ	81 Ⓐ Ⓑ Ⓒ Ⓓ
7 Ⓐ Ⓑ Ⓒ Ⓓ	32 Ⓐ Ⓑ Ⓒ Ⓓ	57 Ⓐ Ⓑ Ⓒ Ⓓ	82 Ⓐ Ⓑ Ⓒ Ⓓ
8 Ⓐ Ⓑ Ⓒ Ⓓ	33 Ⓐ Ⓑ Ⓒ Ⓓ	58 Ⓐ Ⓑ Ⓒ Ⓓ	83 Ⓐ Ⓑ Ⓒ Ⓓ
9 Ⓐ Ⓑ Ⓒ Ⓓ	34 Ⓐ Ⓑ Ⓒ Ⓓ	59 Ⓐ Ⓑ Ⓒ Ⓓ	84 Ⓐ Ⓑ Ⓒ Ⓓ
10 Ⓐ Ⓑ Ⓒ Ⓓ	35 Ⓐ Ⓑ Ⓒ Ⓓ	60 Ⓐ Ⓑ Ⓒ Ⓓ	85 Ⓐ Ⓑ Ⓒ Ⓓ
11 Ⓐ Ⓑ Ⓒ Ⓓ	36 Ⓐ Ⓑ Ⓒ Ⓓ	61 Ⓐ Ⓑ Ⓒ Ⓓ	86 Ⓐ Ⓑ Ⓒ Ⓓ
12 Ⓐ Ⓑ Ⓒ Ⓓ	37 Ⓐ Ⓑ Ⓒ Ⓓ	62 Ⓐ Ⓑ Ⓒ Ⓓ	87 Ⓐ Ⓑ Ⓒ Ⓓ
13 Ⓐ Ⓑ Ⓒ Ⓓ	38 Ⓐ Ⓑ Ⓒ Ⓓ	63 Ⓐ Ⓑ Ⓒ Ⓓ	88 Ⓐ Ⓑ Ⓒ Ⓓ
14 Ⓐ Ⓑ Ⓒ Ⓓ	39 Ⓐ Ⓑ Ⓒ Ⓓ	64 Ⓐ Ⓑ Ⓒ Ⓓ	89 Ⓐ Ⓑ Ⓒ Ⓓ
15 Ⓐ Ⓑ Ⓒ Ⓓ	40 Ⓐ Ⓑ Ⓒ Ⓓ	65 Ⓐ Ⓑ Ⓒ Ⓓ	90 Ⓐ Ⓑ Ⓒ Ⓓ
16 Ⓐ Ⓑ Ⓒ Ⓓ	41 Ⓐ Ⓑ Ⓒ Ⓓ	66 Ⓐ Ⓑ Ⓒ Ⓓ	91 Ⓐ Ⓑ Ⓒ Ⓓ
17 Ⓐ Ⓑ Ⓒ Ⓓ	42 Ⓐ Ⓑ Ⓒ Ⓓ	67 Ⓐ Ⓑ Ⓒ Ⓓ	92 Ⓐ Ⓑ Ⓒ Ⓓ
18 Ⓐ Ⓑ Ⓒ Ⓓ	43 Ⓐ Ⓑ Ⓒ Ⓓ	68 Ⓐ Ⓑ Ⓒ Ⓓ	93 Ⓐ Ⓑ Ⓒ Ⓓ
19 Ⓐ Ⓑ Ⓒ Ⓓ	44 Ⓐ Ⓑ Ⓒ Ⓓ	69 Ⓐ Ⓑ Ⓒ Ⓓ	94 Ⓐ Ⓑ Ⓒ Ⓓ
20 Ⓐ Ⓑ Ⓒ Ⓓ	45 Ⓐ Ⓑ Ⓒ Ⓓ	70 Ⓐ Ⓑ Ⓒ Ⓓ	95 Ⓐ Ⓑ Ⓒ Ⓓ
21 Ⓐ Ⓑ Ⓒ Ⓓ	46 Ⓐ Ⓑ Ⓒ Ⓓ	71 Ⓐ Ⓑ Ⓒ Ⓓ	96 Ⓐ Ⓑ Ⓒ Ⓓ
22 Ⓐ Ⓑ Ⓒ Ⓓ	47 Ⓐ Ⓑ Ⓒ Ⓓ	72 Ⓐ Ⓑ Ⓒ Ⓓ	97 Ⓐ Ⓑ Ⓒ Ⓓ
23 Ⓐ Ⓑ Ⓒ Ⓓ	48 Ⓐ Ⓑ Ⓒ Ⓓ	73 Ⓐ Ⓑ Ⓒ Ⓓ	98 Ⓐ Ⓑ Ⓒ Ⓓ
24 Ⓐ Ⓑ Ⓒ Ⓓ	49 Ⓐ Ⓑ Ⓒ Ⓓ	74 Ⓐ Ⓑ Ⓒ Ⓓ	99 Ⓐ Ⓑ Ⓒ Ⓓ
25 Ⓐ Ⓑ Ⓒ Ⓓ	50 Ⓐ Ⓑ Ⓒ Ⓓ	75 Ⓐ Ⓑ Ⓒ Ⓓ	100 Ⓐ Ⓑ Ⓒ Ⓓ

Practice Questions

100 Questions

Directions: Select the best answer to each of the following questions.

1. log(9) – log(5) is the same as

   (A) log(4)

   (B) $\log\left(\dfrac{9}{5}\right)$ → $\log(9) + \log(5)$

   (C) $\dfrac{\log(9)}{\log(5)}$

   (D) log(45)

   $350 \times 3 + 500 \times 4 + 400 \times 1 =$

2. During an 8-hour flight, a plane flew 350 mph for the first 3 hours, 500 mph for the next 4 hours, and 400 mph for the last hour. What was the plane's average speed for the entire flight?

   (A) 417 mph
   (B) 420 mph
   (C) 431 mph
   (D) 440 mph

   $\dfrac{\text{total distance}}{\text{total time}} = \dfrac{3450}{8} = 431$

For questions 3–5, consider the given graph of the function $y = f(x)$.

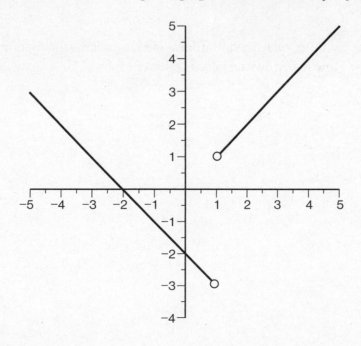

3. $\lim\limits_{x \to 1^+} f(x) =$

(A) 1 and –3
(B) Does not exist
(C) 1 or –3
(D) 1

4. $\lim\limits_{x \to 1^-} f(x) =$

(A) –3
(B) Does not exist
(C) 1 or –3
(D) 1 and –3

5. $\lim\limits_{x \to 1} f(x) =$

(A) 1 and –3
(B) Does not exist
(C) 1 or –3
(D) 1 and –3

6. Simplify the expression $\dfrac{x^2 - 12x + 35}{x - 5}$.

(A) $x + 7$
(B) $x - 19$
(C) $x - 7$
(D) $x + 19$

$$\dfrac{(x - 7)(x - 5)}{(x - 5)}$$

7. John has \$9.00 in quarters and dimes. He has twice as many dimes as quarters. How many quarters does he have?

(A) 25
(B) 30
(C) 35
(D) 20

$$25x + 10(2x) = 900$$
$$25x + 20x = 900$$
$$\dfrac{45x = 900}{45}$$

For questions 8–9, consider the data shown in the table below.

Cause of Death	# of deaths
Accidents and adverse effects	590
Homicide and legal intervention	230
Suicide	142
Malignant neoplasms ✓	55
Diseases of heart ✓	335
Human immunodeficiency virus infection	29
Congenital anomalies	115
Chronic obstructive pulmonary diseases	114
Pneumonia and influenza	111
Cerebrovascular diseases	35
All other causes	244

2000

8. What percentage of deaths were due to heart disease or malignant neoplasms?

$$\frac{55 + 335}{2000} \times 100 =$$

   (A) 15%
   (B) 25%
   (C) 20%
   (D) 30%

9. What percentage of deaths were NOT due to suicide?

   (A) 93%
   (B) 7%
   (C) 86%
   (D) 13%

$$\frac{g \times f' - g' \times f}{g^2}$$

10. Given the function $f(x) = \dfrac{x^2 + 5x + 2}{x^3 + 9}$, compute $\dfrac{dy}{dx}$.

$$\frac{(x^3 + 9)(2x + 5) - (3x^2)(x^2 + 5x + 2)}{(x^3 + 9)^2}$$

   (A) $\dfrac{(x^3 + 9)(2x + 5) + (x^2 + 5x + 2)(3x^2)}{(x^3 + 9)^2}$

   (B) $\dfrac{(x^3 + 9)(2x + 5) - (x^2 + 5x + 2)(3x^2)}{(x^3 + 9)^2}$

   (C) $\dfrac{(x^2 + 5x + 2)(3x^2) - (x^3 + 9)(2x + 5)}{(x^3 + 9)^2}$

   (D) None of the above

4 + 7 = about 11

11. $\sqrt{18} + \sqrt{50} =$

   (A) $8\sqrt{2}$

   (B) $2\sqrt{17}$

   (C) $34\sqrt{2}$

   (D) None of the above

12. Mike can wash a car in 45 minutes. His brother takes twice as long to do the same job. Working together, how many cars can they wash in 6 hours?

   (A) 12

   (B) 10

   (C) 8

   (D) 14

$\frac{6}{.75} = 8$ $1.5 = 4$ 360 min

$45x + 45(2x) = 360$

$45x + 90x$

$135x = 360$

13. If a coin is tossed four times, what is the probability of obtaining tails on the last toss?

   (A) $\frac{1}{2}$

   (B) $\frac{3}{5}$

   (C) $\frac{2}{5}$

   (D) $\frac{5}{8}$

$\frac{1}{2} * \frac{1}{2} * \frac{1}{2} * \frac{1}{2} = \frac{1}{8}$

independent of others

14. A number is chosen at random from the set {1, 2, 3, 4, 5, 6, 7, 8, 9, 10}. What is the probability that the chosen number is divisible by 2 or divisible by 3?

   (A) 20%

   (B) 40%

   (C) 80%

   (D) 70%

1 + 8 = 9

15. $\left(\frac{1}{x}\right)^6 + \left(\frac{2}{x^2}\right)^3 =$ $\left(\frac{2}{x^3}\right)$

   (A) $3x^4$

   (B) $\frac{9}{x^6}$

   (C) $6x$

   (D) $\frac{1}{2x^4}$

16. $\log_5(125) =$

    (A) 3

    (B) $\dfrac{1}{3}$

    (C) 5

    (D) $\dfrac{1}{5}$

$5^x = 125$

17. $-4 + 3\{2 + [3 - (2 + 3) + 2] + 2\} + 4 =$

    (A) −12

    (B) 0

    (C) 2

    (D) 8

2 + 4 + 2 = 8

−4 − 3(8) + 4 =

−4 + −24   −24

4

−4 + 12   +4

= −16 + 4 = −12

18. 8 feet is approximately

    (A) 260 cm

    (B) 244 cm

    (C) 282 cm

    (D) 278 cm

1 ft = 30.5 cm

8 ft × $\dfrac{30.5 cm}{1 ft}$ =

For questions 19 and 20, consider the graph data shown below.

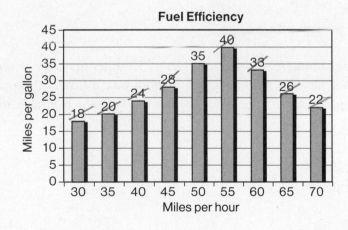

19. What is the mean value for miles per gallon?

    (A) 27.33

    (B) 26

    (C) 29

    (D) 25.24

20. What is the median value for miles per gallon?

    (A) 29
    (B) 24.89
    (C) 26
    (D) 25.24

21. $\int\limits_{\sqrt{e}}^{e}\left(\dfrac{4}{x}\right)dx =$

    (A) 2

    (B) $\dfrac{4}{e} - \dfrac{4}{\sqrt{e}}$

    (C) 6

    (D) $\dfrac{4}{e} + \dfrac{4}{\sqrt{e}}$

22. Event A has a probability of 7/10. What is the probability that event A does NOT occur?

    (A) 10/7
    (B) 3/10
    (C) 10/3
    (D) Not enough information

23. Parks leaves home for work and drives at 30 miles per hour. Twenty minutes later Susan, his wife, realizes he left his tool box at home. If Susan drives at 40 miles per hour, how far must she drive before she overtakes him?

    (A) 20 miles
    (B) 30 miles
    (C) 40 miles
    (D) 60 miles

For questions 24–27, consider the given graph of the function $y = f(x)$.

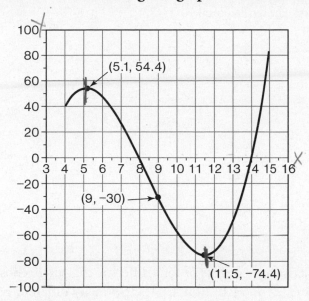

24. Identify the x value(s) at which the slope of the graph equals zero.

    (A) $x = 5.1$, $x = 11.5$
    (B) $x = 8$, $x = 14$
    (C) $x = 9$
    (D) None of the above

25. Identify the x value(s) at which the graph has an inflection point.

    (A) $x = 5.1$, $x = 11.5$
    (B) $x = 8$, $x = 14$
    (C) $x = 9$
    (D) None of the above

26. Identify the interval(s) on which $f'(x) < 0$.

    (A) $(9, 15)$
    (B) $(8, 14)$
    (C) $(4, 9)$
    (D) $(5.1, 11.5)$

    on decreasing interval

27. $\displaystyle \lim_{x \to 5.1} \left(\frac{f(x) - f(5.1)}{x - 5.1} \right) =$

    (A) 11.4
    (B) 0
    (C) 5.1
    (D) Not enough information

28. A pair of fair six-sided dice is thrown. What is the probability that the sum of the numbers shown is equal to 7?

    (A) $\frac{1}{6}$

    (B) $\frac{1}{12}$

    (C) $\frac{1}{3}$

    (D) $\frac{2}{3}$

29. A computer password consists of four different characters chosen from the set {*A, B, C, D, E, F*, 1, 2, 3, 4, 5}. How many different passwords are possible?

    (A) $\frac{11!}{4!}$

    (B) $\frac{11!}{7!}$

    (C) $\frac{11!}{7!4!}$

    (D) $\frac{11!}{7! + 4!}$

30. A box contains apples and oranges in a ratio of 4:5. If the box contains 16 apples, how many oranges does the box contain?

    (A) 17
    (B) 20
    (C) 15
    (D) 12

31. In a student survey, 200 indicated that they would attend Summer Session I, and 150 indicated Summer Session II. If 75 students plan to attend both summer sessions and 275 indicated that they would attend neither session, how many students participated in the survey?

    (A) 550
    (B) 625
    (C) 700
    (D) Not enough information

32. Find the extreme value of the given function and state whether that value represents a maximum or a minimum value for the function.
$$P(x) = -100x^2 + 400x - 200$$

(A) 2, minimum
(B) 2, maximum
(C) 200, minimum
(D) 200, maximum

33. One hundred and forty pounds are equivalent to how many kilograms?

(A) 60.2
(B) 63.6
(C) 65.2
(D) 67.7

34. Find the vertex for the given function.

$$f(x) = 3x^2 - 12x + 5$$

(A) (2,0)
(B) (−2,41)
(C) (−2,0)
(D) (2,−7)

35. A truck is 60 miles from its destination at 4:00 P.M. At what speed must the truck travel to arrive by 4:45 P.M.?

(A) 80 mph
(B) 75 mph
(C) 70 mph
(D) 85 mph

36. Given the following equation:

$$°C = \frac{5}{9}(°F - 32)$$

Convert 50°F to °C.

(A) 10
(B) 14
(C) 12
(D) 16

37. Find all real solutions for the quadratic equation $3x^2 + 2x + 5 = 0$.

    (A) $x = \dfrac{-2 \pm \sqrt{56}}{6}$

    (B) No real solutions

    (C) $x = \dfrac{-2 \pm \sqrt{-56}}{6}$

    (D) $x = \dfrac{-2 \pm \sqrt{60}}{6}$

$\sqrt{2^2 - 4(3)(5)}$

$4 - 4(3)(5)$

$= 4 - 60 = -56$

38. $6^2 \cdot 6^3 =$

    (A) 46,656
    (B) 7,776
    (C) 1,296
    (D) None of the above

39. $\dfrac{8}{9} - \dfrac{1}{2} =$

    (A) $\dfrac{6}{18}$

    (B) $\dfrac{7}{18}$

$\dfrac{16}{18} - \dfrac{9}{18} = \dfrac{7}{18}$

    (C) $\dfrac{3}{18}$

    (D) None of the above

40. Given that 600 milligrams of drug A equals 800 milligrams of drug B, what is the equivalent dose of drug A for a patient taking 500 milligrams of drug B?

    (A) 350 mg
    (B) 325 mg
    (C) 375 mg
    (D) 450 mg

$\dfrac{600A}{800B} = \dfrac{x}{500B}$

41. $3^2 + 3^4 =$

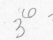

    (A) 729
    (B) 1,296
    (C) 90
    (D) 18

42. A number is chosen at random from the set {1, 2, 3, 4, 5, 6, 7, 8, 9, 10, 11, 12}. What is the probability that the chosen number is NOT divisible by 2 and NOT divisible by 3?

    (A) $\frac{1}{3}$

    (B) $\frac{3}{5}$

    (C) $\frac{3}{4}$

    (D) $\frac{2}{5}$

43. 250 milligrams of aminophylline injection is equivalent to 200 milligrams of theophylline. The strength of aminophylline injection is 25 milligrams per milliliter. How many milliliters of aminophylline injection are needed to provide a dose of 320 milligrams theophylline?

    (A) 10.67
    (B) 12.8
    (C) 16
    (D) 20

44. A patient's creatine clearance rate (CrCl) can be calculated by using the following formula:

    $$CrCl = \frac{140 - \text{age in years}}{72 \cdot SCr} \cdot (\text{ideal body weight in kilograms}).$$

    What is the CrCl for a 74-year-old patient who has a SCr of 3.2 and an ideal body weight of 84 kg?

    (A) 34
    (B) 24
    (C) 28
    (D) 38

45. The graph of a function $y = f(x)$ contains the point (9, 6). Determine which point must be on the graph of $y = 7f(x - 3) + 1$.

    (A) (12, 43)
    (B) (6, 43)
    (C) (12, 85)
    (D) (6, 85)

46. Determine the derivative for the function $f(x) = e^{5x} \cdot \cos(x)$.

   (A) $5e^{5x} \cdot \cos(x) + e^{5x} \cdot \sin(x)$
   (B) $5e^{5x} \cdot \cos(x) - e^{5x} \cdot \sin(x)$
   (C) $e^{5x} \cdot \cos(x) - e^{5x} \cdot \sin(x)$
   (D) $e^{5x} \cdot \cos(x) + e^{5x} \cdot \sin(x)$

For questions 47 and 48, consider the graph below.

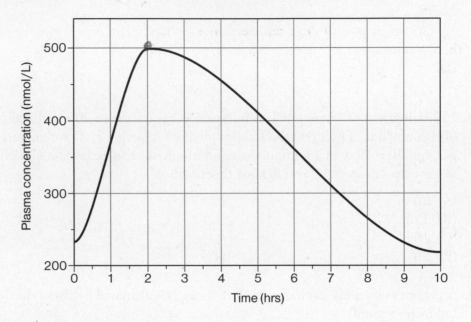

47. What is the maximum plasma concentration?

   (A) 300 nmol/L
   (B) None of these
   (C) 400 nmol/L
   (D) 500 nmol/L

48. When does the maximum plasma concentration occur?

   (A) Approximately 2 hours
   (B) Approximately 4 hours
   (C) Approximately 10 hours
   (D) None of the above

49. Determine the length of the line segment with endpoints (3, 6) and (−2, 5).

   (A) $\sqrt{24}$
   (B) $\sqrt{23}$
   (C) $\sqrt{26}$
   (D) $\sqrt{27}$

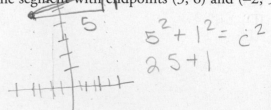

50. Larry's house is 12 miles from the park. Larry rode his bicycle from his house to the park at 12 miles per hour. He then walked the bicycle home from the park at 3 miles per hour. If he took the same route on both trips, what was his average speed?

    (A) 4.8 mph
    (B) 7.5 mph
    (C) 1.6 mph
    (D) 4.0 mph

$$\frac{total\ dis}{total\ time} = \frac{24}{5}$$

$$1 + 4 = 5$$

51. Identify the graph that demonstrates a linear relationship between the variables x and y.

    (A)

    (B)

    (C)

    (D)

52. Find the **radius** of the circle with equation $x^2 + y^2 - 26x + 34y + 11 = 0$.

    (A) $\sqrt{447}$
    (B) 447
    (C) 436
    (D) $\sqrt{436}$

$$(x^2 - 26x + 169)(y^2 + 34y + 289) = -11 + 289 + 169$$

$$\sqrt{447}$$

53. What is the mean of this series of values: 12, 8, 17, 22, 5, 13?

    (A) 16.3
    (B) 12.8
    (C) 14.5
    (D) 14.1

54. Determine the slope of the tangent line to the graph of the function $f(x) = 5x^4 + 6x$ at the point whose x coordinate equals -1.

    (A) -14
    (B) 14
    (C) -1
    (D) 1

    $5 + 6 = 11$

    $f'(x) = 20x^3 + 6$

55. Given that $\ln(a) = 6$ and $\ln(b) = 2$, $\ln(a \cdot b) =$

    (A) 8
    (B) 12
    (C) $\ln(8)$
    (D) $\ln(12)$

    $\ln 6 + \ln 2$

56. Evaluate the integral $\displaystyle\int_{2}^{3}\left(4x^3\right)dx$.

    (A) -65
    (B) 60
    (C) -60
    (D) 65

    x^4

    $3^4 \; 2^4 =$

For questions 57 and 58, consider the given graph of the function $y = f(x)$.

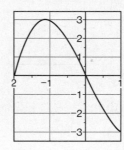

$x = 0$
$y = 0$

shift right

57. Identify the graph of the function $y = f(x - 2)$.

$x = 0$
$y = -2$

(A)
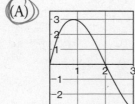

(B)
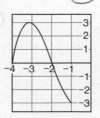

(C)
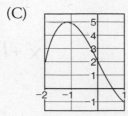

(D)
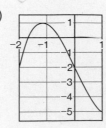

58. Identify the graph of the function $y = f(x) - 2.$

2 down

(A)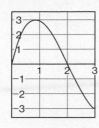

(B)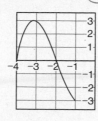

(C)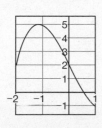

(D)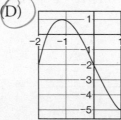

59. Lisa's gas tank is $\frac{2}{3}$ full. She completely filled the tank by putting in an additional 8 gallons. What is the capacity of the gas tank?

(A) 18 gallons
(B) 24 gallons
(C) 26 gallons
(D) 20 gallons

60. A walk-in clinic sees approximately 45% of its daily patients before noon. If the clinic sees a total of 40 patients on a given day, how many patients were seen **after** noon?

(A) 18
(B) 20
(C) 24
(D) 22

$$\frac{45}{55} = \frac{40}{x}$$

61. The height h of a projectile is given by $h(x) = -0.002x^2 + x$, where x is the horizontal distance the projectile travels. The projectile hits the ground after it has traveled a horizontal distance of

(A) 600 feet
(B) 400 feet
(C) 200 feet
(D) 500 feet

$$0 = -0.002x^2 + x$$
$$x(-0.002x + 1)$$
$$x = 0$$
$$-0.002x + 1 = 0$$
$$ -1 \quad -1$$

62. Express the distance from point P to point Q as a function of the x coordinate of point P.

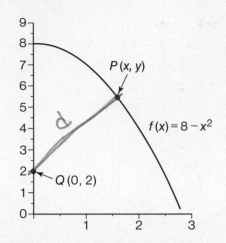

(A) $\sqrt{x^2 - \left(6 - x^2\right)^2}$

(B) $x^2 + \left(6 - x^2\right)^2$

(C) $\sqrt{x^2 + \left(6 - x^2\right)^2}$

(D) $x^2 - \left(6 - x^2\right)^2$

63. If four red balls were placed in a bag with eight black balls, what is the probability of obtaining a red ball?

(A) $\dfrac{1}{3}$

(B) $\dfrac{8}{5}$

(C) 3

(D) 1

$$4 + 8 = 12$$

$$\frac{4}{12} = \frac{1}{3}$$

64. log(4) + log(25) =

(A) log(4)log(25)

(B) log(29)

(C) 2

(D) 10

$$\log(4 \cdot 25)$$

$$\log(100)$$

$$\log(100) = \log(10^2)$$

$$10^x = 10^2$$

$$x = 2$$

65. A jar contains 5 pennies, 4 nickels, and 6 dimes. What is the probability that a randomly chosen coin is a dime?

    (A) 60%
    (B) 40%
    (C) 0.40%
    (D) 0.60%

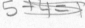

For questions 66–71, consider the given graph of the function $y = f(x)$.

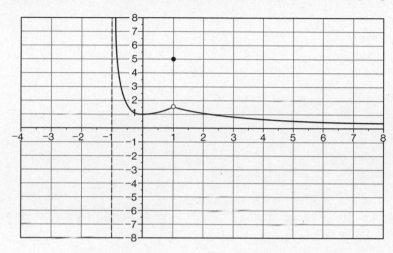

66. $\lim\limits_{x \to -1^+} f(x) =$

    (A) 1.5
    (B) 5
    (C) Undefined
    (D) 0

67. $\lim\limits_{x \to -1^-} f(x) =$

    (A) ∞
    (B) -1
    (C) $-\infty$
    (D) $\pm\infty$

68. $\lim\limits_{x \to \infty} f(x) =$

    (A) ∞
    (B) Undefined
    (C) $-\infty$
    (D) 0

69. The equation of the vertical asymptote is

    (A) $x = -1$.
    (B) $x = \infty$.
    (C) $x = -\infty$.
    (D) $x = 0$.

70. The equation of the horizontal asymptote is

    (A) $y = -1$.
    (B) $y = 0$.
    (C) $y = \infty$.
    (D) $y = -\infty$.

71. $f'(1) =$

    (A) 0
    (B) 1.5
    (C) Undefined
    (D) 5

72. Determine the average rate of change of the function $f(x) = x^2$ on the interval $1 \leq x \leq 3$.

    (A) 4
    (B) 8
    (C) 3
    (D) 6

$1, 4, 9$

$\dfrac{f(3) - f(1)}{3 - 1} = 4$

73. If 500 milligrams of drug A equal 400 milligrams of drug B, what is the equivalent dose of drug B for a patient taking 250 mg of drug A?

    (A) 200 mg
    (B) 240 mg
    (C) 250 mg
    (D) 300 mg

$\dfrac{500 A}{400 B}$

74. Determine the **domain** for the function $f(x) = \dfrac{x-1}{x^2 + 6x - 55}$.

    (A) $\{x : x = -11, x = 5\}$
    (B) $\{x : x = -11, x = -5\}$
    (C) $\{x : x \neq -11, x \neq -5\}$
    (D) $\{x : x \neq -11, x \neq 5\}$

$x^2 + 6x - 55$

$(x + 11)(x - 5)$

$x \neq -11, 5$

75. $\dfrac{\sqrt{36} \cdot \sqrt{16}}{\sqrt{9}}$

$$\dfrac{6 \cdot 4}{3}$$

(A) $\dfrac{6 \cdot 4}{3} = 12$

(B) $\dfrac{6 \cdot 4}{3} = 8$

(C) $\dfrac{4 \cdot 4}{4} = 4$

(D) $\dfrac{4 \cdot 3}{2} = 6$

76. The quadratic equation $ax^2 + bx + c = 0$ has solutions given by

(A) $x = \dfrac{-b \pm \sqrt{b^2 - 4ac}}{2a}$.

(B) $x = \dfrac{b \pm \sqrt{b^2 + 4ac}}{2a}$.

(C) $x = -b \pm \dfrac{\sqrt{b^2 - 4ac}}{2a}$.

(D) $x = -b \pm \dfrac{\sqrt{b^2 + 4ac}}{2a}$.

77. Given the function $f(x) = \begin{cases} 3x^2 & \text{for } x < 2 \\ 1 - 5x & \text{for } x > 2 \end{cases}$, evaluate the limit.

$\lim\limits_{x \to 2} f(x) =$

(A) Undefined
(B) 12
(C) –9
(D) –9 and 12

78. The equation $5(x + 2)(x - 1) = 5x^2 + 6x$ has solution

    (A) $x = 10$.
    (B) $x = -10$.
    (C) $x = -\dfrac{2}{5}$.

    (D) $x = \dfrac{2}{5}$.

$5x^2 + 5x - 10 = 5x^2 + 6x$
$-5x^2 \qquad -5x^2$

$5x - 10 = 6x \qquad -10 =$
$-5x \qquad -5x$

For questions 79 and 80, consider the survey data shown in the table below.

Seat Belt Worn	Probability
Never	0.0262
Rarely	0.0678
Sometimes	0.1156
Most of the time	0.2632
Always	0.5272

$= 1$

79. What is the probability that someone rarely or never wears a seat belt?

    (A) 5.32%
    (B) 2.62%
    (C) 6.78%
    (D) 9.40%

80. If 8,000 people participated in the survey, how many people sometimes wear a seat belt?

    (A) 1,156
    (B) 925
    (C) 116
    (D) 654

81. A pair of six-sided dice is thrown. What is the probability that the sum of the numbers shown is NOT equal to 7?

    (A) $\dfrac{2}{3}$

    (B) $\dfrac{1}{6}$

    (C) $\dfrac{1}{3}$

    (D) $\dfrac{11}{12}$

82. Find the exact value of the shaded area.

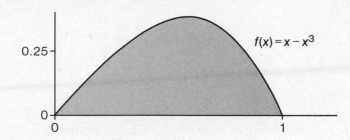

(A) $\dfrac{1}{3}$

(B) $\dfrac{1}{2}$

(C) $\dfrac{1}{4}$

(D) $\dfrac{1}{5}$

$0 \rightarrow 1$

$\displaystyle\int x - x^3$

$= \dfrac{x^2}{2} - \dfrac{x^4}{4}$

$\dfrac{1}{2} - \dfrac{1}{4} = \dfrac{1}{4}$

83. Determine the inverse function for $f(x) = \dfrac{10x}{x+1}$.

(A) $f^{-1}(x) = \dfrac{x+1}{10x}$

(B) $f^{-1}(x) = \dfrac{x}{10-x}$

(C) $f^{-1}(x) = \dfrac{x}{10x-10}$

(D) $f^{-1}(x) = \dfrac{x-1}{10x}$

$2 - 3 = -1$
$-2 + 1 = -3$

84. If $x < 3$, then $\dfrac{x^2 - 2x - 3}{|x - 1|}$ =

    (A) $x + 1$
    (B) ~~x + 1~~
    (C) $x - 1$
    (D) $-x - 1$

$\dfrac{(x - 3)(x + 1)}{|x - 1|}$ ...

85. Event A has a probability of 0.26. Event B has a probability of 0.42. The probability that events A and B both occur is 0.12. What is the probability that either event A or event B occurs?

    (A) 0.68
    (B) 0.44
    (C) 0.56
    (D) 0.32

86. Set A contains 12 elements, set B contains 8 elements, and set $A \cap B$ contains 6 elements. Determine the number of elements in the set $A \cup B$.

    (A) 14
    (B) 20
    (C) 26
    (D) Not enough information

87. Determine the slope of the line passing through the points (5, 3) and (2, −1).

$y = 4$

    (A) $\dfrac{4}{3}$

    (B) $-\dfrac{4}{3}$

    (C) $\dfrac{3}{4}$

    (D) $-\dfrac{3}{4}$

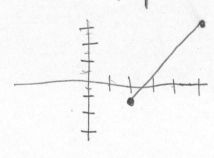

$slope = \dfrac{y}{x}$

88. If $\ln(w + 5x) = 3$, then

(A) $x = \dfrac{e^3 - w}{5}$

(B) $x = \dfrac{e^3 + w}{5}$

(C) $x = \dfrac{3e - w}{5}$

(D) $x = \dfrac{3e + w}{5}$

89. Write the equation of the **circle** with center point $C = (5, -6)$ and containing the point $P = (8, 3)$.

(A) $(x - 5)^2 + (y + 6)^2 = \sqrt{90}$

(B) $(x - 5)^2 + (y + 6)^2 = 90$

(C) $(x + 5)^2 + (y - 6)^2 = 90$

(D) $(x + 5)^2 + (y - 6)^2 = \sqrt{90}$

90. Find the equation of the horizontal asymptote, if any, for the given function.

$f(x) = \dfrac{3x + 1}{5 - 4x}$

(A) $y = -\dfrac{4}{5}$

(B) $y = \dfrac{3}{4}$

(C) $y = \dfrac{4}{5}$

(D) $y = -\dfrac{3}{4}$

91. Write the equation of the line passing through the point (5, –7) that is perpendicular to the line with equation $y = 4$.

    (A) $x = -\dfrac{1}{4}$

    (B) None of these

    (C) $x = 5$

    (D) $x = -7$

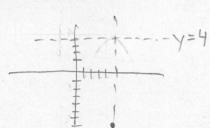

92. How many different ways can a 5-person committee be chosen from a group of 12 people?

    (A) $\dfrac{12!}{7!}$

    (B) $\dfrac{12!}{5!}$

    (C) $\dfrac{12!}{5!\,7!}$

    (D) $\dfrac{12!}{5! + 7!}$

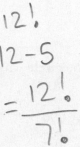

$12!$

$12 - 5$

$= \dfrac{12!}{7!}$

93. Convert 86°F to Kelvin.

    (A) 30
    (B) 243
    (C) 54
    (D) 303

$86 - 32 \left(\dfrac{5}{9}\right) = 30$

$30 + 273 = 303$

94. Determine the domain of the function $f(x) = \ln(4x - 2)$.

    (A) $(-\infty, \infty)$
    (B) $[-\infty, \infty]$
    (C) $[0.5, \infty)$
    (D) $(0.5, \infty)$

95. A rental car company charges \$25 per day, plus 12 cents per mile. Express the total rental cost of a 6-day rental as a function of the number of miles driven, x.

    $150 + .12x$

    (A) $C(x) = 25 + 12x$
    (B) $C(x) = 25 + 0.12x$
    (C) $C(x) = 150 + 12x$
    (D) $C(x) = 150 + 0.12x$

For questions 96–98, consider the given graph of the function $y = f(x)$**.**

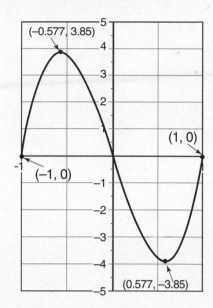

96. Choose the statement that best describes the function $y = f(x)$ with the given graph.

   (A) $y = f(x)$ is an even function.
   (B) $y = f(x)$ is a quadratic function.
   (C) $y = f(x)$ is an odd function.
   (D) $y = f(x)$ is a linear function.

97. Determine the domain of the function $y = f(x)$ with the given graph.

   (A) (−1, 1)
   (B) [−1, 1]
   (C) (−3.85, 3.85)
   (D) [−3.85, 3.85]

98. Determine the range of the function $y = f(x)$ with the given graph.

   (A) (−1, 1)
   (B) [−1, 1]
   (C) (−3.85, 3.85)
   (D) [−3.85, 3.85]

99. Kate had a box of red and blue crayons in a ratio of 5:9. If she had 20 red crayons, how many more blue crayons did she have than red?

   (A) 9
   (B) 16
   (C) 4
   (D) 11

100. $\dfrac{4}{11} - \dfrac{3}{8} =$

$\dfrac{32}{88} - \dfrac{33}{88}$

(A) $\dfrac{1}{3}$

(B) $\dfrac{1}{88}$

$= -\dfrac{1}{88}$

(C) $-\dfrac{1}{3}$

(D) $-\dfrac{1}{88}$

Answer Key
QUANTITATIVE ABILITY

1. **B**	26. **D**	51. **B**	76. **A**
2. **C**	27. **B**	52. **A**	77. **A**
3. **D**	28. **B**	53. **B**	78. **B**
4. **A**	29. **B**	54. **A**	79. **D**
5. **B**	30. **B**	55. **A**	80. **B**
6. **C**	31. **A**	56. **D**	81. **D**
7. **D**	32. **D**	57. **A**	82. **C**
8. **C**	33. **B**	58. **D**	83. **B**
9. **A**	34. **D**	59. **B**	84. **D**
10. **B**	35. **A**	60. **D**	85. **C**
11. **A**	36. **A**	61. **D**	86. **A**
12. **A**	37. **B**	62. **C**	87. **A**
13. **A**	38. **B**	63. **A**	88. **A**
14. **D**	39. **B**	64. **C**	89. **B**
15. **B**	40. **C**	65. **B**	90. **D**
16. **A**	41. **C**	66. **A**	91. **C**
17. **A**	42. **A**	67. **A**	92. **C**
18. **B**	43. **C**	68. **D**	93. **D**
19. **A**	44. **B**	69. **A**	94. **D**
20. **C**	45. **A**	70. **B**	95. **D**
21. **A**	46. **B**	71. **C**	96. **C**
22. **B**	47. **D**	72. **A**	97. **B**
23. **C**	48. **A**	73. **A**	98. **D**
24. **A**	49. **C**	74. **D**	99. **B**
25. **C**	50. **A**	75. **B**	100. **D**

EXPLANATORY ANSWERS

1. **(B)** The *Quotient Rule* for logarithms states that $\log(M) - \log(N) = \log\left(\dfrac{M}{N}\right)$.

2. **(C)** The plane travels $350 \cdot 3 = 1{,}050$ miles during the first 3 hours, $500 \cdot 4 = 2{,}000$ miles during the next 4 hours, and 400 miles during the last hour. So we have

$$\text{avg speed} = \frac{\text{total distance}}{\text{total time}} = \frac{3{,}450}{8 \text{ hrs}} = 431 \text{ mph.}$$

3. **(D)** As x approaches 1 from the right-hand side, the values of $f(x)$ approach 1.

4. **(A)** As x approaches 1 from the left-hand side, the values of $f(x)$ approach -3.

5. **(B)** The left- and right-hand limits are not equal.

6. **(C)** We simplify the expression as follows.

$$\frac{x^2 - 12x + 35}{x - 5} = \frac{(x-5)(x-7)}{x-5} = x - 7$$

7. **(D)** Let x = the number of quarters, and $2x$ = the number of dimes. This yields the equation $25 \cdot x + 10 \cdot 2x = $ money in cents. So we solve $25 \cdot x + 10 \cdot 2x = 900$

$$45x = 900 \Rightarrow x = \frac{900}{45} = 20.$$

8. **(C)** There were 335 deaths due to heart disease and 55 deaths due to malignant neoplasms; $335 + 55 = 390$ deaths due to heart disease or malignant neoplasms.

There were 2,000 total deaths.

Thus, probability $= \dfrac{390}{2{,}000} = 0.195 = 19.5\% \approx 20\%.$

9. **(A)** The percentage of deaths due to suicide was

$$\frac{142}{2{,}000} = 0.071 = 7.1\% \approx 7\%.$$

Thus, the percentage of deaths NOT due to suicide was $1 - 0.07 = 93\%.$

10. **(B)** We use the Quotient Rule for derivatives.

$$\frac{d}{dx}\left(\frac{f(x)}{g(x)}\right) = \frac{g(x) \cdot f'(x) - g'(x) \cdot f(x)}{\left(g(x)\right)^2}$$

11. **(A)** Note that $\sqrt{18} + \sqrt{50} = \sqrt{9 \cdot 2} + \sqrt{25 \cdot 2} = 3\sqrt{2} + 5\sqrt{2} = 8\sqrt{2}$.

12. **(A)** Mike can wash 1 car every 45 minutes = 0.75 hours. Thus, in 6 hours he can wash $\frac{6}{0.75} = 8$ cars. His brother can wash 1 car every 90 minutes = 1.5 hours. Thus, in 6 hours he can wash $\frac{6}{1.5} = 4$ cars. Working together, they can wash 12 cars (8 + 4 = 12 cars) in 6 hours.

13. **(A)** Each time a coin is tossed, there are two possible outcomes, heads and tails. The probability of heads is $\frac{1}{2}$. The outcome of the fourth coin toss is independent of the outcomes of the three earlier tosses.

14. **(D)** There are 7 numbers divisible by 2 or 3; that is, 2, 3, 4, 6, 8, 9, 10. We use the formula: probability $= \frac{7}{10} = 0.70 = 70\%$.

15. **(B)**

$$\left(\frac{1}{x}\right)^6 + \left(\frac{2}{x^2}\right)^3 = \frac{1^6}{x^6} + \frac{2^3}{\left(x^2\right)^3}$$

Rule: $\left(\dfrac{a}{b}\right)^n = \dfrac{a^n}{b^n}$

$$= \frac{1}{x^6} + \frac{8}{x^6}$$

Rule: $\left(a^n\right)^m = a^{n \cdot m}$

$$= \frac{9}{x^6}$$

16. **(A)** Note that $\log_5(125) = x$ is equivalent to the equation $5^x = 125$. This equation has solution $x = 3$.

17. **(A)** Begin with the innermost parentheses, and work outward.
$-4 - 3 \{2 + 1 [3 - (2 + 3) + 2] + 2\} + 4 =$
$-4 - 3 \{2 + 1 [3 - 5 + 2] + 2\} + 4 =$
$-4 - 3 \{2 + 1 \cdot 0 + 2\} + 4 =$
$-4 - 3 \cdot 4 + 4 =$
$-4 - 12 + 4 =$
-12

18. **(B)** We use the conversion 1 foot = 30.5 cm; 1 inch = 2.54 cm; 12 inches = 1 foot, so 8 ft = 96 inches. Therefore, 96 inches = 96 · 2.54 = 244 cm.

19. **(A)** We compute

$$\frac{18 + 20 + 24 + 28 + 35 + 40 + 33 + 26 + 22}{9} = \frac{246}{9} = 27.33.$$

20. **(C)** We list the values in increasing order: 18, 20, 22, 24, 26, 28, 33, 35, 40. The median value occurs at the middle position in the list, that is, the median = 26.

21. **(A)** We use the integration rule

$$\int_{\sqrt{e}}^{e} \left(\frac{4}{x}\right) dx = 4\ln(x)\Big]_{\sqrt{e}}^{e} = 4\ln(e) - 4\ln\left(\sqrt{e}\right) = 4 \cdot 1 - 4 \cdot \frac{1}{2} = 2.$$

22. **(B)** We use the formula $P(\overline{A}) = 1 - P(A) = 1 - \frac{7}{10} = \frac{3}{10}.$

23. **(C)** In 20 min. ($\frac{1}{3}$ hr.), Parks has gone 10 mi. In another hour, he will have covered a total of 40 mi. (10 + 30). Therefore, Susan must drive 40 mi. (for 1 hr.) to catch him.

24. **(A)** The graph has a horizontal tangent line at $x = 5.1$ and $x = 11.5$.

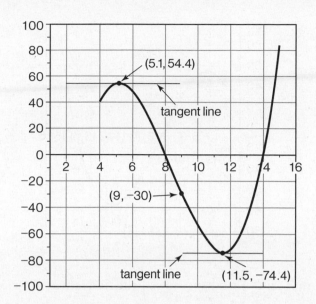

25. **(C)** The graph changes its concavity at $x = 9$. That is, the graph is concave down ("bends downward") for $x < 9$, and the graph is concave up ("bends upward") for $x > 9$.

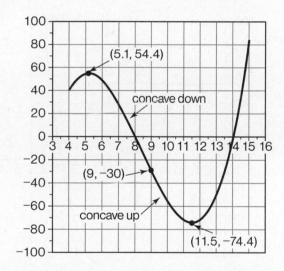

26. **(D)** The graph is decreasing on the interval (5.1, 11.5).

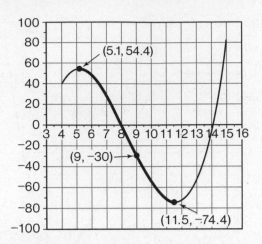

27. **(B)** Note that $\lim\limits_{x \to 5.1}\left(\dfrac{f(x) - f(5.1)}{x - 5.1}\right)$ the derivative of f at $x = 5.1$.

Recall that the derivative gives the slope of the tangent line to the graph at the point of the tangency. Note that the tangent line to the given graph is horizontal at the point where $x = 5.1$. Thus, the slope equals 0 there.

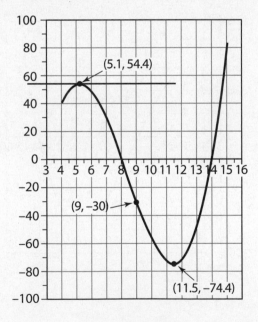

28. **(B)** There are 3 ways that the sum of the numbers shown can equal 7, that is, $1 + 6$, $2 + 5$, and $3 + 4$. Note that there are 6 possible outcomes for each die in the pair. Therefore, to calculate the possible combinations for the pair, we multiple $6 \cdot 6 = 36$.

Thus, probability $= \dfrac{3}{36} = \dfrac{1}{12}$.

29. **(B)** We are choosing 4 elements from an 11-element set, without repetition, such that order matters. Thus, we are counting permutations.

We use the formula $_{11}P_4 = \dfrac{11!}{(11-4)!} = \dfrac{11!}{7!}$.

30. **(B)** We have the ratio $\dfrac{4 \text{ apples}}{5 \text{ oranges}} \Rightarrow \dfrac{4 \cdot 4 \text{ apples}}{4 \cdot 5 \text{ oranges}} = \dfrac{16 \text{ apples}}{20 \text{ oranges}}$.

31. **(A)** Consider the Venn diagram.

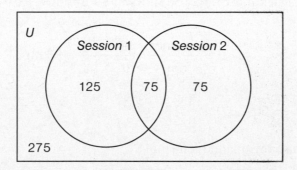

Initially, the solution to this problem seems straightforward. Two hundred students indicated they would attend Session 1, 150 indicated they would attend Session II, and 275 indicated they would not attend either session. If we add these students together, 200 + 150 + 275 = 625. However, there is an overlap (or double count) in the number of students, as 75 indicated they would attend both sessions. To account for the overlap and learn the number of students who will attend only one session, 75 should be subtracted from the number of students attending each session. In this case, 200 − 75 = 125 and 150 − 75 = 75. We then add 125 + 275 + 75 + 75 = 550 to obtain the true number of students who participated in the survey.

32. **(D)** $P(x) = -100x^2 + 400x^2 - 200$ is a quadratic function whose graph opens down.

The maximum value occurs at the vertex, that is, when $x = -\dfrac{400}{-200} = 2$.

Thus, $P(2) = 200$.

33. **(B)** $\dfrac{1 \text{ kg}}{2.2 \text{ lb.}} \cdot 140 \text{ lb.} = 63.6$

34. **(D)** A quadratic function $f(x) = ax^2 + bx + c$ will have its vertex at the point $\left(-\dfrac{b}{2a}, f\left(-\dfrac{b}{2a}\right)\right)$

$$f(x) = 3x^2 - 12x + 5 \Rightarrow x = -\frac{b}{2a} = -\frac{-12}{2(3)} = \frac{12}{6} = 2$$

$$f(2) = 3(2)^2 - 12(2) + 5 = 12 - 24 + 5 = -7$$

Thus, the vertex is (2,–7).

35. **(A)** The truck must travel 60 miles in 45 minutes = 0.75 hour. We have the formula

$$\text{speed} = \frac{\text{distance}}{\text{time}} = \frac{60 \text{ miles}}{0.75 \text{ hr}} = 80 \text{ mph.}$$

36. **(A)** $°C = \dfrac{5}{9}(50 - 32) = \dfrac{5}{9}(18) = 10.$

37. **(B)** We use the quadratic formula.

$$x = \frac{-b \pm \sqrt{b^2 - 4ac}}{2a} = \frac{-2 \pm \sqrt{2^2 - 4 \cdot 3 \cdot 5}}{2 \cdot 3} = \frac{-2 \pm \sqrt{-56}}{6}.$$

Since $\sqrt{-56}$ is not a real number, the equation has no real solutions.

38. **(B)** Note that $6^2 \cdot 6^3 = 6^{2+3} = 6^5 = 7{,}776.$

39. **(B)** The least common denominator for $\dfrac{8}{9}$ and $\dfrac{1}{2}$ is 18. Rewrite the fractions, using the least common denominator: $\dfrac{8 \cdot 2}{18} - \dfrac{1 \cdot 9}{18} = \dfrac{16}{18} - \dfrac{9}{18} = \dfrac{7}{18}.$

40. **(C)** We have the ratio $\dfrac{600 \text{ mg drug A}}{800 \text{ mg drug B}}$. Thus,

$$\frac{600 \text{ mg drug A}}{800 \text{ mg drug B}} \cdot \frac{x}{500 \text{ mg drug B}}$$

$800x = (600 \cdot 500)$
$800x = 300{,}000$

$$x = \frac{300{,}000}{800}$$

$x = 375$

41. **(C)** $3^2 + 3^4 = 9 + 81 = 90$.

42. **(A)** There are four numbers not divisible by either 2 or 3, that is 1, 5, 7, 11.
    Thus, probability $= \dfrac{4}{12} = \dfrac{1}{3}$.

43. **(C)** 250 milligrams of aminophylline injection is equivalent to 200 milligrams
    of theophylline. Thus, aminophylline is 80% theophylline $\left(\dfrac{200}{250} = 80\% \right)$;
    therefore, 25 mg (1 mL) of aminophylline will contain only 20 mg of
    theophylline. Divide 320 mg by 20 mg/mL to obtain 16 mL.

44. **(B)** We plug into the given formula
    $$CrCl = \left(\frac{140 - 74}{72 \cdot 3.2} \right) \cdot (84) = \left(\frac{66}{72 \cdot 3.2} \right) \cdot (84) \approx 24 .$$

45. **(A)** Each point on the graph of $y = 7f(x - 3) + 1$ is obtained by transform-
    ing the points on the graph of $y = f(x)$ as follows. Add 3 to each x coordi-
    nate (in this case, $3 + 9 = 12$); multiply each y coordinate by 7 and then add
    1 (in this case, $7 \cdot 6 = 42 + 1 = 43$). Therefore, the answer is (12, 43).

46. **(B)** We use the Product Rule for derivatives
    $$\frac{d}{dx}\big(f(x) \cdot g(x)\big) = f'(x) \cdot g(x) + f(x) \cdot g'(x)$$
    $\cos = -\sin$

    and the fact that $\dfrac{d}{dx}e^{5x} = 5e^{5x}$ and $\dfrac{d}{dx}\cos(x) = -\sin(x)$.

47. **(D)** The highest point on the graph has y coordinate equal to 500.

48. **(A)** The highest point on the graph occurs when the x coordinate equals 2.

49. **(C)** We calculate the distance using the formula
    $$\sqrt{(x_2 - x_1)^2 + (y_2 - y_1)^2} = \sqrt{(-2 - 3)^2 + (5 - 6)^2} = \sqrt{25 + 1} = \sqrt{26} .$$

50. **(A)** If the house is 12 mi. from the park, at 12 mph Larry needed 1 hr. to
    make the trip. At only 3 mph, he needed 4 hr. to get back home. Thus, he
    traveled 24 mi. ($2 \cdot 12$ mi.) in 5 hr. ($1 + 4$ hr.). Divide 24 by 5 to get an
    average speed of 4.8 mph.

51. **(B)** A linear relationship between two variables yields a graph that is a non-
    vertical line, which is represented in choice (B). The relationships repre-
    sented in the answer choices are as follows: (A) quadratic, (B) linear,
    (C) polynomial, and (D) exponential.

52. **(A)** We complete the square on the given equation as follows.

$$x^2 + y^2 - 26x + 34y + 11 = 0$$
$$x^2 - 26x + 169 + y^2 + 34y + 289 = -11 + 169 + 289$$

$$(x - 13)^2 + (y + 17)^2 = 447$$

$$(x - 13)^2 + (y + 17)^2 = \left(\sqrt{447}\right)^2$$

Now use the fact that a circle with equation $(x - h)^2 + (y - k)^2 = r^2$ has center point (h, k) and radius equal to r. In the given equation, we have $(x - 13)^2 + (y + 17)^2 = \left(\sqrt{447}\right)^2$. Thus, the radius equals $\sqrt{447}$.

53. **(B)** To find the mean, add all the values together $(12 + 8 + 17 + 22 + 5 + 13 = 77)$, then divide the sum by the number of values in the series $(\frac{77}{6} = 12.8)$.

54. **(A)** We compute the derivative $f'(x) = 20^3 + 6$, and then evaluate $f'(-1) = 20(-1)^3 + 6 = -20 + 6 = -14$.

55. **(A)** We use the Product Rule for logarithms. $\ln(a \cdot b) = \ln(a) + \ln(b) = 6 + 2 = 8$

56. **(D)** We use the Fundamental theorem of calculus for integrals.

$$\int_2^3 \left(4x^3\right) dx = \left.\frac{4x^4}{4}\right|_2^3 = \left.x^4\right|_2^3 = 3^4 - 2^4 = 81 - 16 = 65$$

57. **(A)** The original graph is shifted 2 units to the right.

58. **(D)** The original graph is shifted 2 units down.

59. **(B)** Since the tank is already 2/3 full, the additional 8 gallons equals 1/3 of the tank's capacity. Thus, $8 = \frac{1}{3}x \Rightarrow x = 24$.

60. **(D)** The clinic sees 55% of its daily patients after noon. So we have $(0.55)(40) = 22$.

61. **(D)** The projectile hits the ground when the height equals zero. So we solve the equation $-0.002x^2 + x = 0$.

$$-0.002x^2 + x = 0$$
$$x(-0.002x + 1) = 0$$

$$x = 0, \quad -0.002x + 1 = 0 \Rightarrow x = \frac{-1}{-0.002} = 500$$

62. **(C)** We apply the distance formula to points P and Q.

$$\sqrt{(x-0)^2 + (y-2)^2} = \sqrt{x^2 + (8 - x^2 - 2)^2} = \sqrt{x^2 + (6 - x^2)^2}$$

63. **(A)** If four red balls were placed in a bag with eight black balls, the probability of obtaining a red ball would be 4 out of 12 (total number of balls in the bag). After being simplified, the answer is $\frac{1}{3}$.

64. **(C)** The *Product Rule* for logarithms states that

$$\log(M) + \log(N) = \log(M \cdot N).$$

Thus, we have $\log(4) + \log(25) = \log(4 \cdot 25) = \log(100)$.
Note that $\log(100)$ asks the question: Base 10 raised to what power will yield 100?

$$\log(100) = \log(10^2)$$
$$10^x = 10^2$$
$$x = 2$$

65. **(B)** There are 6 possible ways to choose a dime and a total of 15 coins.

We use the formula: $\frac{6}{15} = 0.40 = 40\%$.

66. **(A)** As x approaches 1 from either side, y approaches 1.5.

67. **(A)** As x approaches -1 from the right, y approaches ∞.

68. **(D)** As x approaches ∞, y approaches 0.

69. **(A)** Since $\lim\limits_{x \to -1} f(x) = \pm\infty$, i.e., $x = 1$ represents a vertical line at which the function values become infinite.

70. **(B)** Since $\lim\limits_{x \to \infty} f(x) = 0$.

71. **(C)** The is no tangent line to the graph when $x = 1$, so the derivative does not exist there.

72. **(A)** We compute $\dfrac{f(3) - f(1)}{3 - 1} = \dfrac{9 - 1}{2} = 4$.

73. **(A)** Set up a proportion: $\dfrac{500 \text{ mg drug A}}{100 \text{ mg drug B}} = \dfrac{250 \text{ mg drug A}}{x \text{ mg}}$

    Cross multiply and divide: $500x = 250 \cdot 400$
    $$500x = 10,000$$
    $$x = 200 \text{ mg}$$

74. **(D)** We must exclude any values of x that cause $x^2 + 6x - 55 = 0$.
    Since $x^2 + 6x - 55 = 0 \Rightarrow (x + 11)(x - 5) = 0$, we must exclude $x = -11$, and $x = 5$.

75. **(B)** $\dfrac{\sqrt{36} \cdot \sqrt{16}}{9} = \dfrac{6 \cdot 4}{3} = 8$.

76. **(A)** This is the quadratic formula.

77. **(A)** Since the left-hand limit yields $\lim\limits_{x \to 2^-} f(x) = 3(2)^2 = 12$,

    but the right-hand limit yields $\lim\limits_{x \to 2^+} f(x) = 1 - 5(2) = -9$,

    the overall limit $\lim\limits_{x \to 2} f(x)$ is undefined.

78. **(B)** We solve the equation as follows.

    $$5(x + 2)(x - 1) = 5x^2 + 6x$$
    $$5(x^2 + x - 2) = 5x^2 + 6x$$
    $$5x^2 + 5x - 10 = 5x^2 + 6x$$
    $$5x - 10 = 6x \Rightarrow -10 = x$$

79. **(D)** Using data from the table, add together "Rarely" (0.0678) and "Never" (0.0262). We compute $0.0678 + 0.0262 = 0.094 = 9.4\%$.

80. **(B)** We compute $(0.1156)(8,000) = 924.8 \approx 925$.

81. **(D)** There are 3 ways that the sum of the numbers shown can equal 7, i.e., $1 + 6$, $2 + 5$, $3 + 4$. Note that there are 6 possible outcomes for each die in the pair. Therefore, to calculate the possible combinations for the pair, we multiple $6 \cdot 6 = 36$. So, the probability that the sum of the

numbers shown equals 7 is $\dfrac{3}{36}=\dfrac{1}{12}$. Thus, the probability that the sum

of the numbers shown is NOT equal to 7 is $1-\dfrac{1}{12}=\dfrac{11}{12}$.

82. **(C)** The area bounded above by the curve $y = f(x)$ and below by the x axis

on the interval $a \le x \le b$ is given by the definite integral $\displaystyle\int_a^b f(x)\,dx$.

We use the Fundamental Theorem of Calculus to compute the definite

integral $\displaystyle\int_a^b f(x)\,dx = F(b) - F(a)$, where $F(x)$ is an antiderivative of $f(x)$.

In this problem, we use the Power Rule for antiderivatives,

$\displaystyle\int x^n\,dx = \dfrac{1}{n+1}x^{n+1}$, to get $\displaystyle\int (x - x^3)\,dx = \dfrac{1}{2}x^2 - \dfrac{1}{4}x^4$.

Then we evaluate the expression on the interval $0 \le x \le 1$.

$$\int_0^1 (x - x^3)\,dx = \dfrac{1}{2}x^2 - \dfrac{1}{4}x^4 \Big]_0^1 = \left(\dfrac{1}{2}(1)^2 - \dfrac{1}{4}(1)^4\right) - \left(\dfrac{1}{2}(0)^2 - \dfrac{1}{4}(0)^4\right) = \dfrac{1}{2} - \dfrac{1}{4} = \dfrac{1}{4}$$

83. **(B)** Given the function $f(x) = \dfrac{10x}{x+1}$, we solve for y in the equation

$x = \dfrac{10y}{y+1}$, that is,

$$x = \dfrac{10y}{y+1}$$
$$xy + x = 10y$$
$$x = 10y - xy$$
$$x = y(10 - x) \Rightarrow y = \dfrac{x}{10 - x}.$$

84. **(D)** We simplify the expression as follows.

If $x < 3$, then $x - 3 < 0$. Thus, $|x-3| = -(x-3)$. Therefore,

$$\dfrac{x^2 - 2x - 3}{|x-3|} = \dfrac{(x-3)(x+1)}{-(x-3)} = -(x+1) = -x-1.$$

85. **(C)** With the understanding that the symbol $\cup$ means the set of elements either in A or B or in both, and $\cap$ means the set that contains all those elements that A and B have in common, we use the formula:

$$P(A \cup B) = P(A) + P(B) - P(A \cap B) = 0.26 + 0.42 - 0.12 = 0.56.$$

86. **(A)** With the understanding that the symbol $\cup$ means the set of elements either in A or B or in both, and $\cap$ means the set that contains all those elements that A and B have in common, we use the formula:

$$n(A \cup B) = n(A) + n(B) - n(A \cap B) = 12 + 8 - 6 = 14.$$

87. **(A)** We calculate the slope using the formula $\dfrac{\Delta y}{\Delta x} = \dfrac{3 - (-1)}{5 - 2} = \dfrac{4}{3}$.

88. **(A)** We solve the equation as follows.

$$\ln(w + 5x) = 3$$
$$e^{\ln(w + 5x)} = e^3$$
$$w + 5x = e^3$$
$$5x = e^3 - w \Rightarrow x = \frac{e^3 - w}{5}$$

89. **(B)** We apply the distance formula to points C and P to determine the radius of the circle $r = \sqrt{(5-8)^2 + (-6-3)^2} = \sqrt{9 + 81} = \sqrt{90}$.

Now use the fact that a circle with equation $(x - h)^2 + (y - k)^2 = r^2$ has center point (h, k) and radius equal to r.

90. **(D)** A rational function will have a horizontal asymptote of $y = L$, provided

$$\lim_{x \to \pm\infty} f(x) = L.$$

$$\lim_{x \to \pm\infty} f(x) = \lim_{x \to \pm\infty} \left(\frac{3x + 1}{5 - 4x} \right) \to \frac{3x}{-4x} \to -\frac{3}{4}$$

91. **(C)** The line with equation $y = 4$ is horizontal. So we need the equation of the vertical line passing through the point $(5, -7)$. The answer is $x = 5$.

92. **(C)** We are choosing 5 elements from a 12-element set, without repetition, such that order does not matter. Thus, we are counting combinations.

We use the formula $_{12}C_5 = \dfrac{12!}{5!(12-5)!} = \dfrac{12!}{5!7!}$.

93. **(D)** To convert from °F to °K, you must first convert the temperature from °F to °C. Therefore, the first step is to use

$$T_C = (T_F - 32) \left(\frac{5}{9}\right)$$

to convert the temperature to Celsius. Then, to convert the Celsius temperature to Kelvin, add 273.15.

Step 1:

$$T_C = (T_F - 32) \left(\frac{5}{9}\right)$$

$$= (86 - 32) \left(\frac{5}{9}\right)$$

$$= (54) \left(\frac{5}{9}\right)$$

$$= 30°C$$

Step 2:

$$K = 30 + 273.15 \approx 303$$

94. **(D)** A logarithmic function is undefined unless the input value is strictly greater than zero. Thus, we solve $4x - 2 > 0$ and obtain $x > 0.5$.

95. **(D)** The total rental cost is given by the daily cost plus the mileage cost. Daily cost = ($25 per day)(6 days) = $150. Mileage cost = ($0.12 per mile)(x miles) = $0.12x$.

96. **(C)** The graph has symmetry with respect to the origin.

97. **(B)** The domain is given by the set of x coordinates of the points on the graph.

98. **(D)** The range is given by the set of y coordinates of the points on the graph.

99. **(B)** Since the red and blue crayons are in a 5:9 ratio, we can set up the proportion $\dfrac{5 \text{ red}}{9 \text{ blue}} = \dfrac{20 \text{ red}}{x \text{ blue}}$. Now solve for x and then calculate $20 - x$.

    Step 1:

$$\frac{5}{9} = \frac{20}{x}$$
$$5x = (20)(9)$$
$$5x = 180$$
$$x = 36$$

Step 2:

20 − 36 = 16 more blue crayons than red crayons.

100. **(D)** Note that $\dfrac{4}{11} - \dfrac{3}{8} = \dfrac{8 \cdot 4 - 3 \cdot 11}{11 \cdot 8} = \dfrac{32 - 33}{88} = -\dfrac{1}{88}$.

CHAPTER 8

Reading Comprehension Review and Practice

TIPS FOR THE READING COMPREHENSION SECTION

The reading comprehension section of the PCAT presents relatively short (usually 400–700 words) passages. You are asked to read each passage carefully and then answer questions related to it. For each passage, there are generally 4–8 questions, with a total of 48 questions for the entire section. Keep in mind that the correct answer may be a direct statement taken from the reading passage. You will have 50 minutes to complete the reading comprehension section. Be careful to pace yourself to prevent running out of time.

Practice the reading passages and sample questions in this book. Read the passage first, and then answer the questions. Don't be concerned with how many times you need to refer to the passage to answer questions; just complete the section as quickly as possible, making sure you find the correct answer to every question.

Try to determine where your general strengths and weaknesses as a reader lie. Do you tend to get a quick grasp of the overall sense of a passage but miss the details? Or do you as a reader sometimes fail to see the forest for the trees? In other words, do you remember only the details and find yourself unable to state the basic meaning of the passage as a whole? In either case, take some time to improve your "weak" areas. Be patient with yourself as you practice. With adequate review, you should be able to work at your normal pace when you take the actual PCAT.

Answer Sheet
READING COMPREHENSION

1	Ⓐ Ⓑ Ⓒ Ⓓ	26	Ⓐ Ⓑ Ⓒ Ⓓ
2	Ⓐ Ⓑ Ⓒ Ⓓ	27	Ⓐ Ⓑ Ⓒ Ⓓ
3	Ⓐ Ⓑ Ⓒ Ⓓ	28	Ⓐ Ⓑ Ⓒ Ⓓ
4	Ⓐ Ⓑ Ⓒ Ⓓ	29	Ⓐ Ⓑ Ⓒ Ⓓ
5	Ⓐ Ⓑ Ⓒ Ⓓ	30	Ⓐ Ⓑ Ⓒ Ⓓ
6	Ⓐ Ⓑ Ⓒ Ⓓ	31	Ⓐ Ⓑ Ⓒ Ⓓ
7	Ⓐ Ⓑ Ⓒ Ⓓ	32	Ⓐ Ⓑ Ⓒ Ⓓ
8	Ⓐ Ⓑ Ⓒ Ⓓ	33	Ⓐ Ⓑ Ⓒ Ⓓ
9	Ⓐ Ⓑ Ⓒ Ⓓ	34	Ⓐ Ⓑ Ⓒ Ⓓ
10	Ⓐ Ⓑ Ⓒ Ⓓ	35	Ⓐ Ⓑ Ⓒ Ⓓ
11	Ⓐ Ⓑ Ⓒ Ⓓ	36	Ⓐ Ⓑ Ⓒ Ⓓ
12	Ⓐ Ⓑ Ⓒ Ⓓ	37	Ⓐ Ⓑ Ⓒ Ⓓ
13	Ⓐ Ⓑ Ⓒ Ⓓ	38	Ⓐ Ⓑ Ⓒ Ⓓ
14	Ⓐ Ⓑ Ⓒ Ⓓ	39	Ⓐ Ⓑ Ⓒ Ⓓ
15	Ⓐ Ⓑ Ⓒ Ⓓ	40	Ⓐ Ⓑ Ⓒ Ⓓ
16	Ⓐ Ⓑ Ⓒ Ⓓ	41	Ⓐ Ⓑ Ⓒ Ⓓ
17	Ⓐ Ⓑ Ⓒ Ⓓ	42	Ⓐ Ⓑ Ⓒ Ⓓ
18	Ⓐ Ⓑ Ⓒ Ⓓ	43	Ⓐ Ⓑ Ⓒ Ⓓ
19	Ⓐ Ⓑ Ⓒ Ⓓ	44	Ⓐ Ⓑ Ⓒ Ⓓ
20	Ⓐ Ⓑ Ⓒ Ⓓ	45	Ⓐ Ⓑ Ⓒ Ⓓ
21	Ⓐ Ⓑ Ⓒ Ⓓ	46	Ⓐ Ⓑ Ⓒ Ⓓ
22	Ⓐ Ⓑ Ⓒ Ⓓ	47	Ⓐ Ⓑ Ⓒ Ⓓ
23	Ⓐ Ⓑ Ⓒ Ⓓ	48	Ⓐ Ⓑ Ⓒ Ⓓ
24	Ⓐ Ⓑ Ⓒ Ⓓ	49	Ⓐ Ⓑ Ⓒ Ⓓ
25	Ⓐ Ⓑ Ⓒ Ⓓ	50	Ⓐ Ⓑ Ⓒ Ⓓ

Practice Questions

50 Questions

Passage 1

In the past two decades, people living in the northeastern, north-central, and western United States have unwittingly entered a dangerous enzootic cycle—a cycle of disease that typically is restricted to wildlife. Wild mammals and birds host a wide variety of disease agents, with effects ranging from mild symptoms to mortality, but in most cases the pathogen affects only one or a few host species and never causes disease in humans. However, as a result of a complicated sequence of events, people have become frequent accidental hosts for ticks and the disease agents they carry, including a corkscrew-shaped bacterium called *Borrelia burgdorferi*, the agent of Lyme disease. As of 1995, cases of Lyme disease had been reported in 48 of the 50 states and appear to be increasing, both in numbers of people affected and in geographic distribution.

Where does this disease come from, why has it emerged so rapidly, and what can people do to reduce their risk of exposure? It is possible to address these questions not from a medical point of view, but rather from an ecological one. All living organisms—from the *B. burgdorferi* bacterium and the ticks it infects to the mice and deer on which the ticks feed—form an ecological relationship with their habitats. Understanding the complex interactions between plant and animal species within those habitats may help people to predict the places where they are most likely to encounter disease-bearing ticks and become infected. Thus armed, individuals may ultimately be able to protect themselves from Lyme disease.

Currently, to prevent Lyme disease people wear protective clothing when they are in wooded areas and perform "tick checks" after leaving the woods. One underemphasized means to avoid exposure to Lyme disease, however, is avoiding the most heavily tick-infested habitats at the times of year when ticks are most abundant or dangerous. Recent research has suggested that such habitats can be predicted, often well in advance. Ultimately, it is the hope of ecologists studying this problem that we can use their expertise in pinpointing these habitats to warn the public away from areas that are likely to contain an abundance of disease-carrying ticks.

Excerpted from "The Ecology of Lyme-Disease Risk," by Richard S. Ostfeld, The American Scientist, Vol. 85, p. 338, reprinted by permission of American Scientist, magazine of Sigma Xi, The Scientific Research Society.

1. The agent of Lyme disease is

   (A) an enzootic cycle.
   (B) wild mammals and birds.
   (C) people living in the northeastern, north-central, and western United States.
   (D) a corkscrew-shaped bacterium called *Borrelia burgdorferi*.

2. The aim of understanding Lyme disease from an ecological as well as a medical point of view is

   (A) to help preserve the mice and deer on which the ticks feed.
   (B) to help people predict the places where they are most likely to encounter disease-bearing ticks and become infected.
   (C) to develop a vaccine against the disease.
   (D) to further our understanding of the relationship between ticks and their habitats.

3. To prevent Lyme disease people currently

   (A) receive annual vaccinations.
   (B) perform "tick checks" after leaving the woods.
   (C) wear protective clothing in wooded areas.
   (D) Both B and C

4. Which of the following statements is true?

   (A) Since the ecological approach to Lyme disease was introduced in 1995, cases have been decreasing in the northeastern, north-central, and western United States.
   (B) As of 1995, cases of Lyme disease had been reported in 48 of the 50 states and appear to be increasing, both in numbers of people affected and geographical distribution.
   (C) While cases in the northeastern United States have decreased since 1995, because of alterations in the enzootic cycle, cases are still on the rise in other geographical areas.
   (D) Cases of Lyme disease have remained relatively rare because of the inaccessibility of heavily tick-infested areas, but researchers still hope to keep as many people as possible away from areas where they might become infected.

5. One underemphasized means to avoid exposure to Lyme disease is

   (A) wearing protective clothing.
   (B) avoiding the most heavily tick-infested areas at certain times of the year.
   (C) using insect repellent.
   (D) remembering to get vaccinated before going into areas that are known to be heavily tick-infested.

Passage 2

To the average physician, Lyme disease is suspected when a patient arrives at a clinic or hospital complaining of a strange bull's-eye rash, known as erythema migrans, or EM, together with one or more flulike symptoms, such as fever, chills, muscle aches, or lethargy. The physician will take a blood sample for laboratory confirmation, but will feel quite confident to make a diagnosis of Lyme disease after noting the telltale combination of symptoms, as well as the circumstances surrounding the infection. The patient will undoubtedly have been bitten by the black-legged tick *Ixodes scaplaris*, formerly called the deer tick, or a close relative, which transferred to him or her the *B. burgdorferi* bacterium. Most likely, the physician will prescribe an oral course of antibiotics and will duly report the case to the county or state health department, which will include it in the morbidity statistics for Lyme disease.

Accurate diagnosis and effective treatment of Lyme disease are not always so straightforward, particularly in regions of the country newly invaded by the epidemic. In these regions, health care professionals and the public need to be educated about the confusing and generalized symptoms, the generally poor, but growing, accuracy of lab tests, and the efficacy of various antibiotic treatments. If Lyme disease is left untreated for some time, *B. burgdorferi* may persist in the patient's tissues and can migrate to the central and peripheral nervous systems or to joints and cause more severe late-stage symptoms, which include arthritis and neurological disorders, such as dizziness, memory loss, and disorientation. Vaccines that protect against Lyme disease are now being field tested by pharmaceutical companies, but none has yet been approved by the Food and Drug Administration for public use. Even if an effective vaccine were certified and marketed, the primary means that individuals have of protecting themselves against the disease is avoiding the tick in the first place.

Excerpted from "The Ecology of Lyme-Disease Risk," by Richard S. Ostfeld, The American Scientist, Vol. 85, p. 338, reprinted by permission of American Scientist, magazine of Sigma Xi, The Scientific Research Society.

6. When a patient reports to a clinic or hospital with symptoms of Lyme disease, he or she has undoubtedly been bitten by

   (A) the black-legged tick *Ixodes scaplaris.*
   (B) a tick-bearing wild mammal.
   (C) *B. burgdorferi.*
   (D) none of the above; Lyme disease is generally believed to be spread by an airborne pathogen.

7. Symptoms of Lyme disease include fever, chills, muscle aches, and

   (A) hyperactivity.
   (B) a bull's-eye rash.
   (C) vomiting.
   (D) Both A and B

8. Erythema migrans is best described as

   (A) a benign condition often mistaken for Lyme disease.
   (B) the microorganism believed to be an agent of Lyme disease.
   (C) the black-legged tick.
   (D) a strange, bull's-eye rash characteristic of Lyme disease.

9. In addition to noting the telltale combination of symptoms in a patient with Lyme disease, a physician is likely to

   (A) take a blood sample for laboratory confirmation.
   (B) prescribe an oral course of antibiotics.
   (C) report the case to the county or state health department.
   (D) All of the above

10. If Lyme disease is left untreated for some time,

    (A) health care professionals and the public will not be educated about its confusing and generalized symptoms.
    (B) the accuracy of diagnostic lab tests may be poor.
    (C) *B. burgdorferi* may persist in the patient's tissues and cause more severe late-stage symptoms.
    (D) antibiotic treatments will no longer be effective.

Passage 3

Rabies is a master dissembler. No other disease so completely manipulates its stricken host while barely leaving a trace of its presence. And rabies is preeminently adaptive: even if one host species is eliminated, the virus resurfaces in another. It bides its time, shadowing its victims, waiting for new hosts to emerge as people disrupt habitats and force animals to congregate more densely. Despite the war chest of vaccines designed to stop it and the near certain death of every organism infected by it, rabies persists.

In the United States, on average, fewer than two people a year die of rabies, about the same number as in Western Europe. Vaccination and animal control policies ensure that few, if any, of those cases come from dog bites. Worldwide, between 20,000 and 100,000 people die of rabies in a given year, most of them in developing countries, and some 10 million are treated annually for possible exposures, mostly from dog bites. Compared with the dangers of becoming infected with HIV, tuberculosis, or malaria, each of which strikes millions of people every year, the risk of contracting rabies is vanishingly small. But rabies has had far greater influence on culture and science than its current incidence might suggest. And its devastating effects assure that it is never far from people's minds. Rabies has the highest fatality rate of any known human infection.

Excerpted from "The Deadliest Virus," by Cynthia Mills, from the January/ February 1997 issue of THE SCIENCES, reprinted by permission of The Sciences, 2 East 63rd Street, New York, NY 10021.

11. Rabies persists

    (A) in spite of the vaccines designed to stop it.
    (B) because of its highly adaptive nature.
    (C) because people disrupt habitats, forcing animals to congregate more densely and allowing new hosts to emerge.
    (D) All of the above

12. In the United States, the number of people who die of rabies every year is

    (A) between 2,000 and 10,000.
    (B) comparable to the number who die of rabies in Western Europe.
    (C) increasing in spite of efforts to bring it under control.
    (D) approaching the number in danger of becoming infected with malaria.

13. Which of these statements about rabies may be regarded as true, according to the passage you read?

    (A) It has the lowest fatality rate of any known human infection.
    (B) Although frightening, rabies has had less influence on culture and science than its reputation might suggest.
    (C) Few cases of rabies in the United States and Western Europe, but most cases worldwide, come from dog bites.
    (D) Both A and C

14. Worldwide, the number of people treated annually for possible exposure to rabies is

    (A) between 20,000 and 100,000.
    (B) greater than the number infected with HIV.
    (C) 10 million.
    (D) None of the above

Passage 4

Unlike an electron, a single red blood cell cannot go through two openings at once. Indeed, it is generally true that the physicist seeking to understand the circulation of the blood can ignore most of the perplexities of twentieth-century physics. Given the scale of the circulatory system and the speed of blood flow, neither quantum mechanics nor relativity applies. Instead the flow of blood through the heart and the vascular tree can be adequately described by the familiar mechanics of Newton and Galileo.

If the circulation of the blood obeys the laws of classical mechanics, however, this does not mean that it is simple. An early experimental model of the vascular tree was a system of glass tubes filled with water. But unlike water, blood is not an "ideal" fluid. Instead it is a suspension of cells that, under certain circumstances, can behave in non-Newtonian ways. Moreover, flow through the vascular tree is pulsatile rather than steady; blood vessels taper and are elastic rather than rigid; and flow in any part of the densely interconnected system is affected by flow in neighboring regions. When these factors and the fantastic geometrical complexity of the labyrinthine vascular system are taken into account, the equations of blood flow, while remaining classical in inspiration, quickly become too complex to be solved explicitly.

Confronted with a system of overwhelming complexity, scientists typically resort to the intelligent simplification, that is, to a model. The first mathematical model of the human circulation was the *windkessel,* or compression chamber, model developed by Otto Frank in 1899 to explain how pulsatile flow from the heart is converted into steadier flow in the peripheral circulation. Sophisticated analytical models, the descendants of the windkessel model, still provide insight into the functioning of the circulatory system. But they are increasingly supplemented by numerical models, which exploit the power of the computer to arrive at accurate approximations of values that satisfy systems of equations that would otherwise be unsolvable. The computer can also be used to produce stunning images that allow otherwise cryptic measurements or calculations to be grasped intuitively.

Excerpted from "The Biophysics of Stroke," by George J. Hademenos, The American Scientist, Vol. 85, p. 226, reprinted by permission of American Scientist, magazine of Sigma Xi, The Scientific Research Society.

15. Quantum physics and relativity may be ignored by the physicist seeking to understand the circulation of the blood because

    (A) electrons cannot go through two openings at once in the vascular tree.
    (B) the mechanics of Newton and Galileo do not apply.
    (C) the scale of the circulatory system and the speed of blood flow can be adequately described by the mechanics of Newton and Galileo.
    (D) blood is an "ideal" fluid.

16. An early experimental model of the vascular tree

    (A) revealed that blood cannot behave in non-Newtonian ways.
    (B) consisted of a system of glass tubes filled with water.
    (C) was developed by Galileo.
    (D) yielded equations that although complex, could be solved quickly and explicitly.

17. When scientists are confronted with a system of overwhelming complexity, they typically

    (A) give up.
    (B) resort to intelligent simplification, that is, to a model.
    (C) adjust their most arbitrary assumptions accordingly.
    (D) abandon the mechanics of Galileo and Newton.

18. Otto Frank developed the *windkessel* model in 1899 for the purpose of

    (A) explaining how pulsatile flow from the heart is converted into steadier flow in the peripheral circulation.
    (B) improving on previous mathematical models.
    (C) converting the flow of blood from the heart into steadier flow in the peripheral circulation of human subjects.
    (D) augmenting the mechanics of Galileo and Newton.

19. In the twentieth century

    (A) quantum physics and relativity have given us some useful insights into the functioning of the circulatory system.
    (B) the windkessel model is still in use.
    (C) computers have not proved as useful as physicists had hoped since many systems of equations remain unsolvable.
    (D) computers can be used to produce images that allow cryptic measurements or calculations to be grasped intuitively.

Passage 5

A taxonomist viewing insects or crustaceans tends to see tough, jointed exoskeletons and elaborate limbs as their salient features—so salient, in fact, that the taxonomists who named the phylum to which these animals belong called it Arthropoda, or "jointed foot." The same biologist will also notice that the arthropod body plan is that of a modified worm, where the worm's more-or-less uniform series of segmented units becomes well differentiated along the length of the arthropod body. This gives arthropods distinct head, middle, and tail regions.

As neurobiologists considering evolution from simple to more complex animals, we are interested in the changes in the neural circuits serving locomotion and sensory coding that accompanied the transition from worm to arthropod. Such evolution is crucial to the emergence of advanced mobile animals. Because brains and body plans must have evolved in step from their simpler antecedents, comparative studies of neural development and of the mature nervous systems of animals promise to reveal much about arthropod evolution. In arthropods almost every nerve cell grows in a particular pattern and makes specific synaptic connections to form the elaborate neural circuits that give an animal its mobility and control; these features make each cell a recognizable identity.

Just as vertebrae and ribs are serially repeated, sets of neurons are repeated in each segment of an insect's body, or beneath each facet of the compound eye. Using identified neurons, anatomists can compare the development and structure of nervous systems from different arthropods much as they can compare vertebrate skeletons. In addition, we can record the electrical activity from a single neuron, which allows us to compare physiological function in different lineages. So far, most work has been done on insects, but comparisons can also be made between insects and crustaceans. Such comparisons tell biologists how these arthropods, with their jointed exoskeletons and specialized limbs, evolved from simpler ancestors and how they have subsequently diversified during evolutionary history.

Excerpted from "The Evolution of Anthropod Nervous Systems," by Daniel Ororio, Jonathan P. Bacon, and Paul M. Whitington, The American Scientist, Vol. 85, p. 244, reprinted by permission of American Scientist, magazine of Sigma Xi, The Scientific Research Society.

20. The passage suggests that

    (A) neurobiologists do not agree with taxonomists about the evolution of arthropods from worms.
    (B) the arthropod body plan is that of a modified worm.
    (C) since arthropods evolved from worms, they have no distinct head, middle, and tail regions.
    (D) neurobiologists consider the salient features of insects and crustaceans to be more clearly differentiated than those of arthropods.

21. As worms evolved into arthropods

    (A) their uniform series of segmented units became well differentiated.
    (B) the neural circuits serving locomotion and sensory coding changed.
    (C) they became advanced mobile animals.
    (D) All of the above

22. The name Arthropoda means

    (A) "jointed foot."
    (B) "wormlike."
    (C) "well-differentiated."
    (D) "mobile."

23. The phylum Arthropoda is distinguished by

    (A) a lack of sets of repeated neurons.
    (B) elaborate neural circuits allowing for mobility and control.
    (C) a tough, jointed exoskeleton.
    (D) Both B and C

24. Using identified neurons, anatomists can compare the development and structure of the nervous systems of different arthropods just as they can compare

    (A) sets of nonrepeating neurons.
    (B) vertebrate skeletons.
    (C) exoskeletons and specialized limbs.
    (D) worms and arthropods.

25. The passage suggests that neurobiologists are seeking to discover more about

    (A) how arthropods evolved from simpler ancestors.
    (B) how arthropods have diversified during their evolutionary history.
    (C) how the neural circuits of insects and crustaceans function.
    (D) All of the above

Passage 6

Allergic drug reactions account for 5% to 20% of all observed adverse drug reactions. Adverse drug reactions have been reported to occur in as many as 30% of hospitalized patients, and 3% of all hospitalizations are a result of adverse drug reactions. In a computerized surveillance study of over 36,000 hospitalized patients, 731 adverse events were identified. Of those, 1% were categorized as severe, life threatening, and allergic in nature. The potential morbidity and mortality associated with allergic drug reactions is great even though these outcomes occur infrequently.

In order to appropriately diagnose and treat a patient experiencing an allergic reaction, it is necessary to be able to differentiate allergic reactions from other closely related adverse drug reactions. One method of classification divides adverse reactions into those that are "predictable, usually dose-dependent, and related to the pharmacologic actions of the drug," and those that are "unpredictable, often dose independent, and related to the individual's immunologic response or to genetic differences in susceptible patients." Under this classification scheme, drug allergy or drug hypersensitivity is an unpredictable adverse drug reaction that is immunologically mediated.

Excerpted with permission from "Chapter 6, Anaphylaxis and Drug Allergies," page 6-1, Applied Therapeutics: The Clinical Use of Drugs, Sixth Edition, edited by Lloyd Yee Young and Mary Anne Koda-Kimble, published by Applied Therapeutics, Inc., Vancouver, Washington, © 1995.

26. Which of the following is necessary in order to appropriately diagnose and treat a patient experiencing an allergic reaction to a drug?

    (A) A way to differentiate allergic reactions from other adverse drug reactions
    (B) Determination that the reaction is dose-dependent and related to the pharmacological actions of the drug
    (C) Access to appropriate statistics, such as computerized surveillance studies
    (D) Hospitalization

27. If an adverse reaction is not predictable, dose-dependent, and related to the pharmacologic actions of the drug, then it is likely to be

    (A) adverse but not allergic.
    (B) unrelated to genetic differences in patients
    (C) related to the individual's immunologic response.
    (D) Both B and C

28. Allergic drug reactions account for as many as what percent of all observed adverse drug reactions?

    (A) 1% to 5%
    (B) 5% to 20%
    (C) 30%
    (D) 1%

29. Of 731 adverse drug events identified in a surveillance study of over 36,000 patients, 1% were characterized as

    (A) dose-dependent.
    (B) allergic but not severe or life-threatening.
    (C) severe, life-threatening, and allergic in nature.
    (D) adverse but not allergic.

Passage 7

You have seen the photographs, of course: An apple flaring on two sides as a bullet passes through it; tennis balls flattening themselves against rackets; jagged-edge balloons frozen in mid-pop; droplets in mid-drip; bubbles in mid-burst. They were the work of Harold E. Edgerton, an M.I.T. professor whose invention of the stroboscopic flash in the early 1930s made it possible, for the first time, to capture events as fleeting as a millionth of a second.

For decades chemists and solid-state physicists have yearned for a way of observing even more subtle alterations in matter: chemical reactions, or changes of state such as freezing or evaporation. Those changes depend on the breaking of bonds between atoms, a process that can take place in less than a picosecond—millions of times faster than anything Edgerton ever attempted. A fifth of a picosecond, for instance, is all the time it takes for photons entering your retina to trigger chemical changes in a pigment called rhodopsin—a reaction that makes it possible for you to read this article.

Lasers can flash that quickly. But laser light is too coarse a tool to give sharp closeup pictures of matter. Visible wavelengths are thousands of times longer than the space between the atoms in a solid material. Furthermore, visible light tends to interact with the fuzzy outer electron clouds of an atom—not with the tightly bound inner electrons that give a much better idea of where the atom is. For those reasons, physicists studying atomic structure have long relied on much shorter-wavelength radiation: X-rays. Stroboscopic X-ray crystallography, however, has been a long time coming. Now a team at Lawrence Berkeley National Laboratory in Berkeley, California, has taken a step in that direction by generating the shortest X-ray flash ever.

The main problem with X-rays is that their well known tendency to zip through materials makes them an optical nightmare. "You can't steer them the way you can light. It's difficult. You can't make a good mirror that operates at short wavelengths," says Robert W. Schoenlein, a staff scientist who coheaded the Lawrence Berkeley team. To point their X-rays in the right direction, Schoenlein and his colleagues generated them via Thomson scattering, an effect described early in this century by the English physicist J. J. Thomson. "Fast-moving particles such as electrons," Thomson said, "can transfer energy to photons, much as a Ping-Pong paddle energizes a ball." Thus, if you shoot a laser beam into a stream of high-velocity electrons, some of the photons in the beam may pick up enough energy to turn into X-rays. To produce X-ray flashes, some investigators fire a pulse of electrons head-on into a laser beam. The shorter the pulse, the shorter the flash. So far, however, the X-ray flashes have been too long to be useful.

Excerpted from "Flash Point," by Robert J. Coontz Jr., from the January/ February 1997 issue of THE SCIENCES, reprinted by permission of The Sciences, 2 East 63rd Street, New York, NY 10021.

30. The passage identifies Harold E. Edgerton as

    (A) head of the research team at Lawrence Berkeley National Laboratory.
    (B) an English physicist.
    (C) an M.I.T. professor who invented the stroboscopic flash.
    (D) the discoverer of X-rays in the early 1930s.

31. The time it takes for photons entering your retina to trigger chemical changes in a pigment called rhodopsin is

    (A) about a picosecond.
    (B) a millionth of a second.
    (C) a single pulse.
    (D) a fifth of a picosecond.

32. According to Robert W. Schoenlein, the main problem with X-rays is that

    (A) they tend to zip through materials, making them an optical nightmare.
    (B) they can't be steered the way light can.
    (C) you can't make a good mirror that operates at short wavelengths.
    (D) All of the above

33. Physicists studying atomic structure have relied on X-rays rather than lasers because

    (A) lasers cannot flash quickly enough.
    (B) laser light is too coarse a tool to give good close-up pictures of matter.
    (C) visible light tends to interact with the tightly bound inner electron clouds of an atom.
    (D) Both B and C

34. The main point of this passage is best summarized by which of the following statements?

    (A) Robert W. Schoenlein has invented a technique to transfer energy from electrons to photons, much as a Ping-Pong paddle energizes a ball.
    (B) Lasers have proved to be the most efficient way to produce sharp close-up pictures of matter.
    (C) Robert W. Schoenlein, a staff scientist at Lawrence Berkeley National Laboratory, and his team have succeeded in creating the shortest X-ray flashes ever.
    (D) Robert W. Schoenlein and his research team have succeeded in disproving the Thomson effect.

Passage 8

Sulfasalazine, the most frequently prescribed drug for inflammatory bowel disease therapy, has been used commonly for 50 years for the induction of disease remission in patients with mild acute exacerbations of ulcerative colitis. Initial uncontrolled observations of its efficacy indicated that 80% to 90% of patients improved with the use of this agent. The first placebo-controlled trial using objective parameters of efficacy demonstrated that 80% of the treated group improved as compared to 35% receiving placebo. These data were confirmed subsequently, although improvement may not occur until after four weeks of therapy. Sulfasalazine, 250 to 500 mg four times a day, often is considered the drug of choice in ulcerative colitis exacerbation because its efficacy has been demonstrated and because it has less severe adverse effects than corticosteroids. However, controlled trials have shown that corticosteroids may be more prompt in onset of action than sulfasalazine, alone or in combination with corticosteroid, for the treatment of severe acute ulcerative colitis. While comparative efficacy trials are lacking, the combination of sulfasalazine and prednisone does not appear to be detrimental and often has been used in hope of alleviating patients' symptoms.

Excerpted with permission from "Chapter 24, Inflammatory Bowel Disease," page 24-3, Applied Therapeutics: The Clinical Use of Drugs, Sixth Edition, edited by Lloyd Yee Young and Mary Anne Koda-Kimble, published by Applied Therapeutics, Inc., Vancouver, Washington, © 1995.

35. The most frequently prescribed drug for inflammatory bowel disease therapy is

    (A) prednisone.
    (B) sulfasalazine.
    (C) estrogen.
    (D) All of the above

36. What percent of the patients in the uncontrolled observations improved with sulfasalazine therapy?

    (A) 50% to 60%
    (B) 60% to 70%
    (C) 70% to 80%
    (D) 80% to 90%

37. What percent of the patients in the placebo group in the placebo-controlled trial improved?

    (A) 35%
    (B) 45%
    (C) 55%
    (D) 65%

38. According to the passage, how many times per day is sulfasalazine given?

    (A) Four
    (B) Five
    (C) Six
    (D) Eight

39. The combination of sulfasalazine and prednisone

    (A) appears to be dangerous.
    (B) offers hope.
    (C) shows no benefit.
    (D) Both A and C

Passage 9

Angina pectoris can be defined as a sense of discomfort arising in the myocardium as a result of myocardial ischemia in the absence of infarction. Although angina usually implies severe chest pain or discomfort, its presentation is variable. At one extreme, angina may occur predictably with strenuous exercise; at the other, angina may develop unexpectedly with little or no exertion.

Patients who have a reproducible pattern of angina that is associated with a certain level of physical activity have chronic stable angina or exertional angina. In contrast, patients with unstable angina are experiencing new angina or a change in their angina intensity, frequency, or duration. Both chronic stable angina and unstable angina often reflect underlying atherosclerotic narrowing of coronary arteries. Classic Prinzmetal's variant angina, or vasospastic angina, occurs in patients without coronary heart disease and is due to a spasm of the coronary artery that decreases myocardial blood flow. When coronary vasospasm occurs at the site of a fixed atherosclerotic plaque, mixed angina can result.

Silent myocardial ischemia, which is a transient change in myocardial perfusion, function, or electrical activity, can be detected on an electrocardiogram (ECG) in most angina patients. The patient, however, does not experience chest pain or other signs of angina [e.g., jaw pain, shortness of breath] during these episodes. Silent myocardial ischemia also can occur in patients with no angina history.

Excerpted with permission from "Chapter 13, Ischematic Heart Disease: Anginal Syndromes," pages 13-1 to 13-2, Applied Therapeutics: The Clinical Use of Drugs, Sixth Edition, edited by Lloyd Yee Young and Mary Anne Koda-Kimble, published by Applied Therapeutics, Inc., Vancouver, Washington, © 1995.

40. The term angina usually refers to

    (A) headache.
    (B) chest pain.
    (C) athlete's foot.
    (D) None of the above

41. Angina associated with physical activity is

    (A) Prinzmetal's angina.
    (B) variant angina.
    (C) vasocolonic angina.
    (D) stable angina.

42. Which type of angina occurs in patients without coronary heart disease?

    (A) Variant angina
    (B) Exertional angina
    (C) Prinzmetal's variant angina
    (D) None of the above

43. Silent myocardial ischemia

    (A) is atherosclerotic plaque.
    (B) has no consequences.
    (C) is a permanent change in myocardial perfusion, function, or electrical activity.
    (D) None of the above

44. Of the titles below, which would best describe the passage?

    (A) Angina—the Silent Killer
    (B) The Different Types of Angina
    (C) Chest Pain
    (D) Treating Chest Pain

Passage 10

Many scientists would agree that prions (pronounced PREE-ons) are the most bizarre pathogenic substances ever discovered. The late renowned physician and researcher Dr. Lewis Thomas called them one of the Seven Wonders of the World. Biologists are still arguing as to their composition. Prions had been an elusive, controversial, and well-kept secret in the medical community but this is no longer true.

A new book, *Deadly Feasts*, written by Pulitzer Prize-winning author Richard Rhodes, reveals much of the mystery surrounding these strange and deadly agents. Rhodes believes prions will be responsible for the next worldwide plague. His concern is plausible; prions have been responsible for the deaths of more than 100,000 cows in Great Britain and other countries. The cattle were suspected of carrying bovine spongiform encephalopathy or BSE (also known as "mad cow disease"). This epidemic in English cattle raises concerns about whether Creutzfeldt-Jakob disease, the human counterpart of BSE, will also increase in incidence.

The known prion diseases are sometimes referred to as transmissible spongiform encephalopathies. They are so named because they frequently cause the brain to become riddled with holes. The diseases are distinguished by long incubation periods and failure to produce an inflammatory response.

Dr. Thomas's decision to place these agents on the Seven Wonders list was based on the fact that no nucleic acid had yet been found among the infectious material. Prions have been found to consist of protein and nothing else. (The word *prion* is derived from the words *proteinaceous* and *infectious*. The letters *o* and *i* were transposed by poetic license.) It has been generally accepted that conveyers of transmissible diseases require genetic material, composed of nucleic acid (DNA or RNA), in order to establish an infection in a host. Even viruses, which are among the simplest microbes, rely on such material to direct the synthesis of the proteins needed for survival and replication.

Prions appear to convert normal protein molecules into dangerous ones simply by inducing the benign molecules to change shape. Much of the infectious nature of a prion appears to depend on the similarity of prion protein (PrP) between species. The degree of similarity between bovine and human PrP may therefore be an important determinant of the risk of infection.

Excerpted with permission from "Prions, Bizarre Pathogens," by Max Sherman, R. Ph., U.S. Pharmacist, June, 1997, pages 54-61, © 1997.

45. The passage indicates that Creutzfeld-Jakob disease is

    (A) responsible for the deaths of 100,000 sheep.
    (B) a controversial and well-kept secret.
    (C) the human counterpart of BSE (bovine spongiform encephalopathy).
    (D) "mad cow disease."

46. Dr. Thomas decided to place prions on the Seven Wonders list because

    (A) prions have highly unusual DNA.
    (B) no nucleic acid was found among the infectious material.
    (C) prions have no proteins.
    (D) prions cause the brain to become riddled with holes.

47. Prions appear to convert normal protein molecules into dangerous ones by

    (A) inducing benign molecules to change shape.
    (B) using their DNA to direct the synthesis of dangerous proteins.
    (C) using their RNA to direct the synthesis of dangerous proteins.
    (D) Both B and C

48. The word prion is derived from

    (A) proteinaceous.
    (B) the name of Pulitzer Prize-winning author Richard Prion.
    (C) infectious.
    (D) Both A and C

49. The new book *Deadly Feasts* warns that

    (A) prions will be responsible for the next worldwide plague.
    (B) prions will wipe out cattle herds worldwide.
    (C) prions will become our deadliest viruses.
    (D) prions cannot be defeated until their DNA is understood.

50. The known prion diseases are characterized by

    (A) long incubation periods.
    (B) failure to produce an inflammatory response.
    (C) frequently causing the brain to become riddled with holes.
    (D) All of the above

Answer Key
READING COMPREHENSION

1. D	11. D	21. D	31. D	41. D
2. B	12. B	22. A	32. D	42. C
3. D	13. C	23. D	33. B	43. D
4. B	14. C	24. B	34. C	44. B
5. B	15. C	25. D	35. B	45. C
6. A	16. B	26. A	36. D	46. B
7. B	17. B	27. C	37. A	47. A
8. D	18. A	28. B	38. A	48. D
9. D	19. D	29. C	39. B	49. A
10. C	20. B	30. C	40. B	50. D

EXPLANATORY ANSWERS

The numbers in the margins of the reprinted passages indicate the statements in which the answer to the questions can be found.

PASSAGE 1

In the past two decades, people living in the northeastern, north-central, and western United States have unwittingly entered a dangerous enzootic cycle—a cycle of disease that typically is restricted to wildlife. Wild mammals and birds host a wide variety of disease agents, with effects ranging from mild symptoms to mortality, but in most cases the pathogen affects only one or a few host species and never causes disease in humans. However, as a result of a complicated sequence of events, people have become frequent accidental hosts for ticks and the disease agents they
1   carry, including a <u>corkscrew-shaped bacterium called *Borrelia burgdorferi*, the agent</u>
4   <u>of Lyme disease. As of 1995, cases of Lyme disease had been reported in 48 of the</u>
<u>50 states and appear to be increasing, both in numbers of people affected and in</u>
<u>geographic distribution.</u>

Where does this disease come from, why has it emerged so rapidly, and what can people do to reduce their risk of exposure? It is possible to address these questions not from a medical point of view, but rather from an ecological one. All living organisms—from the *B. burgdorferi* bacterium and the ticks it infects to the mice and deer on which the ticks feed—form an ecological relationship with their habi-
2   tats. <u>Understanding the complex interactions between plant and animal species</u>
<u>within those habitats may help people to predict the places where they are most</u>
<u>likely to encounter disease-bearing ticks and become infected. Thus armed, indi-</u>
<u>viduals may ultimately be able to protect themselves from Lyme disease.</u>

3   <u>Currently, to prevent Lyme disease people wear protective clothing when they are</u>
<u>in wooded areas and perform "tick checks" after leaving the woods. One underem-</u>
5   <u>phasized means to avoid exposure to Lyme disease, however, is avoiding the most</u>
<u>heavily tick-infested habitats at the times of year when ticks are most abundant or</u>
<u>dangerous.</u> Recent research performed in my laboratory, as well as in others, has suggested that such habitats can be predicted, often well in advance. Ultimately, it is the hope of ecologists studying this problem that we can use our expertise in pinpointing these habitats to warn the public away from areas that are likely to contain an abundance of disease-carrying ticks.

1. **(D)** Answer A refers to the enzootic cycle (animal diseases present in a specific locality) in which wild mammals and birds (B) ordinarily participate. People living in specified areas (C) have become participants in this cycle, but the actual agent of Lyme disease is a microorganism, the bacterium *Borrelia burgdorferi* (D).

2. **(B)** While A and D might well be sound ecological goals in other circumstances, when it comes to Lyme disease, ecologists are motivated by a desire to help people predict and avoid the places where they are likely to become infected (B). Although C is an important medical consideration, the development of a vaccine is not the province of ecologists.

3. **(D)** The passage states that both B and C are protective measures. Answer A is not mentioned and is irrelevant.

4. **(B)** Answer B is a true statement, taken directly from the passage. Answer A states the opposite of the truth, and C and D each combine a false statement with a true one.

5. **(B)** Answer B states the main point of the passage. Answer A is mentioned as an often-used, rather than an underemployed protective measure. Answers C and D are irrelevant.

PASSAGE 2

To the average physician, Lyme disease is suspected when a patient arrives at a clinic or hospital complaining of a strange bull's-eye rash, known as erythema migrans, or EM, together with one or more flulike symptoms, such as fever, chills, muscle aches, or lethargy. The doctor will take a blood sample for laboratory confirmation, but will feel quite confident to make a diagnosis of Lyme disease after noting the telltale combination of symptoms, as well as the circumstances surrounding the infection. The patient will undoubtedly have been bitten by the black-legged tick *Ixodes scaplaris*, formerly called the deer tick, or a close relative, which transferred to him or her the *B. burgdorferi* bacterium. Most likely, the doctor will prescribe an oral course of antibiotics and will duly report the case to the county or state health department, which will include it in the morbidity statistics for Lyme disease. 7 8 9 6 9

Accurate diagnosis and effective treatment of Lyme disease are not always so straightforward, particularly in regions of the country newly invaded by the epidemic. In these regions, health care professionals and the public need to be educated about the confusing and generalized symptoms, the generally poor, but growing, accuracy of lab tests, and the efficacy of various antibiotic treatments. If Lyme disease is left untreated for some time, *B. burgdorferi* may persist in the patient's tissues and can migrate to the central and peripheral nervous system or to joints and cause more severe late-stage symptoms, which include arthritis and neurological disorders, such as dizziness, memory loss and disorientation. Vaccines that protect against Lyme disease are now being field tested by pharmaceutical companies, but none has yet been approved by the Food and Drug Administration for public use. Even if an effective vaccine were certified and marketed, the primary means that individuals have of protecting themselves against the disease is avoiding the tick in the first place. 10

6. **(A)** In order for the pathogen *B. burgdorferi* to pass from tick to human, the human must be bitten by the tick—in this case, the black-legged tick, *Ixodes scaplaris*. A tick-bearing mammal (B) might provide the tick, but not the bite. The microbe *B. burgdorferi* is not capable of biting, so C cannot be correct. Answer D is irrelevant (Lyme disease is not airborne).

7. **(B)** The passage mentions B, but not C. A is not true.

8. **(D)** Only the bull's-eye rash is called erythema migrans. Answer A is irrelevant; B refers to *B. burgdorferi*; C refers to scaplaris.

9. **(D)** As stated in the passage, the physician will take a blood sample, prescribe antibiotics, and report the case (A, B, and C).

10. **(C)** Answer A is not addressed in the paragraph. Answer B is false since leaving the disease untreated is not mentioned in the passage as having any effect on lab tests; D is neither stated nor implied in the passage. The result of leaving Lyme disease untreated is clearly described in C.

PASSAGE 3

Rabies is a master dissembler. No other disease so completely manipulates its stricken host while barely leaving a trace of its presence. And rabies is preeminently
11 adaptive: even if one host species is eliminated, the virus resurfaces in another. It bides its time, shadowing its victims, waiting for new hosts to emerge as people disrupt habitats and force animals to congregate more densely. Despite the war chest of vaccines designed to stop it and the near-certain death of every organism infected by it, rabies persists.
12 In the United States, on average, fewer than two people a year die of rabies, about the same number as in Western Europe. Vaccination and animal control policies
13 ensure that few, if any, of those cases come from dog bites. Worldwide, between 20,000 and 100,000 people die of rabies in a given year, most of them in develop-
14 ing countries, and some 10 million are treated annually for possible exposures, mostly from dog bites. Compared with the dangers of becoming infected with HIV, tuberculosis or malaria, each of which strikes millions of people every year, the risk of contracting rabies is vanishingly small. But rabies has had far greater influence on culture and science than its current incidence might suggest. And its devastating effects assure that it is never far from people's minds. Rabies has the highest fatality
13 rate of any known human infection.

11. **(D)** Answers A, B, and C state facts taken directly from the passage.

12. **(B)** Although you might be tempted to complete the statement with an incorrect figure (A), B is actually stated in the passage. Both C and D are false.

13. **(C)** C is true; Both A and B are false and in fact contradict statements in the passage.

14. **(C)** Only one specific figure can be correct in this instance, and the number of people treated for possible exposure is given in the passage as 10 million.

PASSAGE 4

Unlike an electron, a single red blood cell cannot go through two openings at once. <u>Indeed, it is generally true that the physicist seeking to understand the circulation of the blood can ignore most of the perplexities of twentieth century physics.</u> 15 <u>Given the scale of the circulatory system and the speed of blood flow, neither quantum mechanics nor relativity applies. Instead the flow of blood through the heart and the vascular tree can be adequately described by the familiar mechanics of Newton and Galileo.</u>

If the circulation of the blood obeys the laws of classical mechanics, however, this does not mean that it is simple. <u>An early experimental model of the vascular tree was</u> 16 <u>a system of glass tubes filled with water.</u> But unlike water, blood is not an "ideal" fluid. Instead it is a suspension of cells that, under certain circumstances, can behave in non-Newtonian ways. Moreover, flow through the vascular tree is pulsatile rather than steady; blood vessels taper and are elastic rather than rigid; and flow in any part of the densely interconnected system is affected by flow in neighboring regions. When these factors and the fantastic geometrical complexity of the labyrinthine vascular system are taken into account, the equations of blood flow, while remaining classical in inspiration, quickly become too complex to be solved explicitly.

<u>Confronted with a system of overwhelming complexity, scientists typically resort</u> 17 <u>to the intelligent simplification, that is, to a model.</u> <u>The first mathematical model of the human circulation was the *windkessel*, or compression chamber, model devel-</u> 18 <u>oped by Otto Frank in 1899 to explain how pulsatile flow from the heart is converted into steadier flow in the peripheral circulation.</u> Sophisticated analytical models, the descendants of the *windkessel* model, still provide insight into the functioning of the circulatory system. But they are increasingly supplemented by numerical models, which exploit the power of the computer to arrive at accurate approximations of values that satisfy systems of equations that would otherwise be unsolvable. <u>The computer can also be used to produce stunning images that allow</u> 19 <u>otherwise cryptic measurements or calculations to be grasped intuitively.</u>

15. **(C)** The passage states that the mechanics of Newton and Galileo are adequate for describing the circulatory system and blood flow. Answer A is irrelevant; B and D contradict information given in the passage.

16. **(B)** As described in the passage, an early experimental model was a system of glass tubes filled with water. Answer A is irrelevant; C is false; and D is both false and absurd.

17. **(B)** According to the passage, scientists are likely to turn to a model when confronted with a system of overwhelming complexity. Answers A and D are decidedly untrue; in fact, D contradicts information given in the passage.

18. **(A)** As stated in the passage, Frank developed his *windkessel* model of the circulatory system to explain how pulsatile flow from the heart is converted into steadier flow in the peripheral circulation. Since he made use of the model, not human subjects, the answer cannot be C (which is a nonsense statement anyway). His was the first mathematical model, so B cannot be

correct, and Frank was not attempting to augment the mechanics of Galileo and Newton (D).

19. **(D)** As the passage indicates, quantum physics and relativity are not relevant to the study of the circulatory system, so A cannot be the correct answer. Nor is B correct, since the windkessel dates back to 1899 and is no longer in use. Answer C contradicts information stated in the passage. Only D actually occurs as a statement in the passage.

PASSAGE 5

23   A taxonomist viewing insects or crustaceans tends to see tough, jointed exoskeletons and elaborate limbs as their salient features—so salient, in fact, that the tax-
22   onomists who named the phylum to which these animals belong called it Arthropoda, or "jointed foot." The same biologist will also notice that the arthro-
20   pod body plan is that of a modified worm, where the worm's more-or-less uniform series of segmented units becomes well differentiated along the length of the arthropod body. This gives arthropods distinct head, middle and tail regions.
21   As neurobiologists considering evolution from simple to more complex animals, we are interested in the changes in the neural circuits serving locomotion and sensory coding that accompanied the transition from worm to arthropod. Such evolution is crucial to the emergence of advanced mobile animals. Because brains and body plans must have evolved in step from their simpler antecedents, comparative studies of neural development and of the mature nervous systems of animals promise to reveal much about arthropod evolution. In arthropods almost every
23   nerve cell grows in a particular pattern and makes specific synaptic connections to form the elaborate neural circuits that give an animal its mobility and control; these features make each cell a recognizable identity.
       Just as vertebrae and ribs are serially repeated, sets of neurons are repeated in each segment of an insect's body, or beneath each facet of the compound eye. Using iden-
24   tified neurons, anatomists can compare the development and structure of nervous systems from different arthropods much as they can compare vertebrate skeletons.
25   In addition, we can record the electrical activity from a single neuron, which allows us to compare physiological function in different lineages. So far, most work has been done on insects, but comparisons can also be made between insects and crustaceans. Such comparisons tell biologists how these arthropods, with their jointed exoskeletons and specialized limbs, evolved from simpler ancestors and how they have subsequently diversified during evolutionary history.

20. **(B)** The passage states that the arthropod body plan is that of a modified worm (B). A contradicts information given in the passage, as does C; D is a nonsense statement since insects and crustaceans are arthropods.

21. **(D)** The passage lists A, B, and C as changes that took place as worms evolved into arthropods.

22. **(A)** As the passage states, arthropod means "jointed foot." Answers B, C, and D are false.

23. **(D)** Answer A contradicts information given in the passage, but both B and C are accurate.

24. **(B)** The passage draws an analogy between the work done by anatomists who compare neurons to learn more about the development and structure of the nervous systems of different arthropods and the work done by anatomists who compare the skeletons of different vertebrates. Answers A, C, and D do not make sense in the context of the passage.

25. **(D)** The passage directly mentions A, B, and C as subjects that neurobiologists are seeking to discover more about.

PASSAGE 6

Allergic drug reactions account for 5% to 20% of all observed adverse drug reactions. Adverse drug reactions have been reported to occur in as many as 30% of hospitalized patients, and 3% of all hospitalizations are a result of adverse drug reactions. In a computerized surveillance study of over 36,000 hospitalized patients, 731 adverse events were identified. Of those, 1% were categorized as severe, life threatening, and allergic in nature. The potential morbidity and mortality associated with allergic drug reactions is great even though these outcomes occur infrequently.   28   29

In order to appropriately diagnose and treat a patient experiencing an allergic reaction, it is necessary to be able to differentiate allergic reactions from other closely related adverse drug reactions. One method of classification divides adverse reactions into those that are "predictable, usually dose-dependent, and related to the pharmacologic actions of the drug," and those that are "unpredictable, often dose independent, and are related to the individual's immunologic response or to genetic differences in susceptible patients." Under this classification scheme, drug allergy or drug hypersensitivity is an unpredictable adverse drug reaction that is immunologically mediated.   26   27

26. **(A)** As the passage states, allergic reactions must be differentiated from other closely related adverse drug reactions. Answer B describes reactions that are typically adverse but not allergic, and C is irrelevant to diagnosing and treating allergic drug reactions appropriately. While some allergic reactions may require hospitalization (D), this is not necessary to diagnose appropriately and treat all allergic reactions to drugs.

27. **(C)** C appears in the passage. A and B are not true.

28. **(B)** According to the passage, 5% to 20% of all observed drug reactions represent allergic drug reactions.

29. **(C)** That 1% of the 731 adverse drug events were characterized as severe, life-threatening, and allergic in nature is stated in the passage (C). Answer B is only partially true, since the allergic reactions identified were of a severe and life-threatening nature. Both A and D refer to adverse reactions that are not classified as allergic.

PASSAGE 7

You have seen the photographs, of course: An apple flaring on two sides as a bullet passes through it; tennis balls flattening themselves against rackets; jagged-edge balloons frozen in mid-pop; droplets in mid-drip; bubbles in mid-burst. They

30 were the work of Harold E. Edgerton, an M.I.T. professor whose invention of the stroboscopic flash in the early 1930s made it possible, for the first time, to capture events as fleeting as a millionth of a second.

For decades chemists and solid-state physicists have yearned for a way of observing even more subtle alterations in matter: chemical reactions, or changes of state such as freezing or evaporation. Those changes depend on the breaking or forging of bonds between atoms, a process that can take place in less than a picosecond—millions of times faster than anything Edgerton ever attempted. A fifth of a picosec-

31 ond, for instance, is all the time it takes for photons entering your retina to trigger chemical changes in a pigment called rhodopsin—a reaction that makes it possible for you to read this article.

33 Lasers can flash that quickly. But laser light is too coarse a tool to give sharp closeup pictures of matter. Visible wavelengths are thousands of times longer than the space between the atoms in a solid material. Furthermore, visible light tends to interact with the fuzzy outer electron clouds of an atom—not with the tightly bound inner electrons that give a much better idea of where the atom is. For those reasons, physicists studying atomic structure have long relied on much shorter-wavelength radiation: X rays. Stroboscopic X-ray crystallography, however, has been

34 a long time coming. Now a team at Lawrence Berkeley National Laboratory in Berkeley, California, has taken a step in that direction by generating the shortest X-ray flash ever.

32 The main problem with X rays is that their well known tendency to zip through materials makes them an optical nightmare. "You can't steer them the way you can light. It's difficult. You can't make a good mirror that operates at short wavelengths,"

34 says Robert W. Schoenlein, a staff scientist who coheaded the Lawrence Berkeley team. To point their X rays in the right direction, Schoenlein and his colleagues generated them via Thomson scattering, an effect described early in this century by the English physicist J. J. Thomson. "Fast-moving particles such as electrons," Thomson said, "can transfer energy to photons, much as a Ping-Pong paddle energizes a ball." Thus, if you shoot a laser beam into a stream of high-velocity electrons, some of the photons in the beam may pick up enough energy to turn into X rays. To produce X-ray flashes, some investigators fire a pulse of electrons head-on into a laser beam. The shorter the pulse, the shorter the flash. So far, however, the X-ray flashes have been too long to be useful.

30. **(C)** The passage identifies Harold E. Edgerton as an M.I.T. professor who invented the stroboscopic flash.

31. **(D)** A precise figure is required here. According to the passage, the correct answer is a fifth of a picosecond.

32. **(D)** The author of the passage states A, and Schoenlein is quoted in the passage as complaining about B and C.

33. **(B)** The passage reports that physicists have had problems with B, but not A, since lasers do flash quickly enough. C is not true.

34. **(C)** The main thrust of the passage is that Shoenlein and his team have created the shortest X-ray flashes ever (even if they are still not short enough to be truly useful). Answer A is false, since this technique was described in the early 1900's by the English physicist J. J. Thomson. Answer B contradicts information given in the passage, and D is untrue because Schoenlein's research depends on the Thomson effect.

PASSAGE 8

Sulfasalazine, the most frequently prescribed drug for inflammatory bowel disease therapy, has been used commonly for 50 years for the induction of disease remission in patients with mild acute exacerbations of ulcerative colitis. Initial uncontrolled observations of its efficacy indicated that 80% to 90% of patients improved with the use of this agent. The first placebo-controlled trial using objective parameters of efficacy demonstrated that 80% of the treated group improved as compared to 35% receiving placebo. These data were confirmed subsequently, although improvement may not occur until after four weeks of therapy. Sulfasalazine, 250 to 500 mg four times a day, often is considered the drug of choice in ulcerative colitis exacerbation because its efficacy has been demonstrated and because it has less severe adverse effects than corticosteroids. However, controlled trials have shown that corticosteroids may be more prompt in onset of action than sulfasalazine, alone or in combination with corticosteroid, for the treatment of severe acute ulcerative colitis. While comparative efficacy trials are lacking, the combination of sulfasalazine and prednisone does not appear to be detrimental and often has been used in hope of alleviating patients' symptoms.

35

36

37

38

39

35. **(B)** Although prednisone (A) is used to treat inflammatory bowel disease, the first sentence of the passage states clearly that the most frequently prescribed drug for inflammatory bowel disease therapy is sulfasalazine. Ulcerative colitis (C) is a type of inflammatory bowel disease.

36. **(D)** This percentage is given in the passage.

37. **(A)** This percentage is given in the passage.

38. **(A)** Sulfasalazine is given four times per day at doses of 250–500 mg.

39. **(B)** The passage clearly states that the combination of sulfasalazine and prednisone does not appear to be detrimental (dangerous, A) and often has been used in hope of alleviating patients' symptoms.

PASSAGE 9

Angina pectoris can be defined as a sense of discomfort arising in the myocardium as a result of myocardial ischemia in the absence of infarction. <u>Although angina usually implies severe chest pain or discomfort, its presentation is variable</u>. At one extreme, angina may occur predictably with strenuous exercise; at the other, angina may develop unexpectedly with little or no exertion.

40

<u>Patients who have a reproducible pattern of angina that is associated with a certain level of physical activity have chronic stable angina or exertional angina.</u> In contrast, patients with unstable angina are experiencing new angina or a change in their angina intensity, frequency, or duration. Both chronic stable angina and unstable angina often reflect underlying atherosclerotic narrowing of coronary arteries.

41

<u>Classic Prinzmetal's variant angina, or vasospastic angina, occurs in patients without coronary heart disease and is due to a spasm of the coronary artery that decreases myocardial blood flow.</u> When coronary vasospasm occurs at the site of a fixed atherosclerotic plaque, mixed angina can result.

42

<u>Silent myocardial ischemia, which is a transient change in myocardial perfusion, function, or electrical activity, can be detected on an electrocardiogram (ECG) in most angina patients.</u> The patient, however, does not experience chest pain or other signs of angina [e.g., jaw pain, shortness of breath (SOB)] during these episodes. Silent myocardial ischemia also can occur in patients with no angina history.

43

40. **(B)** Although a headache (A) may accompany chest pain (B), angina usually implies severe chest pain. Answer C is absurd in the context of the passage.

41. **(D)** Prinzmetal's and variant angina (A and B) are due to a spasm of the coronary artery. There is no such disorder as vasocolonic angina. Angina that is associated with a certain level of physical activity is called stable angina or exertional angina. `

42. **(C)** The passage states that Prinzmetal's variant angina occurs in patients without coronary heart disease. Answers A, B, and D are untrue.

43. **(D)** Statement C is incorrect because silent myocardial ischemia is a transient (not permanent) change in myocardial perfusion, function, or electrical activity. Silent myocardial ischemia is not atherosclerotic plaque (A), although atherosclerotic plaque may cause ischemia. Myocardial ischemia can cause serious damage (consequences, B). Answers A, B, and C are all false.

44. **(B)** Since the passage does not discuss the mortality rates associated with angina or the treatment of chest pain, answers A and D are incorrect. Chest pain (C) is too broad a title for this passage. Answer B, The Different Types of Angina, best describes the focus of this passage.

PASSAGE 10

Many scientists would agree that prions (pronounced PREE-ons) are the most bizarre pathogenic substances ever discovered. The late, renowned physician and researcher Dr. Lewis Thomas called them one of the Seven Wonders of the World. Biologists are still arguing as to their composition. Prions had been an elusive, controversial, and well-kept secret in the medical community but this is no longer true.

A new book, *Deadly Feasts*, written by Pulitzer Prize-winning author Richard   49
Rhodes, reveals much of the mystery surrounding these strange and deadly agents. Rhodes believes prions will be responsible for the next worldwide plague. His concern is plausible; prions have been responsible for the deaths of more than 100,000 cows in Great Britain and other countries. The cattle were suspected of carrying bovine spongiform encephalopathy or BSE (also known as "mad cow disease"). This epidemic in English cattle raises concerns about whether Creutzfeldt-Jakob   45
disease, the human counterpart of BSE, will also increase in incidence.

The known prion diseases are sometimes referred to as transmissible spongiform encephalopathies. They are so named because they frequently cause the brain to   50
become riddled with holes. The diseases are distinguished by long incubation periods and failure to produce an inflammatory response.

Dr. Thomas's decision to place these agents on the Seven Wonders list was based   46
on the fact that no nucleic acid had yet been found among the infectious material. Prions have been found to consist of protein and nothing else. (The word *prion* is   48
derived from the words *proteinaceous* and *infectious*. The letters *o* and *i* were transposed by poetic license.) It has been generally accepted that conveyers of transmissible diseases require genetic material, composed of nucleic acid (DNA or RNA), in order to establish an infection in a host. Even viruses, which are among the simplest microbes, rely on such material to direct the synthesis of the proteins needed for survival and replication.

Prions appear to convert normal protein molecules into dangerous ones simply   47
by inducing the benign molecules to change shape. Much of the infectious nature of a prion appears to depend on the similarity of prion protein (PrP) between species. The degree of similarity between bovine and human PrP may therefore be an important determinant of the risk of infection.

45   **(C)** Creutzfeldt-Jakob disease is the human counterpart of BSE, according to the passage. Answer A is false (prions killed more than 100,000 cows, not sheep, according to the passage). Answer B refers to prions in general rather than to Creutzfeld-Jakob disease; D is BSE, a disease of animals.

46.   **(B)** Prions are regarded as an oddity because they have no nucleic acid and consist only of protein. Both A and C, therefore, are false. D is definitely a result of diseases caused by prions but is not the reason that Thomas placed them on the Seven Wonders list.

47.   **(A)** That prions appear to induce benign molecules to change shape is the only true statement. Since prions have no nucleic acid, they have neither RNA nor DNA, thereby ruling out B, C, and D.

48. **(D)** The word prion is formed from two adjectives, proteinaceous and infectious. "Richard Prion" is not mentioned in the passage although the passage states that Richard Rhodes is the Pulitzer Prize-winning author of *Deadly Feasts.*

49. **(A)** The passage warns that prions will be responsible for the next worldwide plague. While theoretically possible, B is not mentioned in the passage; C is clearly false (prions are not viruses), and D is false as well (prions have no DNA).

50. **(D)** Prion diseases are characterized by A, B, and C.

The PCAT Essay

CHAPTER 9

PCAT WRITING TEST

The company that administers the PCAT tested an essay component for the exam during the 2004–2005 testing cycle. Based on the results and the grading process utilized, it was determined that the writing test would be included in the PCAT beginning with the 2005–2006 test cycle; a second writing section was added during the 2007–2008 test cycle. The writing section is scored according to two writing rubrics: "Conventions of Language" and "Problem Solving."

The writing sections of the PCAT will present topics that will require you to write short literary compositions as "problem-solving" essays. Each problem-solving essay topic is presented in the form of a statement that poses a problem to be solved. Each essay should present and coherently explain your suggested solution to the problem presented in the statement, as well as possible alternatives to the primary solution being suggested.

You will not be able to use a dictionary or any other reference material(s). You will have 30 minutes to complete each essay. You should allow yourself enough time to determine what your response to the topic will be (brainstorm), to organize and write your essay (you may find that writing a quick outline may help with this), and to edit and proofread your response. The greatest portion of the 30-minute time allotment for each of these PCAT sections should be spent writing the essay; remember to pace yourself and to keep track of time. As with the other sections of the PCAT, each essay will be written on the computer using the computer-based platform provided at the testing center.

TIP

Be sure to present and coherently explain your suggested solution to the problem.

PCAT WRITING SECTION SCORES

As stated previously, you will receive a "Problem Solving" score and a "Conventions of Language" score for the writing test. Please note: you will only be scored on one essay. The other essay is considered experimental and is used to assess potential items for future versions of the PCAT. However, you will not know which of the two essays will be scored so it is important to give your full effort to the composition of each essay. Each of the scores on the writing test will utilize a five-point scale, ranging from 1 = "Weak" to 5 = "Superior." The five score possibilities for each rubric are characterized on the next page, as outlined on the PCAT website (*www.pcatweb.info*).

The writing scores will be included on the score report received by the candidate and sent to those institutions chosen by the candidate. However, the scores are not incorporated into the composite scaled or percentile scores of the PCAT. Some schools do not use the PCAT writing scores at all in their admission processes.

Writing Section Score	Conventions of Language Description
One—"Weak"	The essay response is difficult to understand due to frequent and serious errors in sentence structure, word usage, and grammar.
Two—"Limited"	Several mistakes distract from the essay response that is being presented, and the ability to fully understand the points of the essay may be diminished.
Three—"Adequate"	While there are several mistakes in structure that may interfere with the ease of the essay's interpretation, the general meaning is not compromised.
Four—"Efficient"	Overall, the writer correctly applies the conventions of language. There may be slight errors, but they do not interfere with the understanding of the points intended or the flow of the essay.
Five—"Superior"	Few, if any, errors are made and the writer exhibits good technique in presentation of the essay components.

Writing Section Score	Problem Solving Description
One—"Weak"	The relationship between the problem and the solution is not clear, and the organization is problematic.
Two—"Limited"	Although the solution is related to the problem, support for the solution is problematic, and the structure of the essay detracts from the flow of ideas.
Three—"Adequate"	The essay's solution is clear, but too general in presentation, and organization may be weak.
Four—"Efficient"	The essay shows a clear relationship between problem and solution with solid support and only minor problems in organization.
Five—"Superior"	The essay presents a clear, well-reasoned relationship between problem and solution with convincing support and a powerful argument. Organization has logical flow.

PCAT ESSAY WRITING TIPS

There are many existing guides and tutorials that discuss the construction of an effective essay. For additional guidance on how to write a persuasive essay, refer to *www.hamilton.edu/writing/effective_essays.html* (please note that this website is not specific to the PCAT). You must keep in mind the 30-minute time limit for each of the PCAT writing sections. Below are several tips you can use to help compose an essay.

- The introduction paragraph is the first paragraph of your essay. In your introduction, include some background information and the problem to be solved based on the topic. Use a clear thesis statement to present the topic and inform the reader as to what the essay will be about.
- Follow your introduction with one or more supporting paragraphs to make up the main body of your essay. It is important to develop each point in your essay in a properly structured paragraph. Make sure there is a link between your thesis and the supporting paragraphs. Present applicable and appropriate references based on academic studies or personal experiences.
- Use clear and simple structure to your sentences. Avoid the use of clichés, slang, jargon, and abstract terms that tend to fill space but provide no specific points in your essay. Elaborate on your ideas, leading the reader to your conclusions. You are to present a solution or build a case in support of your viewpoint.
- Use a clear writing style. Avoid redundant words, long sentences, and vague information. Don't use 35 words when five words will efficiently and effectively present your information. Write concisely and cover the topic presented.
- Use appropriate grammar, punctuation, usage, and style. Avoid abbreviations and acronyms when possible.
- Finish with a conclusion, either as a statement or a closing paragraph after the main body of your essay. It is important that your conclusion logically follow the points you have developed in the supporting paragraphs of the essay.
- Always proofread your essay. Glaring or frequent spelling or grammatical errors could be construed as poor writing.

PRACTICE TESTS
AND ANSWERS

Practice Test 1

This sample PCAT is not a copy of an actual PCAT, but it has been designed to closely represent the types of questions that may be included in an actual exam. As in the actual PCAT, this test has seven separate sections—Verbal Ability, Biology, Chemistry, Quantitative Ability, Reading Comprehension, and two Writing sections. The actual PCAT may have additional experimental questions that are being tested for use on future exams. Because the experimental questions do not count toward your actual PCAT score, there are no equivalent questions included in this sample PCAT.

You may find it best to proceed with this practice exam as if you were taking the actual PCAT by adhering to the time allowed for each section in the table below. Your overall strategy should be to answer every question in the time allotted, while getting as many correct answers as possible. Do not leave any questions unanswered, as there will be no penalty for guessing on the actual PCAT. Your score on this sample PCAT will give you a good idea of the subject areas you need to study further. By timing yourself on the sample PCAT, you will also learn whether you need to increase your speed or slow down when you take the actual PCAT.

After completing the sample PCAT, you may grade your exam by using the answer key. Regardless of your score on the sample PCAT, it will benefit you to review all the explanatory answers at the end of the sample PCAT. If your answer to a question was incorrect, the explanation may help you understand where you went wrong. If your answer was correct, the explanation may broaden your understanding of the topic area being tested.

Before starting the exam, please refresh your memory on the test-taking strategies discussed earlier in this book. Good luck on the examination.

Section	Time Allowed*
1. Verbal Ability	30 minutes
2. Biology	30 minutes
3. Chemistry	30 minutes
4. Quantitative Ability	40 minutes
5. Reading Comprehension	50 minutes
6. Writing (Essay)	30 minutes
7. Writing (Essay)	30 minutes

*Please note: The order of the subjects (test sections) may vary from test to test.

VERBAL ABILITY

48 QUESTIONS (#1– #48)

TIME: 30 MINUTES

Directions: Choose the word that **best** completes the analogy.

1. FENCE : ENCLOSE :: DAUB :

   (A) Foil
   (B) Detain
   (C) Smear
   (D) Dry

2. PLACATE : PACIFY :: CONFIRM :

   (A) Ratify
   (B) Invalidate
   (C) Comply
   (D) Reply

3. BOLD : COWARDLY :: OBLIQUE :

   (A) Triangle
   (B) Devious
   (C) Straight
   (D) Timidity

4. VIRUS : COLD :: DEITY :

   (A) Miracle
   (B) Transcendent
   (C) Ubiquitous
   (D) Prayer

5. RIM : VOLCANO :: MARGIN :

   (A) Wound
   (B) Edge
   (C) Probability
   (D) Erupt

6. BOOK : CHAPTER :: CONCERTO :

   (A) Oboe
   (B) Movement
   (C) Applause
   (D) Strings

7. SMALL INTESTINE : DUODENUM :: HAND :

   (A) Finger
   (B) Echidna
   (C) Knee
   (D) Elbow

8. RASPBERRY : KIWI FRUIT :: ROMAINE :

   (A) Papaya
   (B) Horseradish
   (C) Boston lettuce
   (D) Tuber

9. NEEDLE : SEW :: HOSE :

   (A) Lawn
   (B) Down
   (C) Garter
   (D) Siphon

10. UMBRELLA : PEDESTRIAN :: ROOF :

    (A) House
    (B) Stationary
    (C) Dome
    (D) Downpour

11. RECYCLE : PAPER :: INCUBATE :

    (A) Hatch
    (B) Egg
    (C) Sit on
    (D) Return

12. THEORY : REFUTE :: PRESIDENT :

    (A) Impeach
    (B) Elect
    (C) Veto
    (D) Obscure

13. EAR : CORN :: BOLL :

    (A) Weevil
    (B) Stem
    (C) Pod
    (D) Cotton

14. DEBRIS : COMPOST :: RESIN :

(A) Tar
(B) Amber
(C) Industry
(D) Pitchblende

15. SEAL : ROTUND :: CHEETAH :

(A) Fast
(B) Mammal
(C) Protected
(D) Sleek

16. COLD : FLU :: RECESSION :

(A) Temperature
(B) Danger
(C) Depression
(D) Glacier

17. ON : COMMENT :: OUT :

(A) Direction
(B) Pool
(C) Eke
(D) Down

18. PHARMACIST : PHARMACY :: DIPLOMAT :

(A) Ambassador
(B) Embassy
(C) Immunity
(D) Foreign

19. PAINTER : PALETTE :: COOK :

(A) Spices
(B) Chef
(C) Spatula
(D) Bake

20. SENTENCE : ELLIPSIS :: SPEECH :

(A) Applause
(B) Pause
(C) Finale
(D) Silence

21. HAT : PANAMA :: SHARK :

(A) Predator
(B) Skin
(C) Cichlid
(D) Mako

22. DRUMS : BAND :: GOALIE :

(A) Position
(B) Team
(C) Puck
(D) Fans

23. DROPLETS : WATER :: GRAINS :

(A) Pool
(B) Precipitation
(C) Moisture
(D) Sand

24. PROVIDENCE : RHODE ISLAND :: BOISE :

(A) New England
(B) Arizona
(C) Idaho
(D) Capital

25. AREN'T : ARE NOT :: HAVEN'T :

(A) Have not
(B) Has not
(C) Is not
(D) Are

26. LIABLE : RESPONSIBLE :: LIBERAL :

(A) Litigious
(B) Generous
(C) Free
(D) Absolved

27. LIBRETTO : OPERA :: SCREENPLAY :

(A) Director
(B) Film
(C) Operetta
(D) Script

28. ANDES : SOUTH AMERICA :: ALPS :

    (A) Mountains
    (B) Europe
    (C) Switzerland
    (D) Mont Blanc

29. SEEMINGLY : OSTENSIBLY ::
    THOROUGHLY :

    (A) Completely
    (B) Openly
    (C) Divisively
    (D) Ruinously

Directions: Select the word or set of words that makes the most sense when inserted into the sentence and that best fits the meaning of the sentence as a whole.

30. The teacher's harsh words embarrassed the student, especially since he had been _____ in front of the rest of class.

    (A) complemented
    (B) reprimanded
    (C) antagonized
    (D) transformed

31. Because the cell membrane was permeable, the water was able to easily _____ from one side to the other.

    (A) diffuse
    (B) collaborate
    (C) exonerate
    (D) deviate

32. Henry did not rely on his _____ to solve the problem; he used _____ data collected throughout the study.

    (A) curiosity; enigmatic
    (B) influence; cursory
    (C) intuition; empirical
    (D) callousness; compensatory

33. He was a _____ old gentleman who was always complaining and rude. His twin brother, on the other hand, was more _____, always laughing and joking.

    (A) mediocre; inordinate
    (B) cantankerous; mirthful
    (C) formal; militant
    (D) terrific; fastidious

34. In evolution, when a _____ is introduced into a population, it allows for genetic _____ within the population.

    (A) vernacular; utopia
    (B) compilation; concurrence
    (C) mutilation; displacement
    (D) mutation; variation

35. To _____ the success of the fundraiser, we need to _____ the small number of volunteers by asking other organizations around the city to help us.

    (A) facilitate; augment
    (B) assuage; maintain
    (C) encounter; emulate
    (D) justify; repress

36. The history presentations for today will be done in _____ order.

    (A) ecological
    (B) geological
    (C) phenomenal
    (D) chronological

37. The _____ remarks made during the ceremony offended many audience members, and it seemed that _____ damage had been done to the sacred and dignified occasion.

    (A) jovial; reputable
    (B) transitory; unassuming
    (C) irreverent; irreparable
    (D) discrete; figurative

38. The man was _____ concerning his opinions, as everyone thought that he was acting in a stubborn fashion.

    (A) obstinate
    (B) reserved
    (C) conservative
    (D) conceited

39. Even though the shirt was on sale, Karen's mother said it still was too expensive to buy; Karen was frustrated that her mother was so _____.

    (A) peripheral
    (B) patient
    (C) paranoid
    (D) frugal

40. The carelessly discarded match _____ the paper in the trash can; luckily, the damage caused by the fire was not severe because the carpet was made out of fire _____ material.

    (A) ignited; retardant
    (B) maintained; resurgent
    (C) embodied; retraceable
    (D) trapped; conductible

41. Without a doubt, it is _____ that we wait until the solution has completely stabilized. Until _____ is reached, we risk causing a violent chemical reaction.

    (A) immense; illumination
    (B) unfortunate; equivalence
    (C) imperative; equilibrium
    (D) insignificant; consensus

42. In contrast to the other _____ paintings, one painting stood out because of its _____.

    (A) flamboyant; simplicity
    (B) divergent; fortuitousness
    (C) rudimentary; coincidence
    (D) anecdotal; catharsis

43. It is essential that we do not act too hastily; it may be in our best interest to _____ the meeting until next week.

    (A) devour
    (B) shuffle
    (C) modernize
    (D) defer

44. We expected Jack to be more enthusiastic about the trip he had won to Europe and were surprised by his _____ attitude.

    (A) lonesome
    (B) laconic
    (C) indifferent
    (D) rational

45. Although multiple sclerosis was first described over 100 years ago, the cause remains a _____ and a cure is still _____.

    (A) problem; berated
    (B) coercion; obvious
    (C) mystery; undiscovered
    (D) possibility; changed

46. The daredevil thought of himself as _____, as he jumped out of the airplane without a parachute.

    (A) invulnerable
    (B) ironic
    (C) irrefutable
    (D) frenzied

47. During the early _____ period of an individual's lifespan, many of the major organ systems appear and begin to develop.
    (A) enigmatic
    (B) asymmetric
    (C) audacious
    (D) embryonic

48. We must stir the solution for the experiment with a sterile rod to make sure that we do not _____ it.
    (A) impugn
    (B) contaminate
    (C) denounce
    (D) confound

STOP

End of Verbal Ability section. If you have any time left, you may go over your work in this section only.

BIOLOGY

48 QUESTIONS (#49–#96)

TIME: 30 MINUTES

Directions: Choose the **best** answer to each of the following questions.

49. Protists comprise all eukaryotes other than which groups?

    (A) Multicellular forms
    (B) Those with cells containing a cytoskeleton and muscle
    (C) Extinct forms
    (D) Green plants, fungi, and animals

Use Figure 1 to answer question 50.

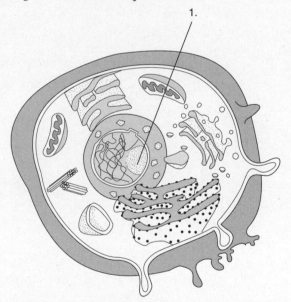

1.

Figure 1.

50. In Figure 1, number 1 is pointing to what part of the cell?

    (A) Nucleolus
    (B) Nuclear envelope
    (C) Ribosomes
    (D) Nucleus

51. As the SPF value increases, the amount of protection from ultraviolet radiation

    (A) increases.
    (B) decreases.
    (C) does not change.
    (D) SPF is unrelated to ultraviolet radiation.

52. The internal cell network that makes cell movement possible is called the

    (A) endoplasmic reticulum.
    (B) mitochondria matrix.
    (C) cytoskeleton.
    (D) endocytosis system.

53. Which of the following organelles have ribosomes attached to them?

    (A) The Golgi apparatus
    (B) Microtubules
    (C) Smooth endoplasmic reticulum
    (D) Rough endoplasmic reticulum

54. By which of the following mechanisms can a cell transport a substance from a lower to a higher concentration:

    (A) Simple diffusion
    (B) Active transport
    (C) Facilitated diffusion
    (D) Extracellular enzymes

55. Which of the following organelles are thought to have arisen from primitive prokaryotes?

    (A) The endoplasmic reticulum and Golgi complex
    (B) Mitochondria and chloroplasts
    (C) Vacuoles and transport vesicles
    (D) Lyposomes

56. DNA replication results in

    (A) two DNA molecules, one with two newly synthesized strands and one with two parental strands.
    (B) two DNA molecules, each with two newly synthesized strands.
    (C) two DNA molecules, each of which has one parental strand and one newly synthesized strand.
    (D) All of the above

57. The chromosome set in Klinefelter's syndrome is

    (A) XYY.
    (B) YXY.
    (C) YYY.
    (D) XXY.

58. A microorganism that obtains its carbon, as well as its energy, from organic compounds is called

    (A) an autotroph.
    (B) a heterotroph.
    (C) a heterozygote.
    (D) a homozygote.

59. If A represents blue (dominant color) and a represents red (recessive color), which of the following crosses would be expected to result in 25% red offspring?

    (A) Aa × aa
    (B) AA × aa
    (C) Aa × Aa
    (D) Aa × AA

60. Which of the following respond(s) to dim light for black and white vision?

    (A) Cones
    (B) Rods
    (C) Iris
    (D) Cornea

61. Normal red blood cells have an average life span of

    (A) 30 days.
    (B) 60 days.
    (C) 120 days.
    (D) 180 days.

62. Which is a sign of infection?

    (A) Increased white blood cell count
    (B) Fever
    (C) Both A and B
    (D) None of the above

63. Which of the following statements is FALSE concerning Monera?

    (A) These organisms are of eukaryotic origin.
    (B) These organisms are mostly single celled.
    (C) These organisms are surrounded by a cell wall.
    (D) These organisms are mostly bacteria.

64. Which of the following modifies materials synthesized in the rough and smooth endoplasmic reticulum?

    (A) Plastids
    (B) Golgi apparatus
    (C) Ribosomes
    (D) Mitochondria

65. In mitosis, at what stage does cytokinesis begin?

    (A) Interphase
    (B) Metaphase
    (C) Prophase
    (D) Anaphase

66. Genes that are capable of relocating from one part of the genome to another are called:

    (A) Mesosomes
    (B) Transposons
    (C) Plasmids
    (D) Fimbriae

67. _____ are gram-positive, spore-forming bacilli. The major diseases associated with these bacteria are caused by exotoxins.

    (A) Acinomyces
    (B) Eubacterium
    (C) Clostridium
    (D) Lactobacillus

68. Which of the following is NOT true concerning the hypothalamus?

    (A) It regulates body temperature.
    (B) It regulates water and electrolyte balance.
    (C) It regulates hunger and control of gastrointestinal activity.
    (D) It regulates the rate and depth of breathing.

69. Which substance is the hardest?

    (A) Nail
    (B) Skin
    (C) Tooth enamel
    (D) Hair

70. Lobes of the cerebrum include all of the following EXCEPT

    (A) frontal.
    (B) permatoral.
    (C) temporal.
    (D) parietal.

71. Which of the following enzymes cut DNA at a highly specific target sequence?

    (A) DNA ligase
    (B) DNA polymerase
    (C) Restriction enzymes
    (D) DNA helicase

72. The _____ connects the middle ear to the throat.

    (A) auricle
    (B) eustachian tube
    (C) tympanic membrane
    (D) cochlea

73. Insulin

    (A) promotes cellular uptake of glucose and formation of glycogen and fat.
    (B) stimulates hydrolysis of glycogen and fat.
    (C) inhibits cellular uptake of glucose and formation of glycogen and fat.
    (D) None of the above

74. The heart wall is composed of three distinct layers. Which of the following is NOT a layer?

    (A) Epicardium
    (B) Asocardium
    (C) Myocardium
    (D) Endocardium

75. Microorganisms that lack cell walls are known as _____; they do not synthesize the precursors of peptidoglycan.

    (A) phototrophic
    (B) archaeobacteria
    (C) mycoplasmas
    (D) plasmids

76. In the cardiac cycle, the relaxation of the heart is referred to as

    (A) systole.
    (B) diastole.
    (C) cardiac rate.
    (D) systemic relaxation.

77. The superficial protective layer of the skin is the

    (A) dermis.
    (B) hypodermis.
    (C) epidermis.
    (D) None of the above

78. What does the term *evolution* mean?

    (A) The characteristics of a population change through time.
    (B) The characteristics of a species become more complex over time.
    (C) The characteristics of an individual change through the course of its life in response to natural selection.
    (D) The strongest individuals produce the most offspring.

79. The adrenal glands produce which two hormones?

    (A) Melatonin and serotonin
    (B) Adrenalin and noradrenaline
    (C) Insulin and glucagon
    (D) None of the above

80. Aldosterone

    (A) promotes potassium retention and sodium loss.
    (B) promotes sodium retention and potassium loss.
    (C) A and B
    (D) Neither A nor B

81. What is the functional unit of the kidney?

    (A) Urinary tubules
    (B) Glomerular capsule
    (C) Loop of Henle
    (D) Nephron

82. In humans, gas exchange takes place in the

    (A) alveoli.
    (B) bronchi.
    (C) trachea.
    (D) bronchioles.

83. Which is FALSE concerning the placenta?

    (A) It develops from the site where the blastocyst implanted.
    (B) It is outside of the uterus.
    (C) It controls the movement and exchange of nutrients between the fetus and the mother.
    (D) It controls the movement and exchange of wastes between the fetus and the mother.

84. In aerobic cellular respiration, most of the ATP is synthesized during

    (A) the Krebs cycle.
    (B) electron transport.
    (C) electron oxidation.
    (D) the citric acid cycle.

85. A normal cell spends approximately 90% of its time in

    (A) prophase.
    (B) metaphase.
    (C) interphase.
    (D) anaphase.

86. In the human respiratory system, there is a net diffusion of carbon dioxide from

    (A) hemoglobin to mitochondria.
    (B) alveoli to blood.
    (C) blood to air in the alveoli.
    (D) All of the above

87. The fat-soluble vitamins include:

    (A) Vitamin A
    (B) Vitamin G
    (C) Vitamin R
    (D) Vitamin B

88. Which of the following would detect the position of your head?

    (A) The cochlea
    (B) The vestibular apparatus
    (C) The pinna
    (D) The organ of Corte

89. The primary defect in a child who has no detectable T or B cells is most likely the result of a defect in:

    (A) The spleen and appendix
    (B) T and B cell interactions
    (C) Bone marrow stem cells
    (D) Failure to produce cytokines

90. The induction of a clinical disease by a virus can result from:

    (A) Killing of virus-infected cells
    (B) Malignant transformation of infected cells
    (C) The development of an immune response to viral-encoded antigens expressed on the surface of an infected cell
    (D) All of the above

91. In the thyroid hormone control network, the source of negative feedback is the

    (A) hypothalamus.
    (B) cerebrum.
    (C) pituitary gland.
    (D) thyroid gland.

92. Why is it difficult to develop a vaccine against viruses with high mutation rates like HIV?

    (A) The vaccines tend to be unstable and deteriorate over time.
    (B) The virus proteins are not recognized by the immune system.
    (C) New viral mutations constantly change the viral proteins.
    (D) The virions contain so many different proteins that the immune system is overwhelmed.

93. Which of the following cell types would engulf and digest bacteria?

    (A) Killer T cells
    (B) B cells
    (C) Natural killer cells
    (D) Macrophages

94. The genomes of viruses may contain

    (A) double-stranded DNA.
    (B) single-stranded RNA.
    (C) single-stranded DNA.
    (D) All of the above

95. A bacteriophage

    (A) is a virus that infects bacteria.
    (B) is a fungus.
    (C) does not contain DNA or RNA.
    (D) B and C

96. Enzyme activity is influenced by

    (A) temperature.
    (B) pH.
    (C) enzyme concentration.
    (D) All of the above

STOP

*End of Biology section. If you have any time left,
you may go over your work in this section only.*

CHEMISTRY

48 QUESTIONS (#97–#144)

TIME: 30 MINUTES

Directions: Choose the **best** answer to each of the following questions.

97. Atoms of the same element having different numbers of neutrons are called

    (A) isotopes.
    (B) isomers.
    (C) allotropes.
    (D) diastereomers.

98. What is the name of the process by which new DNA molecules are synthesized?

    (A) Transcription
    (B) Translation
    (C) Replication
    (D) Translocation

99. The functions of RNA molecules include all of the following EXCEPT

    (A) permanent storage of nucleotide sequence information.
    (B) transporting amino acids to the protein synthesis machinery in the cell.
    (C) providing the information from which proteins are synthesized.
    (D) participating in the construction and function of the ribosomes.

100. In the following reaction:

    $$CS_2 + 2O_2 \rightarrow CO_2 + 2SO_2$$

    38.0 grams of CS_2 (carbon disufide) are reacted with excess O_2 to produce 32.0 grams of SO_2. What is the percent yield of this reaction? (S = 32 amu, O = 16 amu, C = 12 amu, H = 1 amu)

    (A) 50
    (B) 25
    (C) 38
    (D) 13

101. What is the molarity (M) of a solution prepared by dissolving 18.0 grams of sugar, $C_6H_{12}O_6$, in 500 milliliters of solution? (O = 16 amu, C = 12 amu, H = 1 amu)

    (A) 0.130
    (B) 0.230
    (C) 0.200
    (D) 0.910

102. How many milliliters of 4.0 M NaOH solution must be used to prepare 100 milliliters of 2.0 M solution?

    (A) 50
    (B) 13
    (C) 800
    (D) 200

103. What is the density, in grams per liter, of oxygen gas, O_2, if the pressure is 1.00 atmosphere and the temperature is 15°C? (O = 16 amu, R = 0.082 L-atm/K-mole)

    (A) 1.35
    (B) 0.74
    (C) 8.74×10^{-3}
    (D) 1.43

104. A sample of gas contains approximately 56 grams nitrogen, N_2, and 64 grams oxygen, O_2. What is the partial pressure, in atmospheres, of nitrogen if the total pressure of the air is 1.6 atmospheres? (O = 16 amu, N = 14 amu)

    (A) 0.5
    (B) 3.2
    (C) 0.8
    (D) 2.0

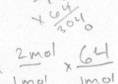

105. The specific heat of copper, Cu, is 0.385 joule per gram °C. If 10.0 joules of heat is absorbed by a 5 g sample of Cu at 25°C, what will be the new temperature?

    (A) 20
    (B) 75
    (C) 30
    (D) 44

106. The amino acid sequence of proteins is determined by the

    (A) nucleotide sequence of the respective mRNA.
    (B) nucleotide sequence of the respective gene.
    (C) codon and anticodon base pairing in translation.
    (D) All of the above

107. Which of the following wavelengths of light will have the highest frequency?

    (A) 0.300 m
    (B) 2.75 mm
    (C) 630 nm
    (D) 0.69 km

    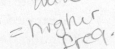
    smaller wave = higher freq.

108. Which statement is true regarding a chloride ion and a sulfide ion?

    (A) They have the same charge.
    (B) They have the same number of valence electrons.
    (C) They have the same number of protons.
    (D) They are diatomic ions.

109. Which of the following is a basic oxide?

    (A) CO_2
    (B) K_2O
    (C) SO_2
    (D) P_2O_5

110. Hydrogen bonding can exist between molecules of all the following EXCEPT

    (A) H_2O H—O—H
    (B) CH_4
    (C) CH_3OH
    (D) NH_3

111. Which of the following is NOT true concerning triglycerides and phospholipids?

    (A) They are esters of glycerol and short-chain carboxylic acids.
    (B) They are found in adipose tissue and cell membranes.
    (C) They contain long-chain fatty acids.
    (D) They contain hydrophilic and hydrophobic regions.

112. The conversion of a gas into a liquid is called

    (A) sublimation.
    (B) evaporation.
    (C) condensation.
    (D) freezing.

113. Gases are usually most soluble in liquids with

    (A) low temperature.
    (B) high temperature.
    (C) low pressure.
    (D) high agitation.

114. Cholesterol is biosynthesized as well as absorbed from dietary fats and is necessary for

    (A) hormone production.
    (B) cell membrane construction.
    (C) DNA synthesis.
    (D) Both A and B.

115. The following reactions have equilibrium constants as indicated below:

$$A + B \leftrightarrow C + D \qquad K^1$$
$$E + F \leftrightarrow G + H \qquad K^2$$

The reactions are added to give the following overall reaction. What will be the overall equilibrium constant for the new equation?

$$A + B + E + F \leftrightarrow C + D + G + H$$

(A) $K^1 + K^2$
(B) $(K^1)(K^2)$
(C) K^1/K^2
(D) K^2/K^1

116. What is the atomic weight of the element $^{35}_{21}X$?

(A) 35
(B) 21
(C) 14
(D) 28

117. Beta sheets and alpha helices are examples of what level of protein structure?

(A) Primary
(B) Secondary
(C) Tertiary
(D) Quarternary

118. In which of the following are the acids listed correctly in decreasing order of strength (i.e., the strongest acid is first and the weakest acid last)?

(A) HF > HCl > HBr > HI
(B) HI > HBr > HCl > HF
(C) HBr > HCl > HI > HF
(D) HCl > HBr > HI > HF

119. Which of the following can be a buffer solution?

(A) H_2SO_4, Na_2SO_4
(B) H_2SO_4
(C) CH_3COOH
(D) CH_3COOH, CH_3COONa

120. The side chain of which of the following amino acids would be completely ionized at physiological pH?

(A) Alanine
(B) Glycine
(C) Lysine
(D) Valine

121. The following reaction:

$$^{90}_{38}Sr \rightarrow {}^{90}_{39}Y + ?$$

can be balanced by adding

(A) ^1_1H
(B) ^1_0n
(C) $^{\ 0}_{-1}e$
(D) ^4_2He

122. Which of the following is a statement of the first law of thermodynamics?

(A) Entropy for a crystalline substance is zero at absolute zero temperature.
(B) Energy can be converted from one form to another but is neither created nor destroyed.
(C) Entropy increases in spontaneous reactions and remains the same in equilibrium systems.
(D) The Gibbs free energy is a measure of the spontaneity of a reaction.

123. If the Gibbs free energy for a certain reaction has a negative value, which of the following statements is true?

(A) The reaction does not take place.
(B) The reaction system is at equilibrium.
(C) The reaction is non-spontaneous.
(D) The reaction is spontaneous.

124. Which statement is true concerning aqueous solutions of Acid A ($Ka = 6 \times 10^{-8}$) and Acid B ($Ka = 3 \times 10^{-5}$)?

   (A) Acid A is stronger than Acid B.
   (B) The pH of the Acid B solution is less than that of Acid A.
   (C) Both solutions are neutral.
   (D) The pKa of Acid B is greater than the pKa of Acid A.

125. What reagent should be used to accomplish the following conversion?

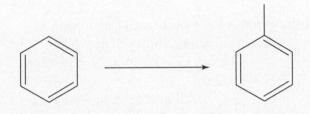

   (A) CH_3COCl, $AlCl_3$
   (B) CH_3Cl, $AlCl_3$
   (C) CH_3CH_3
   (D) CH_3MgCl

126. What is a product of the following reaction?

$$CH_3CO_2CH_3 \xrightarrow{\substack{1.\ LiAlH_4 \\ 2.\ H^+}}$$

   (A) CH_3CH_2OH
   (B) CH_4
   (C) CH_3CO_2H
   (D) $H_2C{=}CH_2$

127. The name the compound symbolized as $CH_3CH_2COOCH_3$ is

   (A) methyl ethyl ester.
   (B) methyl propanoate.
   (C) ethyl ethanoate.
   (D) methyl propyl ether.

128. The reaction of Br_2 with C_2H_6 to produce C_2H_5Br and HBr in the presence of ultraviolet light or heat is an example of

   (A) a nucleophilic substitution reaction.
   (B) a free radical substitution reaction.
   (C) an electrophilic addition reaction.
   (D) an electrophilic elimination reaction.

129. The reaction of Br_2 with C_2H_4 to produce $C_2H_4Br_2$ is an example of

   (A) a nucleophilic substitution reaction.
   (B) a free radical reaction.
   (C) an electrophilic addition reaction.
   (D) an electrophilic elimination reaction.

130. Two molecules that are nonsuperimposable mirror images of each other are called

   (A) diastereomers.
   (B) enantiomers.
   (C) the same compound.
   (D) geometric isomers.

131. What is the organic starting material for the reaction given below performed under basic conditions?

   (A) ⌁CHO
   (B) HCHO
   (C) $CH_2{=}CH_2$
   (D) CH_3CHO

132. For butanone, where would the most significant band be found in the infrared spectrum?

   (A) $3{,}300\ cm^{-1}$
   (B) $1{,}700\ cm^{-1}$
   (C) $2{,}100\ cm^{-1}$
   (D) $1{,}100\ cm^{-1}$

133. Which of the following functional groups is commonly present in lipids?

    (A) Alcohols
    (B) Esters
    (C) Alkyl halides
    (D) Carboxylic acids

134. The reaction of an alcohol with a carboxylic acid will produce

    (A) an aldehyde.
    (B) a ketone.
    (C) an ester.
    (D) an alcohol.

135. What functional group is most commonly present in proteins?

    (A) Alcohol
    (B) Amide
    (C) Ester
    (D) Ketone

136. Which of the following statements about benzene is INCORRECT?

    (A) The benzene molecule has 120° bond angles.
    (B) All bonds in benzene are equivalent in length.
    (C) Hybridization of the carbon atoms is sp^2.
    (D) The benzene molecule is planar.

137. The name of the following compound:

$$CH_3CH_2CHCH_2COOH$$
$$|$$
$$CH_3$$

    is

    (A) 3-methylpentanoic acid.
    (B) 2-methylpentanoic acid.
    (C) 2-methylbutanoic acid.
    (D) 3-methylbutanoic acid.

138. What is the name of the following molecule?

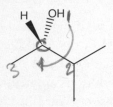

    (A) (S)-isopentanol
    (B) (S)-3-methyl-2-butanol
    (C) (R)-3-methyl-2-butanol
    (D) (R)-2-methyl-3-butanol

139. What is the percentage of hydrogen, H, present in ammonium sulfate, $(NH_4)_2SO_4$? (S = 32 amu, O = 16 amu, N = 14 amu, H = 1 amu)

    (A) 11
    (B) 6
    (C) 3
    (D) 4

140. Oxidation of an aldehyde produces

    (A) a ketone.
    (B) an alcohol.
    (C) a carboxylic acid.
    (D) an amide.

141. A sample of metal weighing 6.0 grams is placed in a graduated cylinder containing 16 milliliters of water. The volume of water increases to 20 milliliters. What is the density, in grams per milliliter, of the metal?

    (A) 1.30
    (B) 1.50
    (C) 2.0
    (D) 2.5

142. What is the final volume in milliliters of a solution prepared by dissolving 18 grams of sugar, $C_6H_{12}O_6$, in sufficient water to produce a 0.5 M solution? (O = 16 amu, C = 12 amu, H = 1 amu)

    (A) 36
    (B) 100
    (C) 200
    (D) 52

    $0.5 = \dfrac{}{x}$

144. If two moles of acetic acid are generated from the cleavage of an organic molecule by ozonolysis followed by reductive work up, what is the name of the organic molecule?

    (A) 1-butyne
    (B) 2-butyne
    (C) 2-butene
    (D) cyclobutyne

143. The reaction of a neutron with a uranium-235 nucleus to generate a strontium atom, a xenon atom, and three neutrons as shown in the equation below is known as

$$^{235}_{92}U + {}^{1}_{0}n \rightarrow {}^{90}_{38}Sr + {}^{143}_{54}Xe + 3{}^{1}_{0}n$$

    (A) radioactive decay
    (B) nuclear fusion
    (C) carbon dating
    (D) nuclear fission

STOP

End of Chemistry section. If you have any time left, you may go over your work in this section only.

QUANTITATIVE ABILITY

48 QUESTIONS (#145–#192)

TIME: 40 MINUTES

Directions: Choose the **best** answer to each of the following questions.

145. $\sqrt{32} + \sqrt{8} =$

    (A) $6\sqrt{2}$

    (B) $2\sqrt{10}$

    (C) $8\sqrt{2}$

    (D) None of the above

146. Given the function, $f(x) = \dfrac{x}{x^2 + 3}$

    compute $\dfrac{dy}{dx}$.

    (A) $\dfrac{3x^2 + 3}{(x^2 + 3)^2}$

    (B) $\dfrac{3 - x^2}{(x^2 + 3)^2}$

    (C) $\dfrac{3 + x^2}{(x^2 + 3)^2}$

    (D) None of the above

147. The quadratic equation $2x^2 + 5x + 1 = 0$ has

    (A) two real roots
    (B) no real root
    (C) one real root
    (D) None of the above

148. A crate of citrus fruit contains 11 limes, 10 oranges, and 4 lemons. What is the probability that a randomly chosen piece of fruit is a lemon?

    (A) 84%
    (B) 16%
    (C) 0.84%
    (D) 0.16%

149. $5^2 + 5^3$

    (A) 3,125
    (B) 1,000
    (C) 150
    (D) 25

150. Determine the inverse function for

    $f(x) = \dfrac{x+1}{10x}$.

    (A) $f^{-1}(x) = \dfrac{10x}{x+1}$

    (B) $f^{-1}(x) = \dfrac{1}{10x - 1}$

    (C) $f^{-1}(x) = \dfrac{1}{10x + 1}$

    (D) $f^{-1}(x) = \dfrac{x-1}{10x}$

151. $\lim\limits_{x \to \infty} \left(\dfrac{8x^6 + 5x^4 - x + 1000}{3x^6 + 21x^3 - 4} \right)$

    (A) ∞

    (B) $\dfrac{8}{3}$

    (C) 1

    (D) $\dfrac{13}{24}$

152. Find the **radius** of the circle with equation
$x^2 + y^2 - 12x + 14y + 9 = 0$.

(A) $\sqrt{76}$

(B) 76

(C) 85

(D) $\sqrt{85}$

153. Find the exact value of the shaded area.

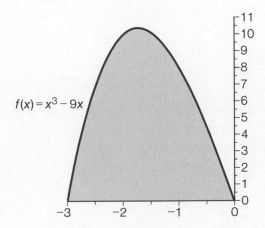

$f(x) = x^3 - 9x$

(A) −20.25

(B) 108

(C) 20.25

(D) −108

154. A number is chosen at random from the set
{1, 2, 3, 4, 5, 6, 7, 8, 9, 10, 11, 12}. What
is the probability that the chosen number is
divisible by 3 or divisible by 4?

(A) 55%

(B) 45%

(C) 60%

(D) 50%

155. Evaluate the integral $\int_{1}^{2} (5x^4)\, dx$.

(A) 32

(B) 140

(C) 180

(D) 31

156. If $x < 6$, then $\dfrac{x^2 - 7x + 6}{|x - 6|} =$

(A) $x + 1$

(B) $-x - 1$

(C) $x - 1$

(D) $-x + 1$

157. Simplify the expression $\dfrac{x^2 - 11x + 24}{x - 8}$.

(A) $x + 3$

(B) $x - 14$

(C) $x - 3$

(D) $x + 14$

158. Find all real solutions for the quadratic
equation $6x^2 + x + 2 = 0$.

(A) $x = \dfrac{-1 \pm \sqrt{23}}{12}$

(B) No real solutions

(C) $x = \dfrac{-1 \pm \sqrt{-23}}{12}$

(D) $x = \dfrac{1 \pm \sqrt{23}}{12}$

159. The graph of a function $y = f(x)$ contains
the point (3, 1). Determine which point
must be on the graph of $y = 5f(x + 2) - 3$.

(A) (1, 2)

(B) (5, 2)

(C) (1, −10)

(D) (5, −10)

160. $\log_7 (49) =$

(A) 2

(B) $\dfrac{1}{2}$

(C) 7

(D) $\dfrac{1}{7}$

161. $\lim\limits_{x \to 4} \left(\dfrac{x^2 - 10x + 24}{4 - x} \right) =$

    (A) Undefined
    (B) 2
    (C) –2
    (D) 1

162. What is the mean of the following numbers: 8, 35, 8, 9, 5, 10, 7, 3, 12?

    (A) 8
    (B) 10.77
    (C) 15.24
    (D) 9

163. A rental car company charges $30 per day, plus 14 cents per mile. Express the total rental cost of a 7-day rental as a function of the number of miles driven, *x*.

    (A) $C(x) = 30 + 14x$
    (B) $C(x) = 30 + 0.14x$
    (C) $C(x) = 210 + 14x$
    (D) $C(x) = 210 + 0.14x$

164. If a coin is tossed four times, what is the probability that the outcome will be all heads?

    (A) $\dfrac{1}{16}$

    (B) $\dfrac{1}{4}$

    (C) $\dfrac{1}{2}$

    (D) $\dfrac{1}{8}$

165. Find the instantaneous rate of change for the function $f(t) = 5e^{t^3 - 1}$ at the moment when $t = 1$.

    (A) $5e$
    (B) 5
    (C) $15e$
    (D) 15

166. Given $f(x) = x^2 + 2x - 1$, and $g(x) = 2x + 1$, what is $(f + g)(x)$?

    (A) $2x^2 + 4x$
    (B) $x^2 - 4x$
    (C) $x^2 + 4x$
    (D) $2x^2 - 4x$

167. The equation $4(x + 3)(x - 2) = 4x^2 + x$ has solution

    (A) $x = -8$
    (B) $x = 8$
    (C) $x = -2$
    (D) $x = 2$

168. If a die is rolled, what is the probability that the number will be odd?

    (A) 50%
    (B) 100%
    (C) 25%
    (D) 0%

169. $\dfrac{5}{9} - \dfrac{3}{10} =$

    (A) $\dfrac{77}{90}$

    (B) $-\dfrac{23}{90}$

    (C) $-\dfrac{77}{90}$

    (D) $\dfrac{23}{90}$

170. Find the mode of the following data set: 3, 6, 29, 8, 6, 4, 2, 6, 8, 6, 9, 3.

    (A) 3
    (B) 6
    (C) 9
    (D) 29

171. A pair of fair six-sided dice is thrown. What is the probability that the sum of the numbers shown is NOT equal to 5?

    (A) $\dfrac{1}{6}$

    (B) $\dfrac{1}{18}$

    (C) $\dfrac{1}{3}$

    (D) $\dfrac{17}{18}$

172. Evaluate $\int (x+2)\,dx$.

    (A) $\dfrac{1}{2}x^2 + 2x + C$

    (B) $\dfrac{1}{x^2} + C$

    (C) $x + C$

    (D) $\dfrac{x}{C}$

173. $\displaystyle\int_{e}^{e^2} \left(\dfrac{6}{x}\right) dx =$

    (A) 6

    (B) $\dfrac{6}{e^2} - \dfrac{6}{e}$

    (C) 18

    (D) $\dfrac{6}{e^2} + \dfrac{6}{e}$

174. Determine the derivative for the function $f(x) = e^{2x} \cdot \sin(x)$.

    (A) $2e^{2x} \cdot \sin(x) - e^{2x} \cdot \cos(x)$
    (B) $2e^{2x} \cdot \sin(x) + e^{2x} \cdot \cos(x)$
    (C) $e^{2x} \cdot \sin(x) + e^{2x} \cdot \cos(x)$
    (D) $e^{2x} \cdot \sin(x) - e^{2x} \cdot \cos(x)$

175. Determine the value(s) of w, if any, for which $\pi x^2 + 8x + w = 0$ has a double root.

    (A) $w = \dfrac{16}{\pi}$

    (B) $w = \dfrac{\pi}{16}$

    (C) $w > \dfrac{16}{\pi}$

    (D) $w > \dfrac{\pi}{16}$

176. Find the domain of the given function.

    $$f(x) = \dfrac{3x - 12}{x^2 + 7x + 10}$$

    (A) $\{x \mid x = -5, x = -2\}$
    (B) $\{x \mid x \neq -5, x \neq -2, x \neq 4\}$
    (C) $\{x \mid x \neq -5, x \neq -2\}$
    (D) $\{x \mid x = -5, x = -2, x = 4\}$

177. $9^3 \cdot 9^{-1} =$

    (A) $\dfrac{1}{729}$

    (B) 81
    (C) −81
    (D) None of the above

178. Five people are chosen at random from a group of 3 boys and 5 girls. What is the probability that 3 girls and 1 boy are chosen?

    (A) $\dfrac{4}{7}$

    (B) $\dfrac{1}{2}$

    (C) $\dfrac{3}{4}$

    (D) $\dfrac{3}{7}$

179. Find the vertex for the given function.
$$f(x) = 9x^2 + 18x - 7$$

   (A) (−1,0)
   (B) (−1,−16)
   (C) (1,20)
   (D) (1,0)

180. Determine the slope of the tangent line to the graph of the function $f(x) = 4x^3 + 7x$ at the point whose x coordinate equals −1.

   (A) 19
   (B) −19
   (C) −11
   (D) 11

181. If $\ln(2w + 9x) = 4$, then

   (A) $x = \dfrac{e^4 - 2w}{9}$

   (B) $x = \dfrac{e^4 + 2w}{9}$

   (C) $x = \dfrac{4e - 2w}{9}$

   (D) $x = \dfrac{4e + 2w}{9}$

182. A box contains apples and oranges in a ratio of 3:7. If the box contains 9 apples, how many oranges does the box contain?

   (A) 13
   (B) 21
   (C) 10
   (D) 18

183. $\dfrac{2 + \sqrt{3}}{2 - \sqrt{3}} =$

   (A) $9 - 5\sqrt{3}$

   (B) $-9 + 5\sqrt{3}$

   (C) $9 + 5\sqrt{3}$

   (D) $-9 - 5\sqrt{3}$

184. In an employee survey, 300 indicated they would attend Workshop I, and 120 indicated Workshop II. If 65 employees plan to attend both workshops and 260 indicated they could not attend either workshop, how many employees participated in the survey?

   (A) 615
   (B) 745
   (C) 550
   (D) Not enough information

185. Given the graph of the function $y = f(x)$.

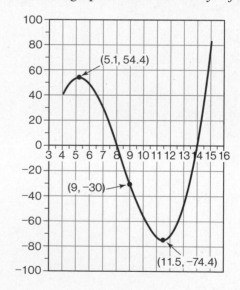

$$\lim_{x \to 11.5} \left(\frac{f(x) - f(11.5)}{x - 11.5} \right) =$$

   (A) −74.4
   (B) 0
   (C) 11.5
   (D) Not enough information

186. Determine the domain of the function $f(x) = \ln(2x - 7)$.

    (A) $(-\infty, \infty)$
    (B) $[-\infty, \infty]$
    (C) $[3.5, \infty)$
    (D) $(3.5, \infty)$

187. Find the extreme value of the given function and state whether that value represents a maximum or a minimum value for the function.

$$P(x) = 50x^2 + 300x - 65$$

    (A) -3, minimum
    (B) -3, maximum
    (C) -515, maximum
    (D) -515, minimum

188. Simplify the expression $\dfrac{\sqrt{x+h} + \sqrt{x}}{h}$.

    (A) $\dfrac{1}{\sqrt{x+h} + \sqrt{x}}$

    (B) 1

    (C) $\dfrac{1}{\sqrt{x+h} - \sqrt{x}}$

    (D) -1

189. $\log(75) - \log(3) =$

    (A) $\dfrac{1}{25}$

    (B) $\log(25)$

    (C) $\dfrac{\log(75)}{3}$

    (D) $\log(72)$

190. A truck is 48 miles from its destination at 5:00 P.M. At what speed must the truck travel to arrive by 5:45 P.M.?

    (A) 64 mph
    (B) 60 mph
    (C) 70 mph
    (D) 74 mph

191. Determine the radius of the circle with equation $(x - 5)^2 + (y - 6)^2 = 9$.

    (A) 5
    (B) 3
    (C) 6
    (D) 9

192. Solve the equation $\dfrac{x}{x+3} + \dfrac{x}{x+2} = 2$.

    (A) $x = \dfrac{12}{5}$

    (B) $x = -\dfrac{5}{12}$

    (C) $x = \dfrac{5}{12}$

    (D) $x = -\dfrac{12}{5}$

STOP

End of Quantitative Ability section. If you have any time left, you may go over your work in this section only.

READING COMPREHENSION

48 QUESTIONS (#193–#240)

TIME: 50 MINUTES

> **Directions:** Read each of the following passages, and choose the one **best** answer to each of the questions that follow each passage.

Passage 1

Although phenytoin may be used to treat cardiac arrhythmias, migraines, and trigeminal neuralgia, the primary use of phenytoin is to treat seizure disorders. Phenytoin, one of the most important agents used to manage seizures, works similarly to those of other hydantoin-derivative anticonvulsants. It decreases seizure activity by stabilizing neuronal membranes and by increasing efflux or decreasing influx of sodium ions across cell membranes in the motor cortex during generation of nerve impulses. Phenytoin is commercially available as oral suspension, tablets, and capsules. It is also available as an injection. The dosage of phenytoin varies according to the frequency of seizures, the type of seizures, and the patient's tolerance for phenytoin. Therefore, it is extremely important to monitor the patient for seizure activity as well as to monitor phenytoin serum concentrations. Phenytoin has a narrow therapeutic window and monitoring of serum concentrations is necessary. Therapeutic serum concentrations of phenytoin are usually 10–20 mcg per mL (millimeter) and depend on the assay method used. Serum concentrations above 20 mcg per mL often result in toxicity. Adverse reactions associated with dose-related toxicities include blurred vision, lethargy, rash, fever, slurred speech, nystagmus, and confusion. In some patients, seizure control is not achieved when plasma concentrations are within the therapeutic concentration range and therefore clinical response of the patient is more meaningful than plasma concentrations. Generally, therapeutic steady state serum concentrations are achieved within 30 days of therapy with an oral dosage of 300 mg daily in adults. Following an intravenous administration of 1000–1500 mg, at a rate not exceeding 50 mg per minute, therapeutic concentrations can be attained within 2 hours. Rapid administration of intravenous phenytoin may result in adverse effects such as decreased blood pressure and other cardiac complications. The use of phenytoin has been associated with osteomalacia, thrombocytopenia, and gastrointestinal upset.

193. According to the passage, which of the following is treated with phenytoin?

    (A) Trigeminal neuralgia
    (B) Arthritis
    (C) Osteomalacia
    (D) Nystagmus

194. The primary use of phenytoin is to treat

    (A) cardiac arrhythmias.
    (B) migraines.
    (C) seizure disorders.
    (D) arthritis.

195. Which of the following best represents the mechanism of action of phenytoin in treating seizures?

    (A) Increases neuronal activity
    (B) Excites peripheral impulses to excite neuronal activity
    (C) Stabilizes neuronal membranes and decreases seizure activity by decreasing the entrance of sodium ions across the cell membranes in the motor cortex during generation of nerve impulses
    (D) Stabilizes neuronal membranes and decreases seizure activity by increasing the entrance of sodium ions across the cell membranes in the motor cortex during generation of nerve impulses

196. Which of the following does (do) NOT affect the dosage of phenytoin?

    (A) Phenytoin serum concentration
    (B) Number of seizures experienced
    (C) Adverse events experienced
    (D) Puncture sites available

197. Which of the following best explains the meaning of the sentence "Phenytoin has a narrow therapeutic window and monitoring of serum concentrations is necessary"?

(A) There is a small difference in the serum concentrations known to produce seizures and the serum concentrations known to produce adverse experiences. Therefore, serum concentrations should be monitored.

(B) There is no difference in the serum concentrations known to produce desirable effects and the serum concentrations known to produce undesirable effects. Therefore, serum concentrations should be monitored.

(C) There is a small difference in the serum concentrations known to control migraines and the serum concentrations known to produce migraines. Therefore, serum concentrations should be monitored.

(D) There is a small difference in the serum concentrations known to control seizures and the serum concentrations known to produce toxicities and adverse effects. Therefore, serum concentrations should be monitored.

198. Which of the following statements describe why phenytoin should NOT be administered at a rate greater than 50 mg per minute?

(A) A higher rate takes longer to achieve adequate plasma concentrations.
(B) A higher rate may lower blood pressure.
(C) A higher rate increases arthritis pain.
(D) A higher rate may cause a rash.

199. According to the passage, which of the following is NOT a common adverse reaction associated with phenytoin toxicity?

(A) Blurred vision
(B) Lethargy
(C) Dysuria
(D) Mental confusion

200. When is the therapeutic steady-state serum concentration generally achieved with an oral dosage of 300 mg daily of phenytoin?

(A) Within 5 days
(B) Within 24 hours
(C) Within 6 days
(D) Within 30 days

Passage 2

Hypercalcemia, increased serum calcium concentrations, occurs in approximately 15% of individuals with cancer. Occurrences of this condition have been reported in most types of malignancies. The most effective management of this life-threatening disease is successful treatment of the malignancy. Unfortunately, successful treatment of the cancer may not be possible. In these cases, treatment goals should include correcting intravascular depletion, enhancing renal excretion of calcium, and inhibiting bone resorption. First line treatment of acute hypercalcemia includes the administration of normal saline and furosemide. Since many patients suffering from acute hypercalcemia are dehydrated, the administration of normal saline is warranted. In addition to treating dehydration, normal saline helps to increase renal excretion of calcium. The optimal administration of normal saline is dependent on the severity of hypercalcemia, the degree of dehydration, and the clinical status of the patient. An infusion rate of 400 mL per hour of normal saline is typical. Furosemide, a diuretic, is useful in the treatment of hypercalcemia due to its ability to enhance urinary excretion and more importantly calcium excretion. Additionally, furosemide protects patients from becoming volume overloaded due to the administration of the normal saline. It is very important that patients be adequately hydrated prior to the administration of furosemide in order to get maximum benefits. Intravenous doses of 100 mg of furosemide every 2 hours may be used. Although normal saline and furosemide are the most commonly used agents to treat acute cancer hypercalcemia, only a modest decrease in calcium levels are achieved from this regimen. The use of normal saline and furosemide may be sufficient for the management of mild to moderate hypercalcemia, but it is commonly insufficient for treating severe hypercalcemia.

201. Hypercalcemia

    (A) does not occur in any type of cancer.
    (B) may occur in most types of cancer.
    (C) may occur in bone cancer only.
    (D) may occur in lung cancer only.

202. Which of the following is the most appropriate title for this passage?

    (A) The Pathogenesis of Cancer-Related Hypercalcemia
    (B) The Uses of Normal Saline and Furosemide
    (C) Hypercalcemia—a Life-Threatening Disorder
    (D) First Line Agents Used to Treat Acute Cancer-Related Hypercalcemia

203. In treating hypercalcemia with a diuretic, it is important to

    (A) use the diuretic every hour.
    (B) administer the diuretic by mouth.
    (C) hydrate the patient before administrating the diuretic.
    (D) give the diuretic before the normal saline.

204. Which of the following is the most effective method of treating cancer-related hypercalcemia?

    (A) The use of normal saline
    (B) The use of furosemide
    (C) The use of dialysis
    (D) Treatment of the malignancy

205. Which of the following is NOT a goal in the treatment of acute hypercalcemia?

    (A) Administration of calcium carbonate
    (B) Enhancing renal excretion of calcium
    (C) Inhibiting bone resorption
    (D) Correcting intravascular depletion

206. In patients who are being treated for acute hypercalcemia, the administration of normal saline is warranted because

    (A) the patients have cancer.
    (B) the patients are dehydrated.
    (C) the patients are seen in the clinic.
    (D) the patients are volume overloaded.

207. The use of normal saline and furosemide is NOT typically sufficient for which type of hypercalcemia?

    (A) Mild cancer-related hypercalcemia
    (B) Mild hypercalcemia
    (C) Moderate hypercalcemia
    (D) Severe hypercalcemia

Passage 3

Gastroesophageal reflux disease (GERD) is a common medical disorder seen by health care practitioners of all specialties. It is generally chronic in nature, and long-term therapy may be required. While the mortality associated with GERD is very low (1 death per 100,000 patients), the quality of life experienced by the patient can be greatly diminished.

GERD refers to any symptomatic clinical condition or histologic alteration that results from episodes of gastroesophageal reflux. Gastroesophageal reflux refers to the retrograde movement of gastric contents from the stomach into the esophagus. Many people experience some degree of reflux, especially after eating, which may be considered a benign physiologic process. When the esophagus is repeatedly exposed to refluxed material for prolonged periods of time, inflammation of the esophagus (i.e., reflux esophagitis) can occur. It is important to realize that gastroesophageal reflux must precede the development of GERD or reflux esophagitis. In severe cases, reflux may lead to a multitude of serious complications including esophageal strictures, esophageal ulcers, motility disorders, perforation, hemorrhage, aspiration, and Barrett's esophagus. While mild disease is often managed with life-style changes and antacids, more intensive therapeutic intervention with histamine (H_2) antagonists, sucralfate, prokinetic agents, or proton pump inhibitors is generally required for patients with more severe disease. In general, response to pharmacologic intervention is dependent on the efficacy of the agent, dosage regimen employed, duration of therapy, and severity of the disease. Following discontinuation of therapy, relapse is common and long-term maintenance therapy may be required. Historically, surgical intervention has been reserved for patients in whom conventional treatment modalities fail. However, the recent development of laparoscopic antireflux surgical procedures has led to a reevaluation of the role of surgery in the long-term management of GERD. Some clinicians have suggested that laparoscopic antireflux surgery may be a cost-effective alternative to long-term maintenance therapy in young patients. However, long-term comparative trials evaluating the cost effectiveness of the various treatment modalities are warranted.

The pathogenesis of gastroesophageal reflux is related to the complex balance between defense mechanisms and aggressive factors. Understanding both the normal protective mechanisms and the aggressive factors that may contribute to or promote gastroesophageal reflux helps one to design rational therapeutic treatment regimens. Gastric acid, pepsin, bile acids, and pancreatic enzymes are considered aggressive factors and may promote esophageal damage upon reflux into the esophagus. Thus, the composition (potency) and volume of the refluxate are aggressive factors that may lead to

esophageal injury. Conversely, normal protective mechanisms include anatomic factors, the lower esophageal sphincter pressure, esophageal clearing, mucosal resistance, and gastric emptying. Rational therapeutic regimens in the treatment of gastroesophageal reflux are designed to maximize normal defense mechanisms and/or attenuate the aggressive factors.

Excerpted with permission from *Pharmacotherapy, A Pathophysiological Approach*, Third Edition, by Joseph T. DiPiro, et al., page 675. Stamford, CT: Appleton & Lange, 1996.

208. Which of the following statements is FALSE?

    (A) GERD is a common medical disorder seen by healthcare practitioners of all specialties.
    (B) Gastroesophageal reflux precedes the development of reflux esophagitis.
    (C) The mortality associated with GERD is very high.
    (D) Mild GERD may be managed with life style changes and antacids.

209. One possible complication of reflux is

    (A) perforation.
    (B) mucosal resistance.
    (C) gastric emptying.
    (D) lower esophageal sphincter pressure.

210. Reflux esophagitis is

    (A) a rational therapeutic treatment regimen.
    (B) a surgical intervention.
    (C) the inflammation of the esophagus due to repeated exposure to refluxed gastric contents for prolonged periods of time.
    (D) a normal defense mechanism.

211. Which of the following statements is true?

    (A) All patients who experience some degree of reflux after eating need intensive therapeutic intervention.
    (B) Pharmacological intervention is not dependent upon the efficacy of the agent, the dosage regimen employed, and the severity of the disease.
    (C) Long-term maintenance therapy may be required to prevent relapse following the discontinuation of therapy.
    (D) GERD is a rare and unique medical disorder but is seen by health care practitioners of ALL specialties.

212. In GERD patients, response to pharmacologic intervention is dependent on the

    (A) dosage regimen employed.
    (B) efficacy of the agent.
    (C) severity of the disease.
    (D) All of the above

213. Long-term comparative trials evaluating the cost effectiveness of various treatment modalities for GERD are

    (A) warranted.
    (B) not feasible.
    (C) premature.
    (D) aggressive.

214. Some clinicians have suggested that a cost-effective alternative therapy for GERD may be

    (A) histamine antagonists.
    (B) prokinetic agents.
    (C) laparoscopic antireflux surgery.
    (D) proton pump inhibitors.

215. Aggressive factors that may promote esophageal damage upon reflux into the esophagus are

    (A) gastric acid and pancreatic enzymes.
    (B) bile acids and esophageal clearing.
    (C) lower esophageal sphincter pressure and gastric emptying.
    (D) None of the above

Passage 4

Many people in the United States are diagnosed with diabetes mellitus. Non-insulin-dependent diabetes mellitus (NIDDM) is the most common type of diabetes and it is associated with a significant amount of morbidities and mortalities. NIDDM is classified as an endocrine disorder characterized by defects in insulin secretion as well as in insulin action. In NIDDM patients a defect also exists in insulin receptor binding. These defects lead to increased serum glucose concentrations or hyperglycemia.

Sulfonylureas are one of the most popular classes of agents used to treat NIDDM. One of the newest agents to treat NIDDM is acarbose, an oral alpha-glucosidase inhibitor. Acarbose interferes with the hydrolysis of dietary disaccharides and complex carbohydrates, thereby delaying absorption of glucose and other monosaccharides. Acarbose is available for oral administration only. To be most effective, it should be taken at the beginning of a meal. The recommended starting dose is 25 mg three times daily and doses as high as 200 mg three times a day have been safely used. The most common adverse experiences associated with the use of acarbose are abdominal cramps, flatulence, diarrhea, and abdominal distension. Most of the adverse effects are due to the unabsorbed carbohydrates undergoing fermentation in the colon. Acarbose has also been associated with decreased intestinal absorption of iron, thereby possibly leading to anemia. The occurrence of hypoglycemia when using acarbose in combination with other agents used to lower serum glucose is great. Glucose should be administered to treat hypoglycemia in patients taking acarbose because sucrose may not be adequately hydrolyzed and absorbed. The effectiveness of this agent to lower serum glucose concentrations in patients with NIDDM has been clearly demonstrated in clinical trials. Acarbose provides another option for treating NIDDM.

216. Which of the following does NOT describe the term *non-insulin-dependent diabetes mellitus?*

    (A) Endocrine in nature
    (B) Hyperglycemia
    (C) May be due to a defect in insulin receptor binding
    (D) Results in iron deficiencies

217. Which of the following is the most common type of agent used to treat NIDDM?

    (A) A sulfonylurea agent
    (B) Glucose
    (C) Sucrose
    (D) Fructose

218. Which of the following statements is false?

    (A) The only effective dose of acarbose is one that is administered intravenously before bedtime.
    (B) Acarbose is a new agent that is used to treat NIDDM.
    (C) Using Acarbose could possibly lead to anemia.
    (D) Diarrhea is a common adverse effect associated with acarbose.

219. According to the passage, which of the following is the most common side effect associated with the use of acarbose?

    (A) Hyperglycemia
    (B) Anemia
    (C) Gastrointestinal discomfort
    (D) Rash

220. Which of the following is the best agent to treat hypoglycemia in patients taking acarbose?

    (A) A sulfonylurea agent
    (B) Glucose
    (C) Sucrose
    (D) Fructose

221. According to the passage, which of the following has NOT been associated with the use of acarbose?

    (A) Low serum glucose concentrations
    (B) Gastrointestinal discomfort
    (C) Decreased iron absorption
    (D) Obstruction of the urinary tract

222. Which of the following used in combination with acarbose increases the risk of experiencing hypoglycemia?

    (A) A sulfonylurea agent
    (B) Glucose
    (C) Iron
    (D) Increased caloric intake

223. Which of the following is the best title for this passage?

    (A) Diabetes in the United States
    (B) Agents Used to Treat Non-Insulin-Dependent Diabetes Mellitus
    (C) The Use of Acarbose in the Treatment of Non-Insulin-Dependent Diabetes Mellitus
    (D) Adverse Effects of Acarbose

Passage 5
Osteoporosis, the most common skeletal disorder associated with aging, is a significant cause of mortality and morbidity among the elderly. The two most common types of osteoporosis are type I (postmenopausal) osteoporosis and type II (senile) osteoporosis. Type I osteoporosis is due to a drastic decline in bone mass during the first five years of menopause and a slower rate of bone loss in subsequent years. Type II osteoporosis is characterized by a gradual, age-related loss of bone in females and males over the age of 65 years. By far, osteoporosis is most prevalent in the postmenopausal population. In addition to menopausal-associated hormonal changes, other risk factors for osteoporosis in women include low calcium intake, medical factors such as oophorectomy, and life-style factors such as inactivity and cigarette smoking. In osteoporosis,

osteoclasts excavate areas in bone that the bone-forming cells, the osteoblasts, are unable to fully reconstitute. Often this defective bone loses compressive strength, thereby leading to an increased risk of fracture. Osteoporosis evolves as a silent disease with no obvious early warning signs. Many patients suffering from osteoporosis are not aware of their condition until a fracture occurs. This disease is responsible for at least 1.5 million fractures in Americans each year, with annual costs to the United States health care system of approximately $10 billion. Other consequences of osteoporosis include pain and spinal deformities such as dorsal kyphosis and dowager's or widow's hump. In addition, a decrease in appetite, fatigue, and weakness may be present. As the population continues to age, the cost of treating osteoporosis and its associated complications is predicted to double over the next 30 years.

224. Osteoporosis is most common in which population?

(A) Postmenopausal women
(B) Young males
(C) Infants
(D) Teenagers

225. Which of the following is NOT a risk factor for osteoporosis?

(A) Age
(B) Low calcium intake
(C) Weight-bearing exercise
(D) Cigarette smoking

226. Which of the following is a direct consequence of osteoporosis?

(A) Height gain
(B) Hypertension
(C) Oophorectomy
(D) Dowager's hump

227. Which of the following statements is FALSE?

(A) There is more than one type of osteoporosis.
(B) Most patients have advanced warning that they have osteoporosis, since there are many early warning signs for the disorder.
(C) Osteoporosis is the most prevalent disease in postmenopausal women.
(D) 1.5 million fractures per year in Americans are attributed to osteoporosis.

228. What is the predicted U.S. cost of treating osteoporosis and its associated complications over the next 30 years?

(A) $5 billion
(B) $7 billion
(C) $10 billion
(D) $20 billion

229. Which cells are responsible for removing bone?

(A) Osteoclasts
(B) Osteoblasts
(C) Osteomasts
(D) Osteotrasts

230. Which cells are responsible for forming bone?

(A) Osteoclasts
(B) Osteoblasts
(C) Osteomasts
(D) Osteotrasts

Passage 6

Bronchial asthma is a common disease of children and adults. Although the clinical manifestations of asthma have been known since antiquity, it is a disease that still defies precise definition. The word *asthma* is of Greek origin and means "panting." More than 2000 years ago, Hippocrates used the word *asthma* to describe episodic shortness of breath; however, the first detailed clinical description of the asthmatic patient was made by Aretaeus in the second century. Since that time *asthma* has been used to describe any disorder with episodic shortness of breath or dyspnea; thus, the terms *cardiac asthma* and *bronchial asthma* have been used to delineate the etiologies of the dyspnea. These terms are now obsolete and *asthma* refers to a disorder of the respiratory system characterized by episodes of difficulty in breathing. An Expert Panel of the National Institutes of Health National Asthma Education Program (NAEP) has defined asthma as a lung disease characterized by (1) airway obstruction that is reversible (but not completely so in some patients) either spontaneously or with treatment; (2) airway inflammation; and (3) increased airway responsiveness to a variety of stimuli. This descriptive definition for asthma is attributed to our lack of knowledge of the precise pathogenic defect that results in the clinical syndrome we recognize as asthma. The current definition does allow for the important heterogeneity of the clinical presentation of asthma. New technologies have added substantially to our understanding of the interrelationships of immunology, biochemistry, and physiology to the clinical presentation of asthma, and further research may yet uncover a specific genetic defect associated with asthma. Until such time, asthma will continue to defy exact definition.

An estimated 10 million persons in the United States have asthma (about 5% of the population). The reported prevalence increased 29% from 1980 to 1987 to 40.1 per 1000 population. African-Americans have a 19% higher incidence of asthma than whites and are twice as likely to be hospitalized. The estimated cost of asthma in the United States in 1990 was $6.2 billion. The largest single direct medical expenditure was for inpatient hospital services (emergency care), reaching almost $1.5 billion, followed by prescription medications ($1.1 billion). The costs of medication increased 54% between 1985 and 1990. In total, 43% of the economic impact was associated with emergency room use, hospitalization, and death. Asthma accounted for 1% of all ambulatory care visits according to the National Ambulatory Medical Care Survey and results in more than 450,000 hospitalizations per year.

Excerpted with permission from *Pharmacotherapy, A Pathophysiological Approach*, Third Edition, by Joseph T. DiPiro, et al., page 553. Stamford, CT: Appleton & Lange, 1996.

231. According to the passage, which of the following statements about the definition of asthma is true?

    (A) Asthma has been defined precisely since the second century.
    (B) Although asthma is a common disease of children and adults, it eludes a precise definition.
    (C) Two opposing views of the etiology of asthma, the cardiac and the bronchial, make it difficult to define the term precisely.
    (D) The NAEP's definition of asthma is widely regarded as exact but does not allow for the heterogeneity of the clinical presentation of asthma.

232. The etiologies of the episodic shortness of breath was once divided into two terms:

    (A) antiquity and panting.
    (B) reversible and spontaneous.
    (C) inpatient and outpatient.
    (D) bronchial asthma and cardiac asthma.

233. According to the NAEP, one way to characterize asthma is by

    (A) the homogeneity of its clinical presentation.
    (B) inflamed airways.
    (C) a decrease in airway responsiveness.
    (D) airway obstruction that is always completely reversible.

234. Which of the following statements is FALSE?

    (A) The cost of asthma in the United States in 1990 was $6.2 billion.
    (B) African-Americans have a 19% higher incidence of asthma than whites.
    (C) The cost of asthma medication decreased 54% between 1985 and 1990.
    (D) Prescription medications for asthma accounted for an expenditure of $1.1 billion in 1990.

235. The passage suggests that in the future researchers are likely to understand more about

  (A) new technologies to treat asthma.
  (B) wheezing and episodes of shortness of breath.
  (C) a specific genetic defect associated with asthma.
  (D) the interrelationship of immunology, biochemistry, and physiology.

236. Asthma results in more than _____ hospitalizations per year.

  (A) 6.2 billion
  (B) 29% of
  (C) 10 million
  (D) 450,000

237. The estimated number of persons in the United States who have asthma is

  (A) 100 million.
  (B) 2.5 million.
  (C) fewer than 2%.
  (D) 10 million.

238. Today, the term *asthma* refers to

  (A) panting.
  (B) dyspnea of cardiac or bronchial etiology.
  (C) Both A and B
  (D) a disorder of the respiratory system characterized by episodes of difficulty in breathing.

239. The word *asthma* has a Greek origin and was used by

  (A) Aretaeus.
  (B) an Expert Panel of the National Institutes of Health.
  (C) Hippocrates.
  (D) the National Ambulatory Medical Care Survey.

240. The passage contains which of the following?

  (A) A descriptive definition of asthma
  (B) Facts about the prevalence of asthma in the United States
  (C) An explanation of the worldwide increase in prevalence of asthma
  (D) Both A and B

STOP

End of Reading Comprehension section. If you have any time left, you may go over your work in this section only.

ESSAY

TIME: 30 MINUTES

Directions: Write a well-constructed essay addressing the statement below.

"More than 50 million U.S. citizens lack health insurance. Discuss solutions to this problem."

_____

_____

_____

_____

_____

_____

_____

_____

_____

_____

_____

_____

_____

_____

_____

_____

_____

_____

_____

_____

_____

ESSAY

TIME: 30 MINUTES

Directions: Write a well-constructed essay addressing the statement below.

"Discuss solutions to the problem of childhood obesity."

_____

_____

_____

_____

_____

_____

_____

_____

_____

_____

_____

_____

_____

_____

_____

_____

_____

_____

_____

_____

_____

_____

_____

_____

Answer Key
PRACTICE TEST 1

VERBAL ABILITY

1. C	13. D	25. A	37. C
2. A	14. B	26. B	38. A
3. C	15. D	27. B	39. D
4. A	16. C	28. B	40. A
5. A	17. C	29. A	41. C
6. B	18. B	30. B	42. A
7. A	19. C	31. A	43. D
8. C	20. B	32. C	44. C
9. D	21. D	33. B	45. C
10. A	22. B	34. D	46. A
11. B	23. D	35. A	47. D
12. A	24. C	36. D	48. B

BIOLOGY

49. B	61. C	73. A	85. C
50. A	62. C	74. B	86. C
51. A	63. A	75. C	87. A
52. C	64. B	76. B	88. B
53. D	65. D	77. C	89. C
54. B	66. B	78. A	90. D
55. B	67. C	79. B	91. D
56. C	68. D	80. B	92. C
57. D	69. C	81. D	93. D
58. B	70. B	82. A	94. D
59. C	71. C	83. B	95. A
60. B	72. B	84. B	96. D

CHEMISTRY

97. A	109. B	121. C	133. B
98. C	110. B	122. B	134. C
99. A	111. A	123. D	135. B
100. A	112. C	124. D	136. B
101. C	113. A	125. B	137. A
102. A	114. D	126. A	138. B
103. A	115. B	127. B	139. B
104. C	116. A	128. B	140. C
105. C	117. B	129. C	141. B
106. D	118. B	130. B	142. C
107. C	119. D	131. D	143. D
108. B	120. C	132. B	144. B

Answer Key
PRACTICE TEST 1

QUANTITATIVE ABILITY

145.	A	157.	C	169.	D	181.	A
146.	B	158.	B	170.	B	182.	B
147.	A	159.	A	171.	D	183.	C
148.	B	160.	A	172.	A	184.	A
149.	C	161.	B	173.	A	185.	B
150.	B	162.	B	174.	B	186.	D
151.	B	163.	D	175.	A	187.	D
152.	A	164.	A	176.	C	188.	C
153.	C	165.	D	177.	B	189.	B
154.	D	166.	C	178.	D	190.	A
155.	D	167.	B	179.	B	191.	B
156.	D	168.	A	180.	A	192.	D

READING COMPREHENSION

193.	A	205.	A	217.	A	229.	A
194.	C	206.	B	218.	A	230.	B
195.	C	207.	D	219.	C	231.	B
196.	D	208.	C	220.	B	232.	D
197.	D	209.	A	221.	D	233.	B
198.	B	210.	C	222.	A	234.	C
199.	C	211.	C	223.	C	235.	C
200.	D	212.	D	224.	A	236.	D
201.	B	213.	A	225.	C	237.	D
202.	D	214.	C	226.	D	238.	D
203.	C	215.	A	227.	B	239.	C
204.	D	216.	D	228.	D	240.	D

EXPLANATORY ANSWERS

1. **(C)** The analogy here is based on words that are synonyms, that is, that have the same or nearly the same meaning. To *fence* something in and to *enclose* it are the same. To *daub* means the same as to *smear*.

2. **(A)** *Placate* and *pacify* have the same or nearly the same meaning, so you need to find the word that is synonymous with *confirm*. The answer is *ratify*.

3. **(C)** In this example, you are looking for a word that means the opposite of *oblique* (indirect or deviating from a straight line), so the correct choice is *straight*. The analogy is one of antonyms.

4. **(A)** This analogy involves causality. A *virus* causes a *cold*, just as a *deity* performs a *miracle*.

5. **(A)** This analogy involves the relationship of part to whole. The *margin* of a wound is the part analogous to the *rim* of a *volcano*.

6. **(B)** Here the analogy is based on the relationship of whole to part. A *book* is divided into parts, each of which is a *chapter*, and a *concerto* is divided into parts, each of which is a *movement*.

7. **(A)** Here the relationship is that of whole to part. The *small intestine* contains a part called the *duodenum*, and the *hand* contains *fingers*. Since an echidna is a spiny anteater, that is clearly not the correct choice. The other alternatives must be rejected as well since neither completes an analogy based on a whole-to-part relationship.

8. **(C)** This is a part-to-part analogy. Both the *raspberry* and *kiwi fruit* are part of the larger group of all fruits, and both *romaine* and *Boston lettuce* are part of the larger group of all kinds of lettuce.

9. **(D)** In this example, the relationship is deceptively simple: purpose or use. We use a *needle* to *sew*, and we use a *hose* to *siphon*. Be careful not to choose the noun *lawn* erroneously; although we water the lawn with a hose, this word is not the correct choice in this case.

10. **(A)** This analogy involves purpose or use. An *umbrella* shelters a *pedestrian* from rain; a *roof* shelters a *house*.

11. **(B)** The correct answer is *egg* because this is an analogy of action to object. We *recycle* (action) *paper* (object), and *incubate* (action) an *egg* (object).

12. **(A)** Just as a *theory* is *refuted*, a *president* is impeached, so *impeach* is the correct choice. This analogy involves object to action.

13. **(D)** This analogy expresses the relationship of part to whole: the *ear* is part of the *corn* plant, and the *boll* is part of the *cotton* plant.

14. **(B)** *Debris* eventually becomes *compost* and can be used as fertilizer; *resin* eventually becomes *amber*. The analogy is one of sequence or time.

15. **(D)** In this analogy of characteristic or description, the *cheetah* is *sleek*, whereas the *seal* is *rotund*.

16. **(C)** A relationship of degree is implied here. The *flu* represents a disease with a much greater degree of severity than a *cold*. Likewise, a *depression* is a much greater economic problem than a recession.

17. **(C)** This is also a grammatical analogy. This time you must find a verb that takes the preposition *out*, just as the verb *comment* takes the preposition *on*. The correct answer can only be *eke*.

18. **(B)** In this analogy of association, the *pharmacist* is associated with a *pharmacy*, and the *diplomat* with an *embassy*.

19. **(C)** An analogy may express the relationship between a worker and tool. In this example, a *painter* uses a *palette*, and a *cook* uses a *spatula*.

20. **(B)** To understand this analogy of definition, it helps to know that an *ellipsis,* usually indicated by three successive dots . . . is an omission of words in a *sentence*. The correct answer is *pause*, a temporary cessation of utterance in a *speech*.

21. **(D)** Since a *Panama* is one of many kinds of *hat*, and a *Mako* is one of many kinds of *shark*, the relationship expressed is part to whole.

22. **(B)** Drums are part of a band; a goalie is part of a team. This is an analogy of part to whole.

23. **(D)** Droplets are a characteristic subdivision of water, and grains are an analogous characteristic subcomponent of sand in this analogy of description.

24. **(C)** In this geographical analogy, Providence is the capital of Rhode Island, and Boise is the capital of Idaho. (Always ask yourself how the first two terms are related, and then look for an analogous relationship between the second two terms.)

25. **(A)** In this grammatical analogy, *are not* and *have not* are the plural verbs and the adverbs from which the contractions are formed. (Remember to take all the relevant factors into account. If you chose B, your answer is incorrect because *has* is third person singular, not plural).

26. **(B)** This is an analogy based on synonyms. Just as *liable* and *responsible* are synonyms, *liberal* and *generous* have the same or nearly the same meaning.

27. **(B)** In this analogy of purpose or use, a libretto is the text for an opera, while a screenplay is the "text" for a film.

28. **(B)** In this geographical analogy, the Andes are a mountain chain in South America, and the Alps are a mountain chain in Europe. (If you chose C, your answer is incorrect because here you need to select a continent rather than a country. D is incorrect because it is the name of a single mountain in the Alps.)

29. **(A)** This grammatical analogy involves pairs of adverbs (*seemingly* and *ostensibly, thoroughly* and *completely*) with the same or nearly the same meaning. This example may also be considered an analogy of synonyms.

30. **(B)** Generally speaking, a teacher's job consists of teaching, correcting, and sometimes disciplining students, which may be viewed at times as admonishment or chastisement. If the teacher disciplines the student in front of the

class (the student's peers), then this could result in the student's embarrassment, as the sentence states. Of the answer choices provided, Answer B (reprimanded) is the best match for this sentence.

31. **(A)** "Permeable" usually describes something that is porous and absorbent, which allows the penetration or passage of an outside substance; thus, we can conclude that this sentence's context is centered on the movement of something from one side of an object to the other. Based on the sentence context, this most likely means that the water can more easily "move" or be transported from one side to the other. The word "diffuse" in Answer A, meaning to spread or disperse, is the correct choice.

32. **(C)** Because what Henry used to solve the problem and what he did NOT rely on seem to be in conflict, then we can conclude that the two correct words for the blanks will be opposing terms. Data collected through scientific study or experimentation are usually heralded as reliable and indisputable. This could be a clue as to why Henry used data to solve the problem and did NOT rely on something that was questionable, subjective, or that did not require the use of concrete reasoning. By reading each of the answer choices back into the sentence, Answer C (intuition and empirical) provides the answer choices that make the most sense.

33. **(B)** The correct answer for the first blank will further describe a gentleman who is always "complaining and rude," indicating that it will be synonymous with "discourteous." Because the phrase "on the other hand" precedes the second blank (or the word we are looking for to replace the blank), we know that the blank will have a meaning that will be the opposite of the first blank. Furthermore, the correct word for the second blank will be synonymous with someone who is always "laughing and joking," also meaning "jovial" or "happy." Based on this, Answer B (cantankerous and mirthful) is the correct answer for this sentence.

34. **(D)** The first blank is associated with evolution, relating to an introduction, development, or emergence of something that was not previously or originally available. After these modifications and deviations from the original state or condition occur (indicated by the first blank), the results can be deemed as dissimilar, irregular, or variant (indicated by the second blank). Based on the sentence's context, "mutation and variation" (Answer D) are the correct answer choices.

35. **(A)** This sentence tells us that "asking other organizations . . . to help" will directly affect the number of volunteers, which also relates to the success of the fundraiser. We can conclude that, since the number of volunteers is small or minimal, asking for help from other organizations will increase or enhance this number. Since the success of the fundraiser is also related to this, we can predict for the first blank that a larger number of volunteers for the fundraiser will promote or encourage its success. If this is true, then the correct word for the second blank must mean to "increase" or "enlarge." Answer A, therefore, best matches our predictions for this sentence's context.

36. **(D)** Generally speaking, history is an account, explanation, or interpretation of past events. It is usually recorded and taught in sequential or

successive order—from past to present. This progression or order in time is known as "chronological" order, which is Answer D.

37. **(C)** The first blank describes the remarks made during a sacred and dignified occasion that were offensive, and therefore probably inappropriate and disrespectful to many audience members. The second blank describes the type of damage these negative remarks potentially caused. Undoubtedly, the disdainful remarks changed the ceremony's solemn and formal tone, but we are not told in the sentence to what extent. It is possible that the damage was irreversible or unalterable, causing the ceremony to be ruined. Based on this and the answer choices provided, Answer C provides the best answer to complete this sentence.

38. **(A)** In this sentence, the word that fits in the blank describes a man whose opinions are directly associated with "acting in a stubborn fashion." Stubborn can also be described as inflexible, headstrong, unyielding, or determined to have one's own way. Answer A (obstinate) is the only answer listed that is synonymous with stubborn.

39. **(D)** Financially speaking, if something is described as "on sale," this makes the particular item less costly or less burdensome to purchase. However, we are told that despite the fact that the shirt was on sale, Karen's mother still thought that spending the money to acquire it would be too excessive. Taking into consideration that this sentence is based on the concept of money and by looking at the answer choices given, only Answer D (frugal) describes a conservative and economical approach to expending or investing monetary funds.

40. **(A)** We know from the wording of the sentence that an action involving the discarded match and the paper in the trash can result in a fire. Since paper is highly flammable (meaning that it burns or is easily set on fire), we know that the word needed for the first blank will be related to the match setting a flame or a spark, causing a fire. Generally speaking, without interference a fire will continue to spread and can lead to significant damage. However, the sentence tells us that this fire's damage was NOT severe because of how the carpet was made, indicated by the word needed for the second blank. There was something in the carpet's material that delayed, hampered, or impeded the fire's progression, resulting in less damage. By reading each of the answer choices back into the sentence, Answer A (ignited and retardant) best matches these projections and the sentence context.

41. **(C)** The word for the first blank is further emphasized by the phrase "Without a doubt." Based on this, we can conclude that waiting until the solution has completely stabilized is of unquestionable importance and is required and mandatory. The word to be placed in the second blank in this sentence provides the connection between a completely stabilized solution and the risk of causing a violent chemical reaction. Until something regarding the solution is attained or achieved (indicated by the word to be placed in the second blank), a violent reaction may result. Based on this, we can conclude that the word in the second blank should be related to the solution being completely stable, balanced, or unchanged. Accordingly, "imperative"

and "equilibrium" (found in Answer C) are the correct answers to complete this sentence.

42. **(A)** Because the word that goes into the first blank is preceded by the phrase "in contrast," we can conclude that the words to be placed in the two blanks describing the paintings in this sentence will have opposite meanings. Of the answer choices given, Answer A—"flamboyant" and "simplicity"—best matches this prediction. By reading each of the answer choices back into the sentence, these words make the most sense and best match the sentence's context.

43. **(D)** The word that goes into the blank in this sentence is in reference to our "best" (or most preferred and most beneficial) interest—in association with NOT acting too hastily. To act hastily means to act rapidly, swiftly, expeditiously, or immediately; therefore, to NOT act hastily means to wait or postpone. Thus, we can conclude that the action for the meeting "until next week" most likely means to "delay" or "reschedule"; Answer D (defer) is the best answer choice.

44. **(C)** It was anticipated that Jack's attitude regarding the trip he had won would be one of enthusiasm and excitement. Based on the element of surprise referred to in the sentence, we know that Jack's attitude in reality must have been the opposite of this. The opposite of excited, emotional, or stimulated is "complacent" and "impassive," which are best matched in Answer C (indifferent).

45. **(C)** In this sentence we are told that the first description of multiple sclerosis was over 100 years ago, which denotes an ample and extended time frame. Because of the word "although," we can assume that something about the cause and cure still exists that should have been resolved or discovered, given the lengthy time period. Answer C (mystery and undiscovered) provides the only two answer choices that make sense for both blanks in this sentence.

46. **(A)** Jumping out of an airplane without a parachute is regarded as dangerous. Under normal circumstances a person would not attempt to do this for fear of serious injury or death. The daredevil most likely does not have any fear or regard for the potential consequences that may result from this perilous act, and he most likely considers himself immune to or unaffected by them. Thus, Answer A (invulnerable) is the correct answer.

47. **(D)** The context clues for the blank in this sentence are the phrases "early" and "begin to develop," which in this sentence describe a period in an individual's life span that is initial or introductory. Answer D (embryonic) most closely denotes a beginning or rudimentary formulation or development; therefore Answer D is the best answer choice.

48. **(B)** The word "sterile" in this sentence provides a clue. Sterile means to be clean, disinfected, or without germs. The sentence states that this is the type of rod that must be used to stir the experiment's solution in order to prevent something—indicated by the blank—from happening. Based on this we can predict that if a rod that is NOT sterile is used to stir the solution, the solution will become dirty, impure, or polluted. All of these words mean the same as "contaminate," which is Answer B.

49. **(B)** Protists do not have cytoskeletons or muscles.

50. **(A)** See figure below.

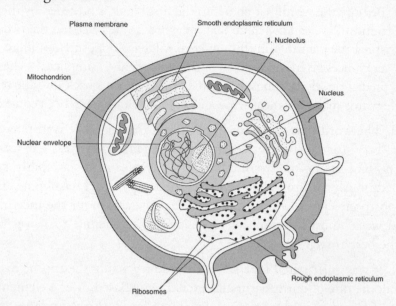

51. **(A)** SPF refers to the ability of a sunscreen to protect users from ultraviolet radiation. As SPF increases, the greater the amount of protection.

52. **(C)** The cytoskeleton is a complex network of protein filaments found in the cytoplasm of all eukaryotic cells and is necessary for cell division and movement.

53. **(D)** The endoplasmic reticulum is a network of interconnected membranes in eukaryotic cells. Ribosomes bind to the rough endoplasmic reticulum and synthesize membrane proteins and proteins destined to be secreted by the cells.

54. **(B)** Active transport is the process in which a cell transports a substance from a lower to a higher graduation. Simple diffusion is the net movement of dissolved particles down their concentration gradients, from a region of higher concentration to a region of lower concentration. Facilitated diffusion, also known as passive transport, is the net movement of dissolved particles down their concentration gradient.

55. **(B)** Mitochondria and chloroplasts are thought to have arisen from primitive prokaryotes. Mitochondria are the sites of cellular respiration by eukaryotic cells. Chloroplasts are the site of photosynthesis in plant cells.

56. **(C)** DNA replication is semi-conservative. The template strand pairs with the newly synthesized strand to produce two daughter molecules that contain one parental and one newly synthesized strand.

57. **(D)** Men with Klinefelter's syndrome have two X chromosomes. Since normal male chromosomes are XY, Klinefelter's syndrome is represented by XXY. This disease occurs in about 1 male in 500. Men with Klinefelter's syndrome are sterile and have a high incidence of mental deficiency.

58. **(B)** A heterotroph (B) is an organism that obtains its carbon, as well as energy, from organic compounds. An autotroph (A) is a microorganism that uses only inorganic materials as its source of nutrients. The other choices, C and D, are irrelevant.

59. **(C)** The cross of Aa and Aa (choice C) will result in 25% red offspring.

	A	a
A	AA	Aa
a	Aa	aa

AA (homozygous blue) and
Aa (heterozygous = blue; aa = red)

This cross will result in 75% blue and 25% red.

60. **(B)** Cones (A) provide daylight color vision and are responsible for visual acuity, while rods (B) respond to dim light for black-and-white vision. The iris (C) surrounds the pupil and regulates its diameter. The cornea (D) is the anterior portion of the outer layer of the eye.

61. **(C)** Normal red blood cells (erythrocytes) have an average life span of 120 days.

62. **(C)** No explanation needed.

63. **(A)** Monera is a taxonomic kingdom including bacteria, blue–green algae, and viruses. They are prokaryotic, not eukaryotic. Prokaryotic cells are small, have a simple internal structure, do not have their genetic material enclosed within a membrane nucleus, and lack organelles. Eukaryotic cells are characterized by the presence of a membrane-bound nucleus and other organelles.

64. **(B)** Of the choices, the Golgi apparatus is the only one that modifies materials synthesized in the rough and smooth endoplasmic reticulum.

65. **(D)** No explanation needed.

66. **(B)** No explanation needed.

67. **(C)** Clostridium are gram-positive, spore-forming bacilli.

68. **(D)** The principal autonomic and limbic functions of the hypothalamus are (1) cardiovascular (heart rate) regulation; (2) body temperature regulation; (3) regulation of water and electrolyte balance; (4) regulation of hunger and control of gastrointestinal activity; (5) regulation of sleeping and wakefulness; (6) regulation of sexual response; (7) regulation of emotions; and (8) control of endocrine functions. The respiratory center of the medulla oblongota controls the rate and depth of breathing.

69. **(C)** No explanation needed.

70. **(B)** Lobes of the cerebrum include the frontal lobe, parietal lobe, temporal lobe, occipital lobe, and insula.

71. **(C)** Enzymes that recognize and cut specific DNA sequences are called restriction enzymes. Helicases unwind DNA, polymerases synthesize nucleic acids, and ligases join two DNA strands together.

72. **(B)** No explanation needed.

73. **(A)** Insulin promotes (A), not inhibits (C), cellular uptake of glucose and formation of glycogen and fat. Glucagon stimulates hydrolysis of glycogen and fat (B).

74. **(B)** No explanation needed.

75. **(C)** Mycoplasmas are microorganisms that lack cell walls and do not synthesize the precursor for peptidoglycan.

76. **(B)** Contraction of the heart is called systole (A), and relaxation of the heart is called diastole (B). Choices C and D are irrelevant.

77. **(C)** No explanation needed.

78. **(A)** Evolution refers to changes that occur in populations over time.

79. **(B)** The adrenal glands produce adrenaline and noradrenaline. The pineal gland produces melatonin and serotonin. The pancreas produces insulin and glucagon.

80. **(B)** Aldosterone promotes sodium retention and potassium loss (B). Choice A is incorrect because it is the exact opposite of choice B.

81. **(D)** No explanation needed.

82. **(A)** Gas exchanges occur in the alveoli. The trachea and bronchi of the lungs carry the air to the alveoli.

83. **(B)** No explanation needed.

84. **(B)** No explanation needed.

85. **(C)** No explanation needed.

86. **(C)** Carbon dioxide is released from blood to the air in the alveoli, the site where gas exchange occurs in the lungs.

87. **(A)** No explanation needed.

88. **(B)** The vestibular apparatus is the collection of receptors and associate structures in the ear that play a central role in maintaining balance in vertebrates.

89. **(C)** The bone marrow in mammals contains stem cells that differentiate to produce T and B cells.

90. **(D)** No explanation needed.

91. **(D)** The thyroid gland produces a hormone that controls the rate at which the body releases energy from food. When the blood levels of these hormones are at low levels, the hypothalamus releases a hormone called thyrotropin-releasing hormone (TRH) in the blood. In response to TRH, the pituitary gland releases thyroid-stimulating hormone (TSH). The thyroid gland responds to TSH by releasing two hormones that then increase the rate of the release of energy from cells. Higher levels of thyroid hormones in the blood shut down the products of TRH and TSH by negative feedback.

92. **(C)** The immune response recognizes sequences in the viral proteins as foreign and makes antibodies specific for that sequence. In viruses, like HIV, frequent mutations change the protein sequences recognized by the immune system.

93. **(D)** Macrophages engulf and destroy bacteria.

94. **(D)** The genetic material of viruses may be double-stranded RNA or double- or single stranded DNA.

95. **(A)** No explanation needed.

96. **(D)** No explanation needed.

97. **(A)** Atoms of the same element having the same number of protons but different numbers of neutrons are called isotopes. Isomers are molecules having the same molecular formula but different structural formulas. Allotropes are different forms of the same element that have significantly different chemical and physical properties, for example, graphite and diamond. The term *diastereomer* is generally used in organic chemistry. Diastereomers are compounds that have two or more stereocenters and differ from each other at at least one of the stereocenters.

98. **(C)** The synthesis of RNA is called transcription, the synthesis of protein is called translation, the synthesis of DNA is called replication, and translocation means the movement of something to a new place (it doesn't refer to a specific biochemical process although there is a step in translation in which the ribosome translocates).

99. **(A)** DNA molecules are the permanent storage of nucleotide sequence information. RNA's are synthesized, used, and degraded.

100. **(A)** The actual yield of the reaction, 32.0 g SO_2, is given. To calculate percent yield you must first calculate the theoretical yield which is the maximum possible yield of the reaction and then use the theoretical yield in the equation below to calculate percent yield.

$$\frac{\text{Actual yield}}{\text{Theoretical yield}} \times 100 = \% \text{ yield}$$

$$CS_2 + 3O_2 \rightarrow CO_2 + 2SO_2$$

$\underline{\text{g } CS_2} \quad \rightarrow \qquad \underline{\text{moles } CS_2} \quad \rightarrow \qquad \underline{\text{moles } SO_2} \quad \rightarrow$

38.0 gm $\qquad \dfrac{38.0 \text{ g}}{76 \text{ g/moles}} \qquad 0.50 \text{ mole } CS_2 \times \dfrac{2 \text{ moles } SO_2}{1 \text{ mole } CS_2}$

$\qquad\qquad\qquad$ 0.50 mole $\qquad\qquad$ 1.00 mole SO_2

$\underline{\text{g } SO_2}$

1.00 mole $SO_2 \times \dfrac{64 \text{ g } SO_2}{1 \text{ mole } SO_2} = 64 \text{ g } SO_2 \qquad \% \text{ yield} = \dfrac{32 \text{ g}}{64 \text{ g}} \times 100 = 50\%$

101. **(C)** Molarity is defined as moles of solute divided by liters of solution.

$$M = \frac{\text{moles of solute}}{\text{liters of solution}} = \frac{\text{g/molecular weight}}{\text{liters of solution}}$$

Sugar, $C_6H_{12}O_6$, has a molecular weight of 180 g/mole. Substituting 18.0 g, 180 g/mole, and 0.500 liter into the above equation gives 0.200 M as the molarity of the solution.

$$M = \frac{18.0 \text{ g}/180 \text{ g/mole}}{0.500 \text{ liter}} = 0.200 \text{ M}$$

102. **(A)** In a dilution problem, the number of moles of solute before dilution equals the number of moles of solute after dilution. Therefore:

Molarity × volume (before dilution) = Molarity × volume (after dilution)

$$2.0 \frac{\text{moles}}{L} (0.100 \text{ L}) = 4.0 \frac{\text{moles}}{L} (\text{volume})$$

0.05 L = volume required

Dilute 50 mL of the 4.0 M solution with water to 100 mL to prepare the 2.0 M solution.

103. **(A)** The density of a gas, O_2 (mol. wt. = 32 g/mole), can be determined by a rearrangement of the ideal gas law.

$$PV = nRT \qquad PV = \frac{\#g}{\text{mol. wt.}} RT \qquad \frac{P(\text{mol. wt.})}{RT} = \frac{\#g}{V} = D$$

$$\frac{1.0 \text{ atm}\left(32 \text{ g/mole}\right)}{0.082 \dfrac{\text{L-atm}}{\text{K-mole}}(273+15)\text{K}} = 1.35 \text{ g/L}$$

The densities of gases are reported as grams per liter because the same value as grams per milliliter would be a very small number. The volume of the gas is in liters because the value of R used is in liters.

104. **(C)** The partial pressure of a gas in a mixture of gases is equal to the mole fraction of the gas times the total pressure of the mixture. First, find the mole fraction of nitrogen and then find the partial pressure of nitrogen.

$$P_{\text{total}} \; x_{\text{nitrogen}} = P_{\text{nitrogen}}$$

$$x_{\text{nitrogen}} = \frac{\#\text{moles N}_2}{\#\text{ moles N}_2 + \#\text{ moles O}_2}$$

$$x_{\text{nitrogen}} = \frac{56/28}{56/28 + 64/32} = 0.50$$

1.6 atm (0.50) = 0.8 atm = P_{nitrogen} = partial pressure of nitrogen

105. **(C)** To solve this problem, let the units of the specific heat help you. The units are J/g°C, so if you multiply the specific heat by grams and °C temperature change, you should get joules. The unknown in this question is temperature change so set up the equation as follows:

$$10 \text{ J} = (5 \text{ g}) (0.385 \text{ J/g°C}) (x \text{ °C})$$

Solving for x gives 5.2°C and since joules of heat were absorbed, the temperature must have increased from 25°C to about 30°C.

106. **(D)** No explanation needed.

107. **(C)** Remember that since the speed of light (c) is a constant, as the wavelength decreases, frequency increases (and vice versa). So the light with the highest frequency will be that with the lowest wavelength. A review of metric prefixes may aid in realizing that nm (nanometers) is the smallest of the units given as possible selections.

108. **(B)** A chloride ion has 8 valence electrons (a chlorine atom has 7 and when it becomes negatively charged by gaining an electron, it would have 8) and a sulfide ion also has 8 (a sulfur atom has 6 but the S^{2-} ion has 8).

109. **(B)** A basic oxide is a compound that, when it reacts with water, produces a base. Another name for a basic oxide is a basic anhydride. The oxide K_2O reacts with water to produce KOH according to the following equation:

$$K_2O + H_2O \rightarrow 2KOH$$

The other oxides, CO_2, SO_2, and P_2O_5, are all acid oxides or acid anhydrides.

$$CO_2 + H_2O \rightarrow H_2CO_3$$
$$SO_2 + H_2O \rightarrow H_2SO_3$$
$$P_2O_5 + 3H_2O \rightarrow 2 H_3PO_4$$

110. **(B)** In order for hydrogen bonding to exist, the hydrogen must be bonded to nitrogen, oxygen, or fluorine: H — N, H — O, H — F. Hydrogen bonding is not possible between molecules of CH_4 because the hydrogen is bonded to carbon, C. Hydrogen bonding is possible, however, between molecules of H_2O, between molecules of CH_3OH, and between molecules of NH_3.

111. **(A)** Both are esters of glycerol and fatty acids, which are long-chain carboxylic acids.

112. **(C)** Condensation is the conversion of a gas into a liquid. Sublimation is the conversion of a solid directly into a gas, for example the conversion of solid carbon dioxide, dry ice, into carbon dioxide vapor. Evaporation is the conversion of a liquid into a gas. Freezing is the conversion of a liquid into a solid.

113. **(A)** Gases are usually most soluble in liquids at low temperature. As the temperature of a liquid increases, the gas molecules dissolved in it move faster and escape more readily from the surface of the liquid. Low pressure on the surface of a liquid will not keep a gas dissolved in the liquid, but rather will allow it to escape from the liquid. High agitation or extreme stirring of the liquid will cause the gas molecules to move faster than they would otherwise move and consequently will decrease the solubility of a gas in a liquid.

114. **(D)** Cholesterol is not used in DNA synthesis. The steroid hormones are made from cholesterol and it is incorporated into some cell membranes.

115. **(B)** When two equilibrium reactions are added to give a third reaction, the equilibrium constant for the third reaction is calculated by multiplying the two equilibrium constants for each original reaction, (K^1) (K^2). Add equations, multiply equilibrium constants.

116. **(A)** In the given symbol, 35 is the atomic weight (number of protons plus number of neutrons), and 21 is the atomic number (number of protons) of element X. Subtracting 21 from 35 gives the number of neutrons, 14.

117. **(B)** With respect to proteins, the primary structure is the sequence of amino acids in the protein, the secondary structure is localized patterns that arise due to hydrogen bonding between peptide bonds in the protein, the tertiary structure is the overall folding pattern of the protein, and the quaternary structure is the association of multiple proteins (not all proteins exhibit quaternary structure). Beta sheets and alpha helices are the most common examples of a secondary structure.

118. **(B)** In determining the acidity of homologous compounds of members of the same family, as in HI, HBr, HCl, and HF, another concept besides electronegativity is invoked. HI is more acidic than HBr, which is more acidic than HCl, which is more acidic than HF. The larger the atom, I versus F, the more readily it can accommodate an extra electron and be stable. Therefore, I^- is more stable than F^- and consequently HI is more acidic than HF. Acidity increases as one progresses from top to bottom in a family, for example, HF < HCl < HBr < HI.

119. **(D)** A small amount of acid or base may be added to a buffer solution; however, the pH of the solution remains approximately the same as before the acid or base was added. A buffer consists of a weak acid and its conjugate base or of a weak base and its conjugate acid. Sulfuric acid, H_2SO_4, is a strong acid and consequently is not a buffer either alone or with one of its salts. Acetic acid, written as either HAc or CH_3COOH, is a weak acid and in combination with an acetate salt is a buffer solution.

120. **(C)** There are just a handful of common amino acids that are essentially 100% ionized at pH 7.4 (physiological pH) and they are lysine (has a primary amine in its side chain that is protonated and thus positively charged), aspartic acid, and glutamic acid (both have carboxylic acids in their side chains that are deprotonated and thus negatively charged).

121. **(C)** In the given reaction $^{90}_{38}Sr \rightarrow \, ^{90}_{39}Y+?$ the total mass has remained the same, 90 for strontium, Sr, and 90 for ytrium, Y. The atomic number, however, has increased, from 38 to 39. The number of protons has increased by 1 because a neutron in the Sr nucleus has been converted into a proton and an electron. The proton has remained in the nucleus while the electron has been expelled from the nucleus. Therefore, the correct answer is the electron, $^{0}_{-1}e$.

122. **(B)** The First Law of Thermodynamics considers the conversion of energy from one form to another form without subsequent formation or loss of any of the energy. The Second Law of Thermodynamics states that entropy, the measure of disorder, increases in spontaneous reactions and remains the same in equilibrium systems. The Third Law of Thermodynamics says that the entropy for a perfect crystal is zero at absolute zero temperature. The statement that the Gibbs Free Energy is a measure of the spontaneity of a reaction is true. Refer to the explanation given to question 123.

123. **(D)** The Gibbs Free Energy measures energy changes which accompany a reaction. If the reaction releases usable energy, i.e. energy available to do work, the Gibbs Free Energy has a negative value and the reaction is spontaneous in the direction written. When the Gibbs Free Energy has a positive value, the reaction is not spontaneous in the direction written but is spontaneous in the opposite direction. When the Gibbs Free Energy equals zero, the reaction system is at equilibrium and no change occurs.

124. **(B)** Both solutes are called acids and have pKa's, so choice (C) is false. The stronger the acid, the larger the Ka and the lower the pKa (since pKa = –log Ka), so choices (A) and (D) are also false. Choice (B) is correct because acid B is the stronger acid (larger Ka) and a solution of it would contain more hydrogen ions lowering the pH (remember pH = –log [H⁺] so as [H⁺] increases, pH decreases).

125. **(B)** Substitution of a methyl group for a hydrogen on an arene is done using Friedel–Craft alkylation. Choice (A) would acylate the ring (place an acetyl group —CH_3CO— on the ring) and nothing would happen with choices (C) and (D).

126. **(A)** $LiAlH_4$ is a hydride reducing agent. When added to an ester, a nucleophilic substitution first occurs converting the ester to an aldehyde, but then the aldehyde is attacked by a second hydride to convert it to the alcohol after protonation.

127. **(B)** The compound $CH_3CH_2COOCH_3$ is called methyl propanoate. An ester may be formed from a carboxylic acid and an alcohol. In this instance the acid is propanoic acid and the alcohol is methanol. The part of the

molecule originating from the alcohol is named first, methyl. The part of the molecule derived from the acid is named by removing *-ic acid* from the name of the acid and adding the suffix *-ate*.

128. **(B)** The formula C_2H_6 is the formula for the alkane ethane. The reaction of Br_2 with C_2H_6 has substituted one of the hydrogen atoms in ethane by a bromine atom. Whenever light or very high temperature is used in a reaction, the reaction usually occurs by a free radical mechanism. The reaction indicated is a free radical substitution reaction.

In a nucleophilic substitution reaction, one nucleophile replaces another in a reaction. In the following example, $Br^{-1} + CH_3I \rightarrow CH_3Br + I^{-1}$, the nucleophilic bromide ion replaces I^{-1}. There is no change in the total number of hydrogen atoms in a nucleophilic substitution reaction while there is such a change in a free radical substitution reaction.

In an electrophilic elimination reaction, a base reacts with a molecule to cause the loss of HZ from the molecule, where Z can be a leaving group. In the following example

$$\underset{\underset{\overset{|}{Br}}{\overset{\overset{CH_3}{|}}{CH_3-C-CH_3}}}{} + \ NaOH \ (in \ alcohol) \ \longrightarrow \ \overset{\overset{CH_3}{|}}{CH_3-C}=CH_2 + H_2O + NaBr$$

the hydroxide ion of sodium hydroxide, NaOH, removes the hydrogen bonded to one of the methyl carbon atoms to form water, H_2O. The sodium and bromide ions combine to form sodium bromide, NaBr. An alkene remains as the organic product. Refer to the answer given to question 129 for an explanation of an electrophilic addition reaction.

129. **(C)** The formula C_2H_4 is the formula for an alkene. The electrophile bromine, Br_2, adds atoms to C_2H_4 to produce the dibromide $C_2H_4Br_2$, 1,2-dibromoethane,

$$CH_2=CH_2 + Br_2 \ \longrightarrow \ \underset{\underset{Br}{|}}{\overset{\overset{Br}{|}}{CH_2-CH_2}}$$

130. **(B)** Enantiomers are a form of stereoisomers, i.e. compounds which have the same groups within the molecules but differ from each other because of the arrangement of groups in the molecules. Enantiomers are two compounds having the same four different groups bonded to the stereocenter(s) in each compound, but because of the different positions in which these groups are placed relative to each other, i.e. because of different configurations, they are nonsuperimposable mirror images. Enantiomers are identical in almost all their physical and chemical properties, Fischer projections of the enantiomers of 1-chloro-1-iodoethane are shown on the next page.

$$
\begin{array}{c}
CH_3 \\
| \\
H - C - Cl \\
| \\
I
\end{array}
\qquad
\begin{array}{c}
CH_3 \\
| \\
Cl - C - H \\
| \\
I
\end{array}
$$

Diastereomers are also a form of stereoisomers. Diastereomers are two compounds, each having at least two different stereocenters. The diastereomers have the arrangement of the four different groups at one of the stereocenters identical in both molecules but the arrangement of another four different groups at the other stereocenter different in both compounds. In other words, diastereomers with two stereocenters have the same configuration at one of the stereocenters but opposite configurations at the other stereocenter. Diastereomers are nonsuperimposable and have different physical and chemical properties. Fischer projections of one pair of diastereomers of 2-bromo-3-chlorobutane are shown below.

$$
\begin{array}{c}
CH_3 \\
| \\
H - C - Cl \\
| \\
H - C - Br \\
| \\
CH_3
\end{array}
\qquad
\begin{array}{c}
CH_3 \\
| \\
H - C - Cl \\
| \\
Br - C - H \\
| \\
CH_3
\end{array}
$$

Geometric isomerism may occur in alkenes. It is not possible to freely rotate around a carbon-carbon double bond as it is around a carbon-carbon single bond. Therefore, when a carbon-carbon double bond is present in a compound, two different compounds, geometric isomers, may exist. In the example shown below:

$$
\begin{array}{ccc}
CH_3 & & CH_3 \\
\diagdown & & \diagup \\
& C = C & \\
\diagup & & \diagdown \\
Cl & & Cl
\end{array}
\qquad
\begin{array}{ccc}
CH_3 & & Cl \\
\diagdown & & \diagup \\
& C = C & \\
\diagup & & \diagdown \\
Cl & & CH_3
\end{array}
$$

the two chlorine atoms are on the same side of the double bond in one compound and on opposite sides of the double bond in the other compound. One could just as easily compare the position of the two methyl groups relative to the carbon-carbon double bond and arrive at the same conclusion. In order that geometric isomerism be present in alkenes, two identical groups cannot be bonded to the same carbon atom.

131. **(D)** Since a beta-hydroxy aldehyde product has been made in the presence of base, an aldol condensation has occurred. The product has 4 carbons so a 2-carbon aldehyde is the reactant.

132. **(B)** In infrared (IR) spectroscopy, the most significant bands are around 3300 cm^{-1} for O—H and N—H, around 2,100 cm^{-1} for triple bonds, and around 1,600–1,700 cm^{-1} for double bonds.

133. **(B)** Lipids have the following general structure where the R groups, which may or may not be the same, are large groups, usually a straight chain of twelve or more carbon atoms.

$$
\begin{array}{c}
\quad\quad\quad O \\
\quad\quad\quad \| \\
CH_2OCR \\
| \quad\quad\quad O \\
\quad\quad\quad \| \\
CHOCR \\
| \\
CH_2OCR \\
\quad\quad \| \\
\quad\quad O
\end{array}
$$

Lipids are triesters of the alcohol 1,2,3–trihydroxypropane.

134. **(C)** The following generalized equation between an alcohol and a carboxylic acid produces an ester and water.

$$
\begin{array}{ccccccc}
O & & & & O & & \\
\| & & & & \| & & \\
RCOH & + & HOR & \longrightarrow & RCOR & + & HOH
\end{array}
$$

135. **(B)** Proteins are polymers of alpha substituted amino acids which have the following generalized structure containing amide linkages.

$$
\begin{array}{c}
\quad\quad O \quad\quad\quad\quad\quad\quad O \quad\; R \quad\quad H \quad\quad O \quad\quad R \\
\quad\quad \| \quad\quad\quad\quad\quad\quad \| \quad\; | \quad\quad | \quad\quad \| \quad\quad | \\
R-CH-C-O-H \;-\!-\!-\!> \; -C-N-CH-C-N-CH-C-N-CH- \\
\quad\quad | \quad\quad\quad\quad\quad\quad\quad\; | \quad\quad\quad \| \quad\; | \quad\quad\quad | \\
\quad\; NH_2 \quad\quad\quad\quad\quad\quad\quad H \quad\quad O \quad\; R \quad\quad H
\end{array}
$$

several molecules of   protein
  alpha amino acid

136. **(B)** It is not true that all bonds in benzene are equivalent in length. All of the C—C bonds are equivalent in length but the C—H bonds are a different length from the C—C bonds. Even though the C—C bonds in benzene may be represented by alternating single and double bonds, all of these C—C bonds are the same length because of delocation of pi electrons, that is, resonance. All of the other statements about benzene are correct.

137. **(A)** The compound is named 3-methylpentanoic acid. The carbonyl carbon is numbered 1, so the carbon atom to which the methyl group is attached is carbon 3. The acid is named by removing the *-e* from pentane and adding *-oic acid*. The formulas for the other answers are shown below.

$$
\begin{array}{ccc}
CH_3CH_2CH_2CHCOOH & CH_3CH_2CHCOOH & CH_3CHCH_2COOH \\
\quad\quad\quad\quad | & \quad\quad\; | & | \\
\quad\quad\quad\; CH_3 & \quad\; CH_3 & CH_3
\end{array}
$$

2-methylpentanoic acid   2-methylbutanoic acid   3-methylbutanoic acid

138. **(B)** To name an alcohol, find the longest carbon chain containing the alcohol carbon, number the carbons of that chain such that the alcohol carbon has the lower number, and then identify any branches off the chain. That leads us to either (B) or (C) as the correct choice. Since there is a chiral center whose 3D arrangement has been specified in the structure, R or S can be designated. Assign priorities to the four groups attached to the chiral center based on atomic number. Here, the OH group would be number 1, the isopropyl group would be number 2, the methyl group would be number 3, and the hydrogen group would be number 4. Orient the molecule such that priority group number 4 is away from you and look at the other three groups. If they are arranged 1, 2, 3 clockwise, it's called R and if counterclockwise, it's S.

139. **(B)** $\% = \dfrac{\text{Part}}{\text{Whole}} \times 100$

$$\frac{8H}{(NH_4)_2\,SO_4} \times 100 = \frac{8}{132} \times 100 = 6.06\%$$

140. **(C)** An aldehyde is very easily oxidized and is converted to a carboxylic acid.

$$\underset{RCH}{\overset{O}{\overset{\|}{}}} \xrightarrow{\;[O]\;} \underset{RCOH}{\overset{O}{\overset{\|}{}}}$$

141. **(B)** Density is defined as mass divided by volume. The density of the sample is its mass, 6.0 g, divided by the volume of water, which is the difference between the final volume and the initial volume, 20 mL – 16 mL, of the water displaced by the object.

$$\frac{6\text{ g}}{4\text{ mL}} = \frac{1.50\text{ g}}{\text{mL}}$$

142. **(C)** Molarity is defined as moles of solute divided by liters of solution.

$$M = \frac{\text{moles of solute}}{\text{liters of solution}} = \frac{\text{g/mol. wt.}}{\text{liters of solution}}$$

Sugar, $C_6H_{12}O_6$, has a molecular weight of 180 g/mole. Substitute 18 g, 180 g/mole, and 0.5 M into the above equation to obtain the volume of the solution.

$$M = \frac{18\text{ g}/180\text{ g /mole}}{x} = 0.5\text{ M}$$

$$x = 0.2\text{ L} = 200\text{ mL}$$

143. **(D)** Nuclear fission is the breakdown of a larger nucleus, usually by bombarding it with neutrons, to produce smaller atoms and more neutrons. A great deal of energy is released in this process, which is the basis for the atomic bomb. Radioactive decay is the spontaneous emission of nuclear particles, eg. alpha and beta particles, as well as gamma rays, by unstable nuclei. Carbon-14 dating is a method of determining the age of an object by comparing the amount of carbon-12 and the amount of radioactive carbon-14 present in the object. Nuclear fusion is the combination of small nucleii to produce a larger atom with the concomitant release of a large amount of energy. Nuclear fusion occurs on the sun. The hydrogen bomb is an example of nuclear fusion.

144. **(B)** Ozonolysis with reductive work up cleaves alkenes and alkynes. For alkenes, the double bond is cleaved and replaced with carbonyl groups on each carbon of the alkene. For alkynes, the triple bond is cleaved and replaced with carboxylic acid groups on each carbon of the alkyne. Acetic acid is CH_3CO_2H, so the reacting organic molecule must have been an alkyne and since two moles of acetic acid resulted, the alkyne must have had a methyl group on each alkyne carbon.

145. **(A)** Note that $\sqrt{32} + \sqrt{8} = \sqrt{16 \cdot 2} + \sqrt{4 \cdot 2} = 4\sqrt{2} + 2\sqrt{2} = 6\sqrt{2}$.

146. **(B)** Use the Quotient Rule for derivatives.

$$\frac{d}{dx}\left(\frac{f(x)}{g(x)}\right) = \frac{g(x) \cdot f'(x) - g'(x) \cdot f(x)}{(g(x))^2} = \frac{(x^2 + 3)(1) - (2x)(x)}{(x^2 + 3)^2}$$

$$= \frac{x^2 + 3 - 2x^2}{(x^2 + 3)^2} = \frac{3 - x^2}{(x^2 + 3)^2}$$

147. **(A)** The discriminant for this quadratic equation is given by $b^2 - 4ac = 5^2 - 4 \cdot 2 = 25 - 8 = 17 > 0$. Thus, there are two real roots.

148. **(B)** There is a total of 25 pieces of fruit, and 4 are lemons.

Thus, we use the formula: Probability $= \dfrac{4}{25} = 0.16 = 16\%$.

149. **(C)** $5^2 + 5^3 = 25 + 125 = 150$.

150. **(B)** Given the function $f(x) = \dfrac{x+1}{10x}$, we solve for y in the equation

$x = \dfrac{y+1}{10y}$, that is, $\qquad x = \dfrac{y+1}{10y}$

$$10xy = y + 1$$

$$10xy - y = 1$$

$$y(10x - 1) = 1 \Rightarrow y = \dfrac{1}{10x - 1}.$$

151. **(B)** To find the limit as x approaches ∞, notice that the expression

$\dfrac{8x^6 + 5x^4 - x + 1000}{3x^6 + 21x^3 - 4}$ has the largest power of x in both the numerator

and the denominator. Thus, as x approaches ∞, the expression

$\dfrac{8x^6 + 5x^4 - x + 1000}{3x^6 + 21x^3 - 4}$ is dominated by these highest powered terms, i.e.,

$\dfrac{8x^6}{3x^6}$. The value of this resulting fraction approaches $\dfrac{8}{3}$ as x approaches ∞.

$$\lim_{x \to \infty} \left(\frac{8x^6 + 5x^4 - x + 1000}{3x^6 + 21x^3 - 4} \right) = \frac{8}{3}$$

152. **(A)** We complete the square on the given equation as follows.

$x^2 + y^2 - 12x + 14y + 9 = 0$
$x^2 - 12x + 36 + y^2 + 14y + 49 = -9 + 36 + 49$
$(x - 6)^2 + (y + 7)^2 = 76$
$(x - 6)^2 + (y + 7)^2 = \left(\sqrt{76} \right)^2$

Now use the fact that a circle with equation $(x - h)^2 + (y - k)^2 = r^2$ has center point (h, k) and radius equal to r. In the given equation,

we have $(x - 6)^2 + (y + 7)^2 = \left(\sqrt{76} \right)^2$. Thus, the radius equals $\sqrt{76}$.

153. **(C)** We compute the definite integral

$$\int_{-3}^{0} \left(x^3 - 9x \right) dx = \frac{1}{4}x^4 - \frac{9}{2}x^2 \bigg]_{-3}^{0} = 0 - \left(\frac{81}{4} - \frac{81}{2} \right) = 20.25.$$

154. **(D)** There are 6 numbers divisible by 3 or 4, that is, 3, 4, 6, 8, 9, and 12.

We use the formula: Probability $= \dfrac{6}{12} = 0.5 = 50\%$.

155. **(D)** We use the fundamental theorem of calculus for integrals.

$$\int_1^2 \left(5x^4\right) dx = \frac{5x^5}{5}\bigg|_1^2 = x^5\bigg|_1^2 = 2^5 - 1^5 = 32 - 1 = 31.$$

156. **(D)** We simplify the expression as follows.

If $x < 6$, then $x - 6 < 0$. Thus, $|x - 6| = -(x - 6)$. Therefore,

$$\frac{x^2 - 7x + 6}{|x - 6|} = \frac{(x-6)(x-1)}{-(x-6)} = -(x-1) = -x + 1.$$

157. **(C)** We simplify the expression as follows.

$$\frac{x^2 - 11x + 24}{x - 8} = \frac{(x-8)(x-3)}{x-8} = x - 3$$

158. **(B)** We use the quadratic formula.

$$x = \frac{-b \pm \sqrt{b^2 - 4ac}}{2a} = \frac{-1 \pm \sqrt{1^2 - 4 \cdot 6 \cdot 1}}{2 \cdot 6} = \frac{-1 \pm \sqrt{-23}}{12}$$

Since $\sqrt{-23}$ is not a real number, the equation has no real solutions.

159. **(A)** Each point on the graph of $y = 5f(x + 2) - 3$ is obtained by transforming the points on the graph of $y = f(x)$ as follows. Subtract 2 from each x coordinate; multiply each y coordinate by 5 and then subtract 3.

160. **(A)** Note that $\log_7(49) = x$ is equivalent to the equation $7^x = 49$. This equation has solution $x = 2$.

161. **(B)** Note that

$$\lim_{x \to 4}\left(\frac{x^2 - 10x + 24}{4 - x}\right) = \lim_{x \to 4}\left(\frac{(x-4)(x-6)}{4 - x}\right) =$$

$$\lim_{x \to 4}\left(\frac{(x-4)(x-6)}{-(x-4)}\right) = \lim_{x \to 4}(-(x-6)) = -(4-6) = 2$$

162. **(B)** Add $8 + 35 + 8 + 9 + 5 + 10 + 7 + 3 + 12 = 97$. Then, divide 97 by 9, which is the total amount of numbers in the set; therefore, $97 \div 9 = 10.77$.

163. **(D)** The total rental cost is given by the daily cost plus the mileage cost. Daily cost = ($30 per day)(7 days) = $210. Mileage cost = ($0.14 per mile)(x miles) = $0.14x$.

164. **(A)** The probability of heads on a coin toss is $\frac{1}{2}$. Since there are four

tosses, each with a probability of $\frac{1}{2}$ for heads, we have:

$$\frac{1}{2} \cdot \frac{1}{2} \cdot \frac{1}{2} \cdot \frac{1}{2} = \frac{1}{16}$$

165. **(D)** We compute the derivative $f'(t) = 15t^2 \cdot e^{t^3-1}$ and then evaluate at $t = 1$.

$f'(1) = 15 \cdot e^0 = 15.$

166. **(C)** To compute $(f+g)(x)$, add the function formulas for f and g, then combine like terms.

$$(f+g)(x) = x^2 + 2x - 1 + 2x + 1 = x^2 + 4x$$

167. **(B)** We solve the equation as follows.

$4(x+3)(x-2) = 4x^2 + x$
$4(x^2 + x - 6) = 4x^2 + x$
$4x^2 + 4x - 24 = 4x^2 + x$
$4x - 24 = x$
$3x = 24 \Rightarrow x = 8$

168. **(A)** Each time a die is rolled, there are two possible outcomes: an even number or an odd number. Therefore, the probability that the die will land on an odd number is 50%.

169. **(D)** Note that $\frac{5}{9} - \frac{3}{10} = \frac{5 \cdot 10 - 3 \cdot 9}{9 \cdot 10} = \frac{50 - 27}{90} = \frac{23}{90}$.

170. **(B)** The mode of a list of numbers is the number that occurs most frequently. The number 6, which occurs four times, is the mode of the given data set.

171. **(D)** There are 2 ways that the sum of the numbers shown can equal 5, that is, $1 + 4$ and $2 + 3$. Note that there are 6 possible outcomes for each die in the pair. Therefore, to calculate the possible combinations for the pair, we multiple $6 \cdot 6 = 36$. So, the probability that the sum of the numbers shown

equals 5 is $\frac{2}{36} = \frac{1}{18}$. Thus, the probability that the sum of the numbers

shown is NOT equal to 5 is $1 - \frac{1}{18} = \frac{17}{18}$.

172. **(A)** We can use the *Power Rule* for integrals to integrate term-by-term.

$$\int (x+2)\,dx = \int x\,dx + \int 2\,dx$$
$$= \int x\,dx + 2\int x^0\,dx$$
$$= \frac{1}{2}x^2 + 2x + C$$

173. **(A)** We use the integration rule

$$\int_e^{e^2}\left(\frac{6}{x}\right)dx = 6\ln(x)\Big]_e^{e^2} = 6\ln(e^2) - 6\ln(e) = 6\cdot 2 - 6\cdot 1 = 6.$$

174. **(B)** We use the Product Rule for derivatives

$$\frac{d}{dx}\big(f(x)\cdot g(x)\big) = f'(x)\cdot g(x) + f(x)\cdot g'(x)$$

and the fact that $\dfrac{d}{dx}e^{2x} = 2e^{2x}$ and $\dfrac{d}{dx}\sin(x) = \cos(x)$.

175. **(A)** The quadratic equation $\pi x^2 + 8x + w = 0$ has a double root when the discriminant equals zero. So we solve $b^2 - 4ac = 64 - 4\pi w = 0$, which yields $w = \dfrac{16}{\pi}$.

176. **(C)** To find the domain of a rational function, we must make sure that the expression in the denominator is never equal to 0.

$f(x) = \dfrac{3x-12}{x^2+7x+10}$ requires that $x^2 + 7x + 10 \neq 0$.

Note that $x^2 + 7x + 10 = 0$ when $(x+5)(x+2) = 0$.

Thus the domain is $\{x \mid x \neq -5,\ x \neq -2\}$.

177. **(B)** Note that $9^3 \cdot 9^{-1} = 9^{3-1} = 9^2 = 81$.

178. **(D)** The total number of ways to choose 3 girls and 1 boy is given by

the formula $\underbrace{{}_5C_3}_{\substack{\text{choose}\\\text{3 girls}}} \cdot \underbrace{{}_3C_1}_{\substack{\text{choose}\\\text{1 boy}}} = \dfrac{5!}{3!2!} \cdot \dfrac{3!}{1!2!} = 10\cdot 3 = 30$. The total number of

ways to choose 4 people is given by the formula ${}_8C_4 = \dfrac{8!}{4!4!} = \dfrac{1680}{24} = 70$.

Thus, probability $= \dfrac{30}{70} = \dfrac{3}{7}$.

179. **(B)** A quadratic function $f(x) = ax^2 + bx + c$ will have its vertex at the

point $\left(-\dfrac{b}{2a}, f\left(-\dfrac{b}{2a} \right) \right)$.

$f(x) = 9x^2 + 18x - 7 \Rightarrow = -\dfrac{b}{2a} = -\dfrac{18}{2(9)} = -\dfrac{18}{18} = -1$

$f(-1) = 9(-1)^2 + 18(-1) - 7 = 9 - 18 - 7 = -16$

Thus, the vertex is $(-1, -16)$.

180. **(A)** We compute the derivative $f'(x) = 12x^2 + 7$, and then evaluate $f'(-1) = 12(-1)^2 + 7 = 12 + 7 = 19$.

181. **(A)** We solve the equation as follows.

$\ln(2w + 9x) = 4$

$e^{\ln(2w + 9x)} = e^4$

$2w + 9x = e^4 \Rightarrow 9x = e^4 - 2w \Rightarrow x = \dfrac{e^4 - 2w}{9}$

182. **(B)** We have the ratio $\dfrac{3 \text{ apples}}{7 \text{ oranges}} \Rightarrow \dfrac{3 \cdot 3 \text{ apples}}{7 \cdot 3 \text{ oranges}} = \dfrac{9 \text{ apples}}{21 \text{ oranges}}$.

183. **(C)** Note that $\dfrac{2 + \sqrt{3}}{2 - \sqrt{3}} \cdot \dfrac{3 + \sqrt{3}}{2 + \sqrt{3}} = \dfrac{6 + 5\sqrt{3} + 3}{4 - 3} = \dfrac{9 + 5\sqrt{3}}{1} = 9 + 5\sqrt{3}$.

184. **(A)** Consider the Venn diagram.

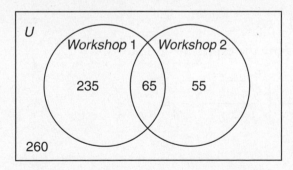

The total number of employees = $260 + 235 + 65 + 55 = 615$.

185. **(B)** Note that $\lim\limits_{x \to 11.5}\left(\dfrac{f(x) - f(11.5)}{x - 11.5}\right)$ = the derivative of f at $x = 11.5$.

Recall that the derivative gives the slope or the tangent line to the graph at the point of tangency. Note that the tangent line to the given graph is horizontal at the point where $x = 11.5$. Thus the slope equals 0 there.

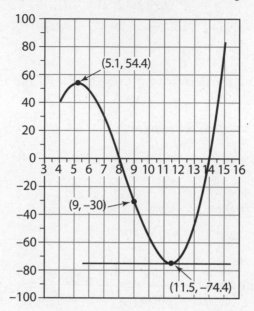

186. **(D)** A logarithmic function is undefined unless the input value is strictly greater than zero. Thus, we solve $2x - 7 > 0$ and obtain $x > 3.5$.

187. **(D)** $P(x) = 50x^2 + 300x - 65$ is a quadratic function whose graph opens up.

The minimum value occurs at the vertex, that is, when $x = -\dfrac{300}{100} = -3$.

Thus, $P(-3) = -515$.

188. **(C)** We simplify the expression as follows.

$$\frac{\sqrt{x+h} + \sqrt{x}}{h} \cdot \left(\frac{\sqrt{x+h} - \sqrt{x}}{\sqrt{x+h} - \sqrt{x}}\right) =$$

$$\frac{x + h - x}{h\left(\sqrt{x+h} - \sqrt{x}\right)} = \frac{h}{h\left(\sqrt{x+h} - \sqrt{x}\right)} = \frac{1}{\sqrt{x+h} - \sqrt{x}}$$

189. **(B)** The *Quotient Rule* for logarithms states that

$$\log(M) - \log(N) = \log\left(\frac{M}{N}\right)$$

$$\log(75) - \log(3) = \log\left(\frac{75}{3}\right)$$

$$= \log(25)$$

190. **(A)** The truck must travel 48 miles in 45 minutes = 0.75 hour.
We have the formula

$$\text{speed} = \frac{\text{distance}}{\text{time}} = \frac{48 \text{ miles}}{0.75 \text{ hr}} = 64 \text{ mph}$$

191. **(B)** A circle with equation $(x - h)^2 + (y - k)^2 = r^2$ has radius equal to r.
In the given equation, we have $(x - 5)^2 + (y - 6)^2 = (3)^2$.
Thus, the radius equals 3.

192. **(D)** We solve the equation as follows.

$$\frac{x}{x+3} + \frac{x}{x+2} = 2$$

$$\frac{x(x+2) + x(x+3)}{(x+3)(x+2)} = 2$$

$$x(x+2) + x(x+3) = 2(x+3)(x+2)$$

$$x^2 + 2x + x^2 + 3x = 2x^2 + 10x + 12$$

$$5x = 10x + 12$$

$$-5x = 12 \Rightarrow x = -\frac{12}{5}$$

The numbers in the margins of the reprinted passages indicate the statements in which the answer to the questions can be found.

Passage 1

193 Although phenytoin may be used to treat cardiac arrhythmias, migraines, and
194 trigeminal neuralgia, the primary use of phenytoin is to treat seizure disorders. Phenytoin, one of the most important agents used to manage seizures, works similarly to those of other hydantoin-derivative anticonvulsants. It decreases seizure activ-
195 ity by stabilizing neuronal membranes and by increasing efflux or decreasing influx of sodium ions across cell membranes in the motor cortex during generation of nerve impulses. Phenytoin is commercially available as oral suspension, tablets, and capsules. It is also available as an injection. The dosage of phenytoin varies according to
196 the frequency of seizures, the type of seizures, and the patient's tolerance for phenytoin. Therefore, it is extremely important to monitor the patient for seizure activity
197 as well as to monitor phenytoin serum concentrations. Phenytoin has a narrow therapeutic window and monitoring of serum concentrations is necessary. Therapeutic serum concentrations of phenytoin are usually 10–20 mcg per mL (millimeter) and depend on the assay method used. Serum concentrations above 20 mcg per mL often
199 result in toxicity. Adverse reactions associated with dose-related toxicities include blurred vision, lethargy, rash, fever, slurred speech, nystagmus, and confusion. In some patients, seizure control is not achieved when plasma concentrations are within the therapeutic concentration range and therefore clinical response of the patient is
200 more meaningful than plasma concentrations. Generally, therapeutic steady state serum concentrations are achieved within 30 days of therapy with an oral dosage of 300 mg daily in adults. Following an intravenous administration of 1000–1500 mg, at a rate not exceeding 50 mg per minute, therapeutic concentrations can be attained
198 within 2 hours. Rapid administration of intravenous phenytoin may result in adverse effects such as decreased blood pressure and other cardiac complications. The use of phenytoin has been associated with osteomalacia, thrombocytopenia, and gastrointestinal upset.

193. **(A)** Trigeminal neuralgia is treated with the phenytoin. Arthritis (B) is not mentioned in the passage; osteomalacia (C) is mentioned as a possible adverse effect; and nystagmus (D) is mentioned as an adverse reaction associated with toxicity.

194. **(C)** The first sentence clearly states that phenytoin is most commonly used to treat seizure disorders. Cardiac arrythmias (A) and migraines (B) are mentioned as other possible uses; arthritis (D) is not mentioned in the passage.

195. **(C)** Neither answer A nor answer B appears in the passage, and answer D states the opposite of the correct answer.

196. **(D)** Although phenytoin serum concentration (A), number of seizures (B), and adverse events (C) are listed as factors that affect the dosage of phenytoin, puncture sites available are not mentioned in the passage.

197. **(D)** Answer A incorrectly implies that phenytoin produces seizures; answer B incorrectly states that there is no known difference between the serum concentrations known to produce desirable and undesirable effects; and answer C refers to migraines rather than to seizures.

198. **(B)** A higher rate of administration may lower blood pressure. Answer A is irrelevant; answer C is inaccurate; and answer D refers to a condition (rash) that may be associated with phenytoin toxicity but not with the rapid administration of intravenous phenytoin.

199. **(C)** Blurred vision (A), lethargy (B), and mental confusion (D) are mentioned in the passage as adverse reactions associated with drug-related toxicities. There is no reference to dysuria.

200. **(D)** The passage states only that the therapeutic steady state serum concentration may be achieved within 30 days with an oral dosage of 300 mg daily of phenytoin. Therefore, 5 days (A), 24 hours (B), and 6 days (C) are all inaccurate.

Passage 2

Hypercalcemia, increased serum calcium concentrations, occurs in approximately 15% of individuals with cancer. Occurrences of this condition have been reported in most types of malignancies. The most effective management of treating this life-threatening disease is successful treatment of the malignancy. Unfortunately, successful treatment of the cancer may not be possible. In these cases, treatment goals should include correcting intravascular depletion, enhancing renal excretion of calcium, and inhibiting bone resorption. First line treatment of acute hypercalcemia includes the administration of normal saline and furosemide. Since many patients suffering from acute hypercalcemia are dehydrated, the administration of normal saline is warranted. In addition to treating dehydration, normal saline helps to increase renal excretion of calcium. The optimal administration of normal saline is dependent on the severity of hypercalcemia, the degree of dehydration, and the clinical status of the patient. An infusion rate of 400 mL per hour of normal saline is typical. Furosemide, a diuretic, is useful in the treatment of hypercalcemia due to its ability to enhance urinary excretion and, more importantly, calcium excretion. Additionally, furosemide protects patients from becoming volume overloaded due to the administration of the normal saline. <u>It is very important that patients be adequately hydrated prior to the administration of furosemide in order to get maximum benefits.</u> Intravenous doses of 100 mg of furosemide every 2 hours may be used. Although normal saline and furosemide are the most commonly used agents to treat acute cancer hypercalemia, only a modest decrease in calcium levels are achieved from this regimen. <u>The use of normal saline and furosemide may be sufficient for the management of mild to moderate hypercalcemia, but it is commonly insufficient for treating severe hypercalcemia.</u>

201. **(B)** Hypercalcemia has been reported in most types of malignancies. Answer A is clearly incorrect, since it states the inverse of B; answers C and D are incorrect because they refer only to specific kinds of malignancies.

202. **(D)** The passage is not concerned with the pathogenesis of cancer-related hypercalcemia (A); it does not cover all the uses of normal saline and furosemide (B); nor does it deal with the general characteristics or severity of cancer-related hypercalcemia (C). The focus is first line agents (normal saline and furosemide) used to manage acute cancer-related hypercalcemia.

203. **(C)** To obtain maximum benefits from the administration of furosemide, it is important to hydrate the patient before administering the diuretic. Answers A, B, and D are not mentioned in the passage.

204. **(D)** The passage states that cancer-related hypercalcemia is most effectively managed by successful treatment of the malignancy. Both normal saline (A) and furosemide (B) are agents used in first line treatment of cancer-related hypercalcemia when successful treatment of the cancer may not be possible. Dialysis (C) is not mentioned in the passage.

205. **(A)** The passage states that treatment goals should include enhancing renal excretion of calcium (B), inhibiting bone resorption (C), and correcting intravascular depletion (D). However, administrating calcium carbonate (A) is not mentioned in the passage.

206. **(B)** The passage states that since many patients suffering from acute hypercalcemia are dehydrated, the administration of normal saline is warranted.

207. **(D)** The last sentence of the passage clearly states that a normal saline-furosemide regimen alone is insufficient for treating severe hypercalcemia. However, it is usually effective in mild cancer-related hypercalcemia (A), mild hypercalcemia (B), and moderate hypercalcemia (C).

Passage 3

Gastroesophageal reflux disease (GERD) is a common medical disorder seen by health care practitioners of all specialties. It is generally chronic in nature, and long-term therapy may be required. <u>While the mortality associated with GERD is very low (1 death per 100,000 patients), the quality of life experienced by the patient can be greatly diminished.</u>

GERD refers to any symptomatic clinical condition or histologic alteration that results from episodes of gastroesophageal reflux. Gastroesophageal reflux refers to the retrograde movement of gastric contents from the stomach into the esophagus. Many people experience some degree of reflux, especially after eating, which may be considered a benign physiologic process. When the esophagus is repeatedly exposed 210 to refluxed material for prolonged periods of time, inflammation of the esophagus (i.e., reflux esophagitis) can occur. It is important to realize that gastroesophageal reflux must precede the development of GERD or reflux esophagitis. In severe cases, reflux may lead to a multitude of serious complications including esophageal stric- 209 tures, esophageal ulcers, motility disorders, perforation, hemorrhage, aspiration, and Barrett's esophagus. While mild disease is often managed with life-style changes and antacids, more intensive therapeutic intervention with histamine (H$_2$) antago- nists, sucralfate, prokinetic agents, or proton pump inhibitors is generally required for patients with more severe disease. In general, response to pharmacologic inter- 212 vention is dependent on the efficacy of the agent, dosage regimen employed, duration of therapy, and severity of the disease. Following discontinuation of ther- 211 apy, relapse is common and long-term maintenance therapy may be required. Historically, surgical intervention has been reserved for patients in whom conven- tional treatment modalities fail. However, the recent development of laparoscopic antireflux surgical procedures has led to a reevaluation of the role of surgery in the long-term maintenance of GERD. Some clinicians have suggested that laparoscopic 214 antireflux surgery may be a cost-effective alternative to long-term maintenance ther- apy in young patients. However, long-term comparative trials evaluating the cost 213 effectiveness of the various treatment modalities are warranted.

The pathogenesis of gastroesophageal reflux is related to the complex balance between defense mechanisms and aggressive factors. Understanding both the nor- mal protective mechanisms and the aggressive factors that may contribute to or pro- mote gastroesophageal reflux helps one to design rational therapeutic treatment regimens. Gastric acid, pepsin, bile acids, and pancreatic enzymes are considered aggressive factors and may promote esophageal damage upon reflux into the esoph- 215 agus. Thus, the composition (potency) and volume of the refluxate are aggressive factors that may lead to esophageal injury. Conversely, normal protective mecha- nisms include anatomic factors, lower esophageal sphincter pressure, esophageal clearing, mucosal resistance, and gastric emptying. Rational therapeutic regimens in the treatment of gastroesophageal reflux are designed to maximize normal defense mechanisms and/or attenuate the aggressive factors.

208. **(C)** Answers A, B, and D all consist of true statements taken directly from the passage. Answer C, however, is a false statement: the mortality associ- ated with GERD is very low, not high.

209. **(A)** One possible complication of reflux is perforation. Mucosal resistance (B), gastric emptying (C), and lower esophageal sphincter pressure (D) are all cited in the passage as normal protective mechanisms.

210. **(C)** The passage states when the esophagus is repeatedly exposed to refluxed material for prolonged periods of time, inflammation of the esophagus (i.e., reflux esophagitis) can occur.

211. **(C)** The passage states that following discontinuation of therapy, relapse is common and long-term maintenance therapy may be required.

212. **(D)** Dosage regimen employed (A), efficacy of the agent (B), and severity of the disease (C) all play a part in GERD patients' response to pharmacologic intervention.

213. **(A)** The passage states that long-term comparative trials evaluating the cost effectiveness of various treatment modalities for GERD are warranted.

214. **(C)** The passage states that laparoscopic antireflux surgery has been suggested as a possible cost-effective alternative therapy.

215. **(A)** Gastric acid and pancreatic enzymes are aggressive factors and may promote esophageal damage upon reflux into the esophagus. The factors in answer C are protective, and the factors in answer B are a combination of aggressive (bile acids) and protective (esophageal clearing).

Passage 4

Many people in the United States are diagnosed with diabetes mellitus. Non-insulin-dependent diabetes mellitus (NIDDM) is the most common type of diabetes and it is associated with a significant amount of morbidities and mortalities. NIDDM is classified as an endocrine disorder characterized by defects in insulin secretion as well as in insulin action. In NIDDM patients a defect also exists in insulin receptor binding. These defects lead to increased serum glucose concentrations or hyperglycemia.

Sulfonylureas are one of the most popular classes of agents used to treat NIDDM. One of the newest agents to treat NIDDM is acarbose, an oral alpha-glucosidase inhibitor. Acarbose interferes with the hydrolysis of dietary disaccharides and complex carbohydrates, thereby delaying absorption of glucose and other monosaccharides. Acarbose is available for oral administration only. To be most effective, it should be taken at the beginning of a meal. The recommended starting dose is 25 mg three times daily and doses as high as 200 mg three times a day have been safely used. The most common adverse experiences associated with the use of acarbose are abdominal cramps, flatulence, diarrhea, and abdominal distension. Most of the adverse effects are due to the unabsorbed carbohydrates undergoing fermentation in the colon. Acarbose has also been associated with decreased intestinal absorption of iron thereby possibly leading to anemia. The occurrence of hypoglycemia when using acarbose in combination with other agents used to lower serum glucose is great. Glucose should be administered to treat hypoglycemia in patients taking acarbose because sucrose may not be adequately hydrolyzed and absorbed. The effectiveness of this agent to lower serum glucose concentrations in patients with NIDDM has been clearly demonstrated in clinical trials. Acarbose provides another option for treating NIDDM.

216. **(D)** Whereas "endocrine in nature" (A), "hyperglycemia" (B), and "may be due to a defect in insulin receptor binding" (C) are stated in, or may be inferred from, the passage, "results in iron deficiencies" is not listed as a

characteristic of insulin-dependent diabetes. Rather, it is mentioned as a possible adverse effect of acarbose.

217. **(A)** The passage states that a sulfonylurea agent is one of the most popular classes of agents used to treat NIDDM. Glucose (B), sucrose (C), and fructose (D) all represent types of sugar.

218. **(A)** The passage states that Acarbose is available for oral administration only, and to be most effective, it should be taken at the beginning of a meal.

219. **(C)** Hyperglycemia (A) is a characteristic of NIDDM; anemia (B) is a possible adverse effect of acarbose, but not one of the most common side effects; rash (D) is not mentioned in the passage. Gastrointestinal discomfort is stated to be the most common side effect of acarbose.

220. **(B)** The passage states that glucose is the best choice for patients taking acarbose. A sulfurylurea agent (A) is the most popular class of agents used to treat NIDDM. Sucrose (C) is mentioned in the passage as a sugar that the patient may not be able to adequately hydrolyze and absorb, and fructose (D) is not mentioned at all.

221. **(D)** Although low serum glucose concentration (A), gastrointestinal discomfort (B), and decreased iron absorption (C) are all described in the passage as possible adverse effects associated with the use of acarbose, obstruction of the urinary tract is not mentioned.

222. **(A)** The passage states that sulfonylureas are one of the most popular classes of agents used to treat NIDDM and that using acarbose in combination with other agents may lead to hypoglycemia. Glucose (B), iron (C), and increased caloric intake (D) are not described as having this effect.

223. **(C)** Since the passage does not cover the topic of diabetes in the United States, answer A cannot be the correct choice. Nor does the passage deal with all the various agents used to treat NIDDM, so answer B is ruled out. Answer D is too specific; the passage does deal with some adverse effects of acarbose, but it covers much more than that. The best title for the passage is The Use of Acarbose in the Treatment of Non-Insulin-Dependent Diabetes Mellitus.

Passage 5

Osteoporosis, the most common skeletal disorder associated with aging, is a significant cause of mortality and morbidity among the elderly. The two most common types of osteoporosis are type I (postmenopausal) osteoporosis and type II (senile) osteoporosis. Type I osteoporosis is due to a drastic decline in bone mass during the first five years of menopause and a slower rate of bone loss in subsequent years. Type II osteoporosis is characterized by a gradual, age-related loss of bone in females and males over the age of 65 years. <u>By far, osteoporosis is most prevalent in the post-</u> 224
<u>menopausal population. In addition to menopausal-associated hormonal changes,</u> 225
<u>other risk factors for osteoporosis in women include low calcium intake, medical</u>
<u>factors such as oophorectomy, and life-style factors such as inactivity and cigarette</u>

229 smoking. In osteoporosis, osteoclasts excavate areas in bone that the bone forming
230 cells, the osteoblasts, are unable to fully reconstitute. Often this defective bone loses compressive strength, thereby leading to an increased risk of fracture. Osteoporosis
227 evolves as a silent disease with no obvious early warning signs. Many patients suffering from osteoporosis are not aware of their condition until a fracture occurs. This disease is responsible for at least 1.5 million fractures in Americans each year,
228 with annual costs to the United States health care system of approximately $10 billion. Other consequences of osteoporosis include pain and spinal deformities such
226 as dorsal kyphosis and dowager's or widow's hump. In addition, a decrease in appetite, fatigue, and weakness may be present. As the population continues to age, the cost of treating osteoporosis and its associated complications are predicted to
228 double over the next 30 years.

224. **(A)** Since the passage states that osteoporosis is associated with aging, infants (C) and teenagers (D) are clearly incorrect. Young males (B) is also incorrect; males with osteoporosis are described as over the age of 65. Postmenopausal women are the population in whom osteoporosis most commonly occurs.

225. **(C)** Age (A), low calcium intake (B), and cigarette smoking (D) are all mentioned or implied as risk factors; however, weight-bearing exercises is not. In fact, answer C is the opposite of one of the stated risk ractors, inactivity.

226. **(D)** The passage mentions dowager's hump as a consequence of osteoporosis. Height gain (A) is clearly not the best choice, since a decline in bone mass is more likely to lead to height loss. Oophorectomy (C) is mentioned in the passage as a risk factor for osteoporosis; hypertension (B) is irrelevant.

227. **(B)** The passage states that osteoporosis evolves as a silent disease with no obvious early warning signs, and that many patients who suffer from osteoporosis are not aware of their condition until a fracture occurs.

228. **(D)** The passage states that the current cost of treating osteoporosis is approximately $10 billion. The last sentence in the passage states that the cost of treating osteoporosis and its associated complications is predicted to double over the next 30 years; thus $20 billion is the correct answer.

229. **(A)** The passage states that osteoclasts excavate areas in bone. Osteoblasts (B) are also discussed in the passage, but they are the cells that form bone. The other two choices, osteomasts (C) and osteotrasts (D) are not mentioned in the passage and are therefore irrelevant.

230. **(B)** Osteoblasts are responsible for forming bone. As stated in the explanation for question 269, osteoclasts remove bone. Again, osteomasts (C) and osteotrasts (D) are irrelevant.

Passage 6

Bronchial asthma is a common disease of children and adults. Although the clinical 231
manifestations of asthma have been known since antiquity, it is a disease that still
defies precise definition. The word *asthma* is of Greek origin and means "panting."
More than 2000 years ago, Hippocrates used the word *asthma* to describe episodic 239
shortness of breath; however, the first detailed description of the asthmatic patient
was made by Aretaeus in the second century. Since that time *asthma* has been used
to describe any disorder with episodic shortness of breath or dyspnea; thus, the terms 232
cardiac asthma and *bronchial asthma* have been used to delineate the etiologies of the
dyspnea. These terms are now obsolete and asthma refers to a disorder of the respi- 238
ratory system characterized by episodes of difficulty in breathing. An Expert Panel of
the National Institutes of Health National Asthma Education Program (NAEP) has
defined asthma as a lung disease characterized by (1) airway obstruction that is
reversible (but not completely so in some patients) either spontaneously or with
treatment; (2) airway inflammation; and (3) increased airway responsiveness to a 233
variety of stimuli. This descriptive definition for asthma is attributed to our lack of
knowledge of the precise pathogenic defect that results in the clinical syndrome we
recognize as asthma. The current definition does allow for the important heterogeneity of the clinical presentation of asthma. New technologies have added substantially 235
to our understanding of the interrelationships of immunology, biochemistry, and
physiology to the clinical presentation of asthma, and further research may yet
uncover a specific genetic defect associated with asthma. Until such time, asthma will
continue to defy exact definition.

An estimated 10 million persons in the United States have asthma (about 5% of 237
the population). The reported prevalence increased 29% from 1980 to 1987 to 40.1
per 1000 population. African-Americans have a 19% higher incidence of asthma
than whites and are twice as likely to be hospitalized. The estimated cost of asthma
in the United States in 1990 was $6.2 billion. The largest single direct medical
expenditure was for inpatient hospital services (emergency care), reaching almost
$1.5 billion, followed by prescription medications ($1.1 billion). The costs of medication increased 54% between 1985 and 1990. In total, 43% of the economic 234
impact was associated with emergency room use, hospitalization, and death.
Asthma accounted for 1% of all ambulatory care visits according to the National
Ambulatory Medical Care Survey and results in more than 450,000 hospitalizations 236
per year.

231. **(B)** Answer B sums up the main point of the first paragraph of the passage.
Answer A is not true, since the passage states that the term *asthma* has been
defined precisely. Answer C is incorrect since *cardiac asthma* and *bronchial
asthma* are simply two terms that are no longer in use, although they were
used for a long time to delineate the etiologies of the dyspnea associated
with asthma. Answer D is incorrect because the statement that the NAEP's
definition of asthma does *not* allow for the heterogeneity of the clinical
presentation of the disease is false; in fact, the definition does allow for this.

232. **(D)** The passage states *cardiac asthma* and *bronchial asthma* are now two
obsolete terms that delineated the etiologies of dyspnea.

233. **(B)** The passage states that the NAEP defines asthma as a lung disease characterized by: (1) airway obstruction that is reversible, but not completely in some patients either spontaneously or with treatment; (2) airway inflammation; and (3) increased airway responsiveness to a variety of stimuli.

234. **(C)** Answers A, B, and D are true statements taken directly from the passage. In actuality, however, the cost of asthma medication *increased* (not decreased) 54% between 1985 and 1990.

235. **(C)** Wheezing and episodes of shortness of breath (B) and the interrelationship of immunology, biochemistry, and physiology (D) are already understood, and answer A is irrelevant. Researchers hope to uncover a specific genetic defect in asthma.

236. **(D)** No explanation necessary.

237. **(D)** The passage states that the estimated number of persons in the United States who have asthma is 10 million.

238. **(D)** Answers A, B, and C are incorrect choices, since "panting" (A) and dyspnea of cardiac or bronchial etiology (B) are obsolete definitions. Answer D represents the current definition of asthma.

239. **(C)** The passage states that more than 2,000 years ago Hippocrates used the word *asthma* to describe episodic shortness of breath.

240. **(D)** The passage does not go into the reasons for the worldwide increase in the prevalence of asthma. However, it does provide a descriptive definition of the disease (A) and also some facts about the prevalence of asthma in the United States (B).

Practice Test 2

This second sample PCAT is not a copy of an actual PCAT, but it has also been designed to closely represent the types of questions that may be included in an actual exam. Proceed with this practice exam as if you were taking the actual PCAT, adhering to the time allowed for each section in the table below.

Section	Time Allowed*
1. Verbal Ability	30 minutes
2. Chemistry	30 minutes
3. Biology	30 minutes
4. Reading Comprehension	50 minutes
5. Quantitative Ability	40 minutes
6. Writing (Essay)	30 minutes
7. Writing (Essay)	30 minutes

*Please note: The order of the subjects (test sections) may vary from test to test.

Answer Sheet
PRACTICE TEST 2

Verbal Ability (1–48)

1 Ⓐ Ⓑ Ⓒ Ⓓ　　13 Ⓐ Ⓑ Ⓒ Ⓓ　　25 Ⓐ Ⓑ Ⓒ Ⓓ　　37 Ⓐ Ⓑ Ⓒ Ⓓ
2 Ⓐ Ⓑ Ⓒ Ⓓ　　14 Ⓐ Ⓑ Ⓒ Ⓓ　　26 Ⓐ Ⓑ Ⓒ Ⓓ　　38 Ⓐ Ⓑ Ⓒ Ⓓ
3 Ⓐ Ⓑ Ⓒ Ⓓ　　15 Ⓐ Ⓑ Ⓒ Ⓓ　　27 Ⓐ Ⓑ Ⓒ Ⓓ　　39 Ⓐ Ⓑ Ⓒ Ⓓ
4 Ⓐ Ⓑ Ⓒ Ⓓ　　16 Ⓐ Ⓑ Ⓒ Ⓓ　　28 Ⓐ Ⓑ Ⓒ Ⓓ　　40 Ⓐ Ⓑ Ⓒ Ⓓ
5 Ⓐ Ⓑ Ⓒ Ⓓ　　17 Ⓐ Ⓑ Ⓒ Ⓓ　　29 Ⓐ Ⓑ Ⓒ Ⓓ　　41 Ⓐ Ⓑ Ⓒ Ⓓ
6 Ⓐ Ⓑ Ⓒ Ⓓ　　18 Ⓐ Ⓑ Ⓒ Ⓓ　　30 Ⓐ Ⓑ Ⓒ Ⓓ　　42 Ⓐ Ⓑ Ⓒ Ⓓ
7 Ⓐ Ⓑ Ⓒ Ⓓ　　19 Ⓐ Ⓑ Ⓒ Ⓓ　　31 Ⓐ Ⓑ Ⓒ Ⓓ　　43 Ⓐ Ⓑ Ⓒ Ⓓ
8 Ⓐ Ⓑ Ⓒ Ⓓ　　20 Ⓐ Ⓑ Ⓒ Ⓓ　　32 Ⓐ Ⓑ Ⓒ Ⓓ　　44 Ⓐ Ⓑ Ⓒ Ⓓ
9 Ⓐ Ⓑ Ⓒ Ⓓ　　21 Ⓐ Ⓑ Ⓒ Ⓓ　　33 Ⓐ Ⓑ Ⓒ Ⓓ　　45 Ⓐ Ⓑ Ⓒ Ⓓ
10 Ⓐ Ⓑ Ⓒ Ⓓ　　22 Ⓐ Ⓑ Ⓒ Ⓓ　　34 Ⓐ Ⓑ Ⓒ Ⓓ　　46 Ⓐ Ⓑ Ⓒ Ⓓ
11 Ⓐ Ⓑ Ⓒ Ⓓ　　23 Ⓐ Ⓑ Ⓒ Ⓓ　　35 Ⓐ Ⓑ Ⓒ Ⓓ　　47 Ⓐ Ⓑ Ⓒ Ⓓ
12 Ⓐ Ⓑ Ⓒ Ⓓ　　24 Ⓐ Ⓑ Ⓒ Ⓓ　　36 Ⓐ Ⓑ Ⓒ Ⓓ　　48 Ⓐ Ⓑ Ⓒ Ⓓ

Chemistry (49–96)

49 Ⓐ Ⓑ Ⓒ Ⓓ　　61 Ⓐ Ⓑ Ⓒ Ⓓ　　73 Ⓐ Ⓑ Ⓒ Ⓓ　　85 Ⓐ Ⓑ Ⓒ Ⓓ
50 Ⓐ Ⓑ Ⓒ Ⓓ　　62 Ⓐ Ⓑ Ⓒ Ⓓ　　74 Ⓐ Ⓑ Ⓒ Ⓓ　　86 Ⓐ Ⓑ Ⓒ Ⓓ
51 Ⓐ Ⓑ Ⓒ Ⓓ　　63 Ⓐ Ⓑ Ⓒ Ⓓ　　75 Ⓐ Ⓑ Ⓒ Ⓓ　　87 Ⓐ Ⓑ Ⓒ Ⓓ
52 Ⓐ Ⓑ Ⓒ Ⓓ　　64 Ⓐ Ⓑ Ⓒ Ⓓ　　76 Ⓐ Ⓑ Ⓒ Ⓓ　　88 Ⓐ Ⓑ Ⓒ Ⓓ
53 Ⓐ Ⓑ Ⓒ Ⓓ　　65 Ⓐ Ⓑ Ⓒ Ⓓ　　77 Ⓐ Ⓑ Ⓒ Ⓓ　　89 Ⓐ Ⓑ Ⓒ Ⓓ
54 Ⓐ Ⓑ Ⓒ Ⓓ　　66 Ⓐ Ⓑ Ⓒ Ⓓ　　78 Ⓐ Ⓑ Ⓒ Ⓓ　　90 Ⓐ Ⓑ Ⓒ Ⓓ
55 Ⓐ Ⓑ Ⓒ Ⓓ　　67 Ⓐ Ⓑ Ⓒ Ⓓ　　79 Ⓐ Ⓑ Ⓒ Ⓓ　　91 Ⓐ Ⓑ Ⓒ Ⓓ
56 Ⓐ Ⓑ Ⓒ Ⓓ　　68 Ⓐ Ⓑ Ⓒ Ⓓ　　80 Ⓐ Ⓑ Ⓒ Ⓓ　　92 Ⓐ Ⓑ Ⓒ Ⓓ
57 Ⓐ Ⓑ Ⓒ Ⓓ　　69 Ⓐ Ⓑ Ⓒ Ⓓ　　81 Ⓐ Ⓑ Ⓒ Ⓓ　　93 Ⓐ Ⓑ Ⓒ Ⓓ
58 Ⓐ Ⓑ Ⓒ Ⓓ　　70 Ⓐ Ⓑ Ⓒ Ⓓ　　82 Ⓐ Ⓑ Ⓒ Ⓓ　　94 Ⓐ Ⓑ Ⓒ Ⓓ
59 Ⓐ Ⓑ Ⓒ Ⓓ　　71 Ⓐ Ⓑ Ⓒ Ⓓ　　83 Ⓐ Ⓑ Ⓒ Ⓓ　　95 Ⓐ Ⓑ Ⓒ Ⓓ
60 Ⓐ Ⓑ Ⓒ Ⓓ　　72 Ⓐ Ⓑ Ⓒ Ⓓ　　84 Ⓐ Ⓑ Ⓒ Ⓓ　　96 Ⓐ Ⓑ Ⓒ Ⓓ

Answer Sheet

PRACTICE TEST 2

Biology (97–144)

97 Ⓐ Ⓑ Ⓒ Ⓓ	109 Ⓐ Ⓑ Ⓒ Ⓓ	121 Ⓐ Ⓑ Ⓒ Ⓓ	133 Ⓐ Ⓑ Ⓒ Ⓓ
98 Ⓐ Ⓑ Ⓒ Ⓓ	110 Ⓐ Ⓑ Ⓒ Ⓓ	122 Ⓐ Ⓑ Ⓒ Ⓓ	134 Ⓐ Ⓑ Ⓒ Ⓓ
99 Ⓐ Ⓑ Ⓒ Ⓓ	111 Ⓐ Ⓑ Ⓒ Ⓓ	123 Ⓐ Ⓑ Ⓒ Ⓓ	135 Ⓐ Ⓑ Ⓒ Ⓓ
100 Ⓐ Ⓑ Ⓒ Ⓓ	112 Ⓐ Ⓑ Ⓒ Ⓓ	124 Ⓐ Ⓑ Ⓒ Ⓓ	136 Ⓐ Ⓑ Ⓒ Ⓓ
101 Ⓐ Ⓑ Ⓒ Ⓓ	113 Ⓐ Ⓑ Ⓒ Ⓓ	125 Ⓐ Ⓑ Ⓒ Ⓓ	137 Ⓐ Ⓑ Ⓒ Ⓓ
102 Ⓐ Ⓑ Ⓒ Ⓓ	114 Ⓐ Ⓑ Ⓒ Ⓓ	126 Ⓐ Ⓑ Ⓒ Ⓓ	138 Ⓐ Ⓑ Ⓒ Ⓓ
103 Ⓐ Ⓑ Ⓒ Ⓓ	115 Ⓐ Ⓑ Ⓒ Ⓓ	127 Ⓐ Ⓑ Ⓒ Ⓓ	139 Ⓐ Ⓑ Ⓒ Ⓓ
104 Ⓐ Ⓑ Ⓒ Ⓓ	116 Ⓐ Ⓑ Ⓒ Ⓓ	128 Ⓐ Ⓑ Ⓒ Ⓓ	140 Ⓐ Ⓑ Ⓒ Ⓓ
105 Ⓐ Ⓑ Ⓒ Ⓓ	117 Ⓐ Ⓑ Ⓒ Ⓓ	129 Ⓐ Ⓑ Ⓒ Ⓓ	141 Ⓐ Ⓑ Ⓒ Ⓓ
106 Ⓐ Ⓑ Ⓒ Ⓓ	118 Ⓐ Ⓑ Ⓒ Ⓓ	130 Ⓐ Ⓑ Ⓒ Ⓓ	142 Ⓐ Ⓑ Ⓒ Ⓓ
107 Ⓐ Ⓑ Ⓒ Ⓓ	119 Ⓐ Ⓑ Ⓒ Ⓓ	131 Ⓐ Ⓑ Ⓒ Ⓓ	143 Ⓐ Ⓑ Ⓒ Ⓓ
108 Ⓐ Ⓑ Ⓒ Ⓓ	120 Ⓐ Ⓑ Ⓒ Ⓓ	132 Ⓐ Ⓑ Ⓒ Ⓓ	144 Ⓐ Ⓑ Ⓒ Ⓓ

Reading Comprehension (145–192)

145 Ⓐ Ⓑ Ⓒ Ⓓ	157 Ⓐ Ⓑ Ⓒ Ⓓ	169 Ⓐ Ⓑ Ⓒ Ⓓ	181 Ⓐ Ⓑ Ⓒ Ⓓ
146 Ⓐ Ⓑ Ⓒ Ⓓ	158 Ⓐ Ⓑ Ⓒ Ⓓ	170 Ⓐ Ⓑ Ⓒ Ⓓ	182 Ⓐ Ⓑ Ⓒ Ⓓ
147 Ⓐ Ⓑ Ⓒ Ⓓ	159 Ⓐ Ⓑ Ⓒ Ⓓ	171 Ⓐ Ⓑ Ⓒ Ⓓ	183 Ⓐ Ⓑ Ⓒ Ⓓ
148 Ⓐ Ⓑ Ⓒ Ⓓ	160 Ⓐ Ⓑ Ⓒ Ⓓ	172 Ⓐ Ⓑ Ⓒ Ⓓ	184 Ⓐ Ⓑ Ⓒ Ⓓ
149 Ⓐ Ⓑ Ⓒ Ⓓ	161 Ⓐ Ⓑ Ⓒ Ⓓ	173 Ⓐ Ⓑ Ⓒ Ⓓ	185 Ⓐ Ⓑ Ⓒ Ⓓ
150 Ⓐ Ⓑ Ⓒ Ⓓ	162 Ⓐ Ⓑ Ⓒ Ⓓ	174 Ⓐ Ⓑ Ⓒ Ⓓ	186 Ⓐ Ⓑ Ⓒ Ⓓ
151 Ⓐ Ⓑ Ⓒ Ⓓ	163 Ⓐ Ⓑ Ⓒ Ⓓ	175 Ⓐ Ⓑ Ⓒ Ⓓ	187 Ⓐ Ⓑ Ⓒ Ⓓ
152 Ⓐ Ⓑ Ⓒ Ⓓ	164 Ⓐ Ⓑ Ⓒ Ⓓ	176 Ⓐ Ⓑ Ⓒ Ⓓ	188 Ⓐ Ⓑ Ⓒ Ⓓ
153 Ⓐ Ⓑ Ⓒ Ⓓ	165 Ⓐ Ⓑ Ⓒ Ⓓ	177 Ⓐ Ⓑ Ⓒ Ⓓ	189 Ⓐ Ⓑ Ⓒ Ⓓ
154 Ⓐ Ⓑ Ⓒ Ⓓ	166 Ⓐ Ⓑ Ⓒ Ⓓ	178 Ⓐ Ⓑ Ⓒ Ⓓ	190 Ⓐ Ⓑ Ⓒ Ⓓ
155 Ⓐ Ⓑ Ⓒ Ⓓ	167 Ⓐ Ⓑ Ⓒ Ⓓ	179 Ⓐ Ⓑ Ⓒ Ⓓ	191 Ⓐ Ⓑ Ⓒ Ⓓ
156 Ⓐ Ⓑ Ⓒ Ⓓ	168 Ⓐ Ⓑ Ⓒ Ⓓ	180 Ⓐ Ⓑ Ⓒ Ⓓ	192 Ⓐ Ⓑ Ⓒ Ⓓ

Answer Sheet
PRACTICE TEST 2

Quantitative Ability (193–240)

193 (A) (B) (C) (D)	205 (A) (B) (C) (D)	217 (A) (B) (C) (D)	229 (A) (B) (C) (D)
194 (A) (B) (C) (D)	206 (A) (B) (C) (D)	218 (A) (B) (C) (D)	230 (A) (B) (C) (D)
195 (A) (B) (C) (D)	207 (A) (B) (C) (D)	219 (A) (B) (C) (D)	231 (A) (B) (C) (D)
196 (A) (B) (C) (D)	208 (A) (B) (C) (D)	220 (A) (B) (C) (D)	232 (A) (B) (C) (D)
197 (A) (B) (C) (D)	209 (A) (B) (C) (D)	221 (A) (B) (C) (D)	233 (A) (B) (C) (D)
198 (A) (B) (C) (D)	210 (A) (B) (C) (D)	222 (A) (B) (C) (D)	234 (A) (B) (C) (D)
199 (A) (B) (C) (D)	211 (A) (B) (C) (D)	223 (A) (B) (C) (D)	235 (A) (B) (C) (D)
200 (A) (B) (C) (D)	212 (A) (B) (C) (D)	224 (A) (B) (C) (D)	236 (A) (B) (C) (D)
201 (A) (B) (C) (D)	213 (A) (B) (C) (D)	225 (A) (B) (C) (D)	237 (A) (B) (C) (D)
202 (A) (B) (C) (D)	214 (A) (B) (C) (D)	226 (A) (B) (C) (D)	238 (A) (B) (C) (D)
203 (A) (B) (C) (D)	215 (A) (B) (C) (D)	227 (A) (B) (C) (D)	239 (A) (B) (C) (D)
204 (A) (B) (C) (D)	216 (A) (B) (C) (D)	228 (A) (B) (C) (D)	240 (A) (B) (C) (D)

Writing

For the essay portions of the test, please compose your responses on separate sheets of paper.

VERBAL ABILITY

48 QUESTIONS (#1–#48)

TIME: 30 MINUTES

Directions: Select the word that **best** completes the analogy.

1. SHALLOW : DEPTH :: APATHETIC :

   (A) Monopoly
   (B) Apology
   (C) Trying
   (D) Caring

2. GLUE : FASTEN :: ELEVATOR :

   (A) Launch
   (B) Service
   (C) Lift
   (D) Camp

3. ORACLE : FORESIGHT :: SAGE :

   (A) Wisdom
   (B) Talent
   (C) Wealth
   (D) Clarity

4. FLOWERS : FLORIST :: RINGS :

   (A) Tiara
   (B) Jeweler
   (C) Thorns
   (D) Roses

5. MECHANIC : WRENCH :: GARDENER :

   (A) Lawn
   (B) Grass seed
   (C) Annuals
   (D) Trowel

6. BUILDING : BLUEPRINT :: REPORT :

   (A) Outline
   (B) Canvas
   (C) Table
   (D) Artist

7. ANTISEPTIC : GERMS :: WATER :

   (A) Sterilized
   (B) Disinfectant
   (C) Thirst
   (D) Cook

8. SLUGGISH : ENERGY :: SATIATED :

   (A) Dissatisfied
   (B) Slothful
   (C) Wary
   (D) Hunger

9. LIBRARY : BOOK :: STABLE :

   (A) Horse
   (B) Automobile
   (C) Boat
   (D) Magazine

10. NEOPHYTE : EXPERIENCED :: INVALID :

    (A) Sickly
    (B) Healthy
    (C) Compliant
    (D) Wealthy

11. BUS : PASSENGERS :: FREIGHTER :

    (A) Requirement
    (B) Tires
    (C) Plane
    (D) Cargo

12. VERIFICATION : CONFIRM :: CONCILIATION :

    (A) Application
    (B) Appease
    (C) Reiteration
    (D) Affirm

13. EMBARGO : TRADE :: HELMET :

    (A) Injury
    (B) Respite
    (C) Football
    (D) Hearing

14. RESOLUTE : DETERMINATION ::
SKEPTICAL :

(A) Doubt
(B) Mutiny
(C) Hostility
(D) Certainty

15. METER : LENGTH :: POUND :

(A) Inch
(B) Yard
(C) Heavy
(D) Weight

16. ROSE : FLOWER :: ELM :

(A) Street
(B) Tree
(C) Plant
(D) Dew

17. HUMIDITY : SWAMP :: ARIDITY :

(A) Air-conditioning
(B) Desert
(C) Sea level
(D) Beach

18. ANACONDA : SNAKE :: BASKETBALL :

(A) Serve
(B) Sport
(C) Shorts
(D) Ball

19. BRUISE : SKIN :: STAIN :

(A) Muscle
(B) Bone
(C) Fabric
(D) Veneer

20. SPHYGMOMANOMETER : BLOOD
PRESSURE :: THERMOMETER :

(A) Temperature
(B) Fahrenheit
(C) Ampere
(D) Air

21. EBB : FLOW :: REGRESS :

(A) Advance
(B) Retard
(C) Shrink
(D) Backslide

22. OEDIPUS COMPLEX : FREUD ::
UNCERTAINTY PRINCIPLE :

(A) Hindenberg
(B) Heisenberg
(C) Jung
(D) Newton

23. HINDENBERG : BLIMPS :: TITANIC :

(A) Tragedies
(B) Oceans
(C) Icebergs
(D) Ocean liners

24. PHOENIX : ARIZONA :: ATLANTA :

(A) Georgia
(B) Fulton County
(C) Southeast United States
(D) North Carolina

25. ANTHROPOMORPHIC : HUMAN ::
THERIOMORPHIC :

(A) Inhuman
(B) Evolution
(C) Egypt
(D) Animal

26. BLUES : MISSISSIPPI :: BLUEGRASS :

    (A) Kentucky
    (B) Appalachia
    (C) Folk
    (D) Country

27. NUCLEAR MEMBRANE : CELL ::
    HYPOTENUSE :

    (A) Algebra
    (B) Hippocrates
    (C) Triangle
    (D) Pythagoras

28. BASS : TREBLE :: ACME :

    (A) Pitch
    (B) Rhythm
    (C) Peak
    (D) Nadir

29. IMPERCEPTIBLE : TANGIBLE :: MILD :

    (A) Tiny
    (B) Severe
    (C) Bland
    (D) Magnified

Directions: Select the word or set of words that makes the most sense when inserted into the sentence and that best fits the meaning of the sentence as a whole.

30. Since it had been lifeless for several years, there was a green film on the surface of the _____ pond.

    (A) turbulent
    (B) stalemate
    (C) stagnant
    (D) fermented

31. If you are able to write with either hand, you are most likely to be called _____.

    (A) amoral
    (B) ambidextrous
    (C) ambiguous
    (D) ambivalent

32. By planning ahead, you may be able to _____ some of the _____ events that may spoil your camping trip.

    (A) circumvent; unforeseen
    (B) circumscribe; suggested
    (C) oppose; progressive
    (D) misconstrue; catastrophic

33. Marey's Law states that if blood pressure falls, then the heart will beat faster. This type of relationship is _____ proportional.

    (A) indecisively
    (B) directly
    (C) inversely
    (D) inadvertently

34. Had it not been for her generous _____, she may not have been able to afford the expenses of college on her own.

    (A) antecedent
    (B) malefactor
    (C) beneficiary
    (D) benefactor

35. One example of _____ is Greek mythology because it was _____ on the belief that many gods exist.

    (A) polytheism; established
    (B) triennial; extended
    (C) monotheism; legalized
    (D) truancy; admitted

36. Not all tree fungi are detrimental to trees; there are some instances where both the fungi and the tree live together in a _____ existence where both organisms _____.

    (A) psychotic; succumb
    (B) triangular; synchronize
    (C) symbiotic; benefit
    (D) superimposed; cooperate

37. The new toy will _____ the baby for a little while; afterwards he may start crying again.

    (A) allude
    (B) ratify
    (C) enable
    (D) pacify

38. The new manuscript guidelines had a 150-page limit, which _____ the previous maximum page limit of 50.

    (A) conceded
    (B) preceded
    (C) superceded
    (D) receded

39. The puzzled and impatient listener _____ a question before the speaker could _____ the presentation.

    (A) interjected; conclude
    (B) projected; preclude
    (C) postponed; transmit
    (D) interceded; supervise

40. You don't have to _____ the message exactly as it was spoken; you may _____ it in your own words.

    (A) delegate; convene
    (B) communicate; paraphrase
    (C) suggest; eradicate
    (D) provide; devalue

41. Synapses allow one-way _____ of impulses in the nervous system of the body.

    (A) conduction
    (B) induction
    (C) covalence
    (D) convalescence

42. When the facilitator asked her to make a few _____ remarks about the conference's festivities, she was _____.

    (A) sporadic; illuminated
    (B) indecisive; thorough
    (C) impromptu; unprepared
    (D) devised; equipped

43. When we saw the manager hanging the "Standing Room Only" sign, we _____ that the theater seating capacity was filled.

    (A) interfered
    (B) implied
    (C) impressed
    (D) inferred

44. The puddles of water on the ground let us know that the ground was _____ from an _____ of rain.

    (A) saturated; overabundance
    (B) satisfied; anticipation
    (C) divested; indulgence
    (D) sufficed; occlusion

45. She had a contemptuous and _____ attitude toward the volunteers, and it seemed as though she thought of them as _____ and inferior.

    (A) submissive; superficial
    (B) condescending; substandard
    (C) perceptive; incriminating
    (D) contentious; cosmopolitan

46. Do not include _____ and irrelevant information; please keep your reports as _____ as possible.

    (A) rhetorical; sufficient
    (B) incessant; ideological
    (C) extraneous; succinct
    (D) affable; sardonic

47. One of the _____ aspects of his dynamic presentation was his ability to _____ the listless children so that they wanted to fully participate.

    (A) sanctimonious; compel
    (B) luminous; chastise
    (C) absolute; acquire
    (D) salient; captivate

48. This initial class is _____; it is imperative that you complete it so that you will be able to _____ to the next class.

    (A) malignant; transfer
    (B) inevitable; propagate
    (C) mandatory; advance
    (D) undetermined; transcend

STOP

End of Verbal Ability section. If you have any time left, you may go over your work in this section only.

CHEMISTRY

48 QUESTIONS (#49–#96)

TIME: 30 MINUTES

Directions: Choose the **best** answer to each of the following questions.

49. In the synthesis of protein from the nucleotide sequence in the mRNA, what is the term used to describe the group of three nucleotides that corresponds to an amino acid?

    (A) rRNA
    (B) codon
    (C) tRNA
    (D) anticodon

50. When a solute is dissolved in a solvent, which of the following is true concerning the solution?

    (A) The boiling point will increase.
    (B) The freezing point will increase.
    (C) The osmotic pressure will decrease.
    (D) The solution will conduct electricity if the solute is a nonelectrolyte.

51. How many protons are indicated in the following symbol for the lithium ion, $^{7}_{3}Li^{+1}$?

    (A) 3
    (B) 7
    (C) 10
    (D) 4

52. DNA and RNA are both polymers of nucleotides including

    (A) a purine or pyrimidine.
    (B) a cyclized glucose.
    (C) a triphosphate group.
    (D) All of the above

53. The class of biomolecules that is primarily characterized by its hydrophobicity is

    (A) proteins.
    (B) nucleic acids.
    (C) carbohydrates.
    (D) lipids.

54. What is the name of the following compound?

    (A) (1S, 3S)-3-methyl-1-chlorocyclohexane
    (B) (1S, 3R)-3-methyl-1-chlorocyclohexane
    (C) (1R, 3S)-3-methyl-1-chlorocyclohexane
    (D) (1R, 3R)-3-methyl-1-chlorocyclohexane

55. What is the product of the following reaction?

    (A)

    (B)

    (C)

    (D)

56. How many moles of carbon dioxide, CO_2, are present in 22 grams CO_2? (O = 16 amu, C = 12 amu)

    (A) 0.80
    (B) 0.50
    (C) 2.00
    (D) 1.30

57. What is the percentage yield of the following reaction if 1.0 gram of hydrogen, H_2, reacts with excess chlorine, Cl_2, to produce 18.3 grams of hydrogen chloride, HCl? (Cl = 35.5 amu, H = 1 amu)
    $$H_2 + Cl_2 \rightarrow 2\ HCl$$

    (A) 100%
    (B) 75%
    (C) 50%
    (D) 25%

58. How many moles of copper, Cu, are present in 1.2×10^6 atoms of Cu? (Avogadro's Number = $6 \times 10^{+23}$, Cu = 63.5 amu)

    (A) $5.0 \times 10^{+17}$
    (B) $2.0 \times 10^{+4}$
    (C) 5.3×10^{-5}
    (D) 2.0×10^{-18}

59. What functional group results from the following reaction?

    $$(CH_3)_2NH + CH_3CH_2COCl \rightarrow$$

    (A) Amine
    (B) Enamine
    (C) Amide
    (D) Imine

60. Which of the following reactions is a neutralization reaction?

    (A) $Mg + 2HCl \rightarrow MgCl_2 + H_2$
    (B) $2HCl + CaCO_3 \rightarrow CaCl_2 + H_2O + CO_2$
    (C) $BaCl_2 + Na_2SO_4 \rightarrow BaSO_4 + 2NaCl$
    (D) $2KClO_3 \rightarrow 2KCl + 3O_2$

61. What is the oxidation number of phosphorus, P, in PO_4^{-3}?

    (A) −8
    (B) −3
    (C) +8
    (D) +5

62. Protein function is destroyed by denaturation that

    (A) causes the cleavage of peptide bonds.
    (B) results in the loss of secondary structure.
    (C) does not affect hydrogen bonding.
    (D) digests the protein.

63. How many grams of sodium hydroxide, NaOH, are required to produce 800 milliliters of a 2.0 molar, 2.0 M, solution? (Na = 23 amu, O = 16 amu, H = 1 amu)

    (A) 8.0
    (B) 64
    (C) $1.6 \times 10^{+3}$
    (D) $6.4 \times 10^{+4}$

64. An autoclave has an initial pressure of 1.0 atmosphere and initial temperature of 27°C. The autoclave is heated until the final pressure inside the autoclave equals 5.0 atmospheres. What is the final temperature in degrees Celsius of the oven?

    (A) 1500
    (B) 1227
    (C) 135
    (D) 1000

65. To which biomolecular class does the following molecule belong?

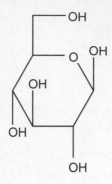

(A) Nucleic acids
(B) Proteins
(C) Lipids
(D) Carbohydrates

Use the periodic table below in order to answer questions 66–73.

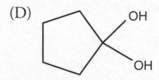

66. What is the electron configuration of the magnesium atom, Mg?

(A) $1s^2 2s^2 2p^6 3s^2$
(B) $1s^2 2s^2 2p^6$
(C) $1s^2 2s^2 2p^6 3s^2 3p^4$
(D) $1s^2 2s^2$

67. Which reagent would accomplish the following conversion?

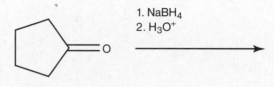

(A) H_2SO_4
(B) $K^+ {}^-OC(CH_3)_3$
(C) NH_3
(D) $LiAlH_4$

68. What is the product of the following reaction?

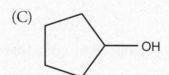

(A)

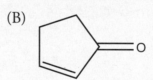

(B)

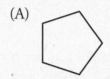

(C)

(D)

69. Which of the following compounds is NOT ionic?

(A) NaCl
(B) ICl
(C) CsF
(D) LiBr

70. Which structure for a substance with the formula $C_5H_{10}O_2$ is consistent with the following ^1H NMR data?

    δ 1.2 ppm, doublet, 6H
    δ 2.0 ppm, singlet, 3H
    δ 5.0 ppm, septet, 1H

    (A)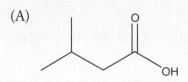

    (B)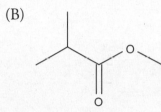

    (C)

    (D)

71. Which is a resonance structure of the following ion?

    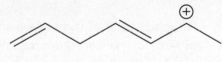

    (A)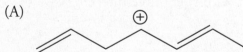

    (B)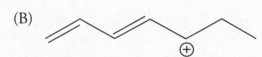

    (C)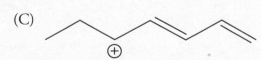

    (D)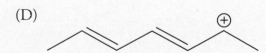

72. Which of the following bonds is a nonpolar covalent bond?

    (A) C — C
    (B) Li — Cl
    (C) H — F
    (D) B — C

73. Which of the following compounds has the highest boiling temperature?

    (A) HCl
    (B) H_2O
    (C) HF
    (D) NaCl

74. What is the molality of a solution that is 12 M (formula weight of solute is 33) and has a density of 1.2 g/ml?

    (A) 15 m
    (B) 12 m
    (C) 10 m
    (D) Cannot be determined

75. Lipids are involved in all of the following biological processes or structures EXCEPT

    (A) cell membrane construction.
    (B) hormones.
    (C) protein synthesis.
    (D) storage of carbon chains.

76. How would 100 mL of a 1.5 M NaBr solution be prepared? (Na = 23 amu, Br = 80 amu)

    (A) Dissolve 103 g of NaBr in 100 mL of water
    (B) Dissolve 15.5 g of NaBr in 100 mL of water
    (C) Dissolve 1.5 g of NaBr in enough water to make a final volume of 100 mL
    (D) Dissolve 15.5 g of NaBr in enough water to make a final volume of 100 mL

77. Phosholipids are found in cell membranes and are characterized by

   (A) a triester of glucose.
   (B) the presence of a nonpolar phosphate group.
   (C) their arrangement in a bilayer that has a nonpolar interior.
   (D) extensive arrangements in alpha helices.

78. In an aqueous environment, proteins assume an overall conformation driven by

   (A) their nucleotide sequence.
   (B) the positioning of hydrophilic side chains toward the interior of the conformation.
   (C) a variety of forces including hydrogen bonding.
   (D) All of the above

79. Which is expected to have the lowest boiling point?

   (A)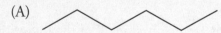

   (B)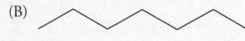

   (C)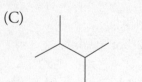

   (D)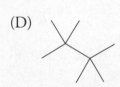

80. What is the molecular geometry of BCl_3?

   (A) Trigonal planar
   (B) Trigonal pyramid
   (C) Linear
   (D) Tetrahedron

81. What is the geometry of the ammonium ion, NH_4^{+1}?

   (A) Linear
   (B) Bent
   (C) Tetrahedral
   (D) Trigonal planar

82. Which reagent(s) will accomplish the following conversion?

   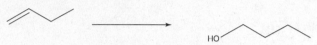

   (A) 1. $Hg(OAc)_2$, H_2O
       2. $NaBH_4$

   (B) 1. BH_3
       2. H_2O_2, OH^-

   (C) MCPBA

   (D) 1. OsO_4
       2. $NaHSO_3$

83. What is the hybridization state of the carbon, C, atom in $H_2C = CH_2$?

   (A) sp
   (B) sp^2
   (C) sp^3
   (D) sp^3d^2

84. What is the pH of a solution in which the hydrogen ion concentration equals 1×10^{-5} M (moles/liter)?

   (A) 5
   (B) 9
   (C) 6
   (D) 7

85. Which of the following statements about the behavior of gases is NOT true?

    (A) Gases generally behave the same way regardless of their identity.
    (B) If the volume of a gas is increased, the pressure will decrease if the temperature remains constant.
    (C) If the temperature of a gas is decreased, the molecular motion of the gas particles will increase.
    (D) The average kinetic energy of gas particles is directly proportional to the Kelvin temperature.

86. A solution of the following salt, sodium acetate, CH_3COONa, in water will be

    (A) acidic
    (B) basic
    (C) nearly neutral
    (D) independent of pH

87. Which of the following solutions is a buffer solution?

    (A) Hydrochloric acid and sodium chloride, $HCl + NaCl$
    (B) Acetic acid and sodium acetate, $CH_3COOH + CH_3COONa$
    (C) Nitric acid and sodium nitrate, $HNO_3 + NaNO_3$
    (D) Sulfuric acid and sodium sulfate, $H_2SO_4 + Na_2SO_4$

88. How many sigma bonds are present in the ethylene molecule shown below?

$$\begin{array}{ccc} H & & H \\ | & & | \\ C & = & C \\ | & & | \\ H & & H \end{array}$$

    (A) 1
    (B) 2
    (C) 4
    (D) 5

89. According to the kinetic molecular theory, in which of the following states of matter do atoms or molecules have the greatest freedom of motion?

    (A) Solid
    (B) Gas
    (C) Liquid
    (D) All states have the same freedom of motion.

90. Which compound could be used to react with ethyl magnesium bromide followed by protonation to form 3-pentanol?

    (A)

    (B)

    (C)

    (D)

91. Which of the following is methyl 2-methylbutanoate?

    (A)

    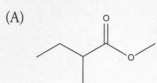

    (B)

    (C)

    (D)

92. The process by which protein is synthesized in the cell involves

    (A) mRNA.
    (B) rRNA.
    (C) tRNA.
    (D) All of the above

93. In the thermodynamic reaction

    $$\Delta G = \Delta H - T \Delta S$$

    ΔG represents the change in free energy in a reaction, ΔH the change in enthalpy, and ΔS the change in entropy. The reaction is spontaneous when ΔG is

    (A) +
    (B) −
    (C) 0
    (D) The sign of ΔG has no significance.

94. Which of the following reactions shows an increase in entropy?

    (A) $2KClO_3 \ (s) \rightarrow 2KCl \ (s) + 3O_2 \ (g)$
    (B) $H_2O \ (g) \rightarrow H_2O \ (l)$
    (C) $2H_2 \ (g) + O_2 \ (g) \rightarrow 2H_2O \ (l)$
    (D) $PCl_3 \ (l) + Cl_2 \ (g) \rightarrow PCl_5 \ (s)$

95. A change in which of the following factors causes a change in the equilibrium constant of the reversible reaction shown?

    $$A + B \leftrightarrow C + D \qquad K = \frac{[C][D]}{[A][B]}$$

    (A) Temperature
    (B) Volume
    (C) Concentration
    (D) Catalyst

96. Which of the following types of radiation is the most dangerous?

    (A) Alpha particles
    (B) Beta particles
    (C) Gamma rays
    (D) All the above types of radiation are equally dangerous.

End of Chemistry section. If you have any time left, you may go over your work in this section only.

Practice Test 2

BIOLOGY

48 QUESTIONS (#97–#144)

TIME: 30 MINUTES

Directions: Choose the **best** answer to each of the following questions.

97. The three types of cellular RNA polymerases in eukaryote cells transcribe different types of genes. What does RNA polymerase II produce?

    (A) Transfer RNA
    (B) Messenger RNA
    (C) Ribosomal RNA
    (D) Satellite RNA

98. Which statement is not true concerning the plasma membrane?

    (A) It controls exchange of materials between the inside and outside of the cell.
    (B) It is the outermost layer of animal cells.
    (C) It regulates cell's chemical composition.
    (D) It is the power plant of the cell.

99. Which of the following is a form of skin cancer?

    (A) Squamous cell carcinoma
    (B) Basal cell carcinoma
    (C) Malignant melanoma
    (D) All of the above

100. In animal x, black hair (B) is dominant over white hair (b). If a homozygous black-hair is crossed with a white-hair, the hair color of white is expected in what percent of the offspring?

    (A) 0%
    (B) 25%
    (C) 75%
    (D) 100%

101. The chromosome number is reduced from diploid to haploid in cell division by

    (A) meiosis.
    (B) mitosis.
    (C) hapnosis.
    (D) triosis.

102. Tetanus is associated with which type of pathogen?

    (A) Virus
    (B) Bacteria
    (C) Fungus
    (D) Protozoa

103. Which of the following represent the proper sequence for the stages of mitosis?

    (A) Prophase, Metaphase, Anaphase, Telophase
    (B) Prophase, Anaphase, Telophase, Metaphase
    (C) Anaphase, Telophase, Prophase, Metaphase
    (D) Anaphase, Prophase, Telophase, Metaphase

104. Serious health conditions associated with the use of smokeless tobacco are

    (A) tooth abrasion.
    (B) gum recession.
    (C) Both A and B
    (D) Neither A nor B

105. An endocrine gland

    (A) lacks a duct.
    (B) depends on the blood for transport of its secretions.
    (C) releases its hormone into the surrounding interstitial fluid.
    (D) All of the above

106. Oxytocin is responsible for

    (A) preventing milk release from the mammary glands.
    (B) causing contraction of the uterus.
    (C) preventing goiter.
    (D) maintaining normal thyroid and calcium levels.

107. During development, different embryonic cells express different sets of genes resulting in

    (A) gene mutation.
    (B) developmental abnormalities.
    (C) genetic recombination.
    (D) the formation of different cell types.

108. Calcitonin

    (A) is produced by the pancreas.
    (B) levels increase when blood calcium levels decrease.
    (C) causes blood calcium levels to decrease.
    (D) is produced by the gallbladder.

109. Parathyroid hormone secretion increases in response to

    (A) a decrease in blood calcium.
    (B) increased production of parathyroid-stimulating hormone from the anterior pituitary.
    (C) increased secretion of parathyroid-releasing hormone from the hypothalamus.
    (D) All of the above

110. The adrenal medulla

    (A) is formed from a modified portion of the sympathetic nervous system.
    (B) has epinephrine as its major secretory product.
    (C) increases its secretions during exercise.
    (D) All of the above

111. Which type of blood is the universal recipient?

    (A) O
    (B) B
    (C) A
    (D) AB

112. The valve between the right atrium and right ventricle is

    (A) Bicuspid (mitral) valve
    (B) Tricuspid valve
    (C) Atrioventricular valve
    (D) Chamber valve

113. Given these blood vessels below:

    1. aorta
    2. inferior vena cava
    3. pulmonary trunk
    4. pulmonary vein

    Choose the arrangement that lists the vessels in the order a red blood cell would encounter them in going from the systemic veins back to the systemic arteries.

    (A) 1, 3, 4, 2
    (B) 2, 3, 4, 1
    (C) 2, 4, 3, 1
    (D) 3, 2, 1, 4

114. Oxygen is mostly transported in the blood

    (A) in white blood cells.
    (B) bound to albumin.
    (C) bound to gamma globulins.
    (D) bound to the heme portion of hemoglobin.

115. Which of these structures function to increase the mucosal surface of the small intestine?

    (A) The length of the small intestine
    (B) Villi
    (C) Microvilli
    (D) All of the above

116. Which of the following statements are true concerning vitamins?

    (A) They function as coenzymes.
    (B) Most can be synthesized by the body.
    (C) They are normally broken down before they can be used by the body.
    (D) A, D, E, and K are water-soluble vitamins.

117. Functions of the kidney involve

    (A) maintaining blood volume.
    (B) disposing nitrogenous wastes.
    (C) maintaining electrolyte balance.
    (D) All of the above

118. In the reaction versus substrate concentration graph below, the curve plateaus because

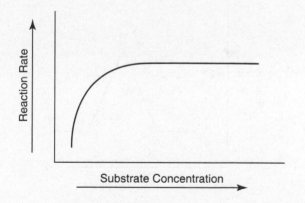

    (A) a noncompetitive inhibitor is present.
    (B) a competitive inhibitor is present.
    (C) the active site is saturated with substrate.
    (D) all the substrate has been converted to product.

119. In a heterozygous monohybrid cross, the dominant trait would be expressed _____ of the time.

    (A) 0 percent
    (B) 25 percent
    (C) 75 percent
    (D) 100 percent

120. Which of the following is the specialized absorptive structure in the intestine?

    (A) Alveoli
    (B) Villi
    (C) Bowman's capsule
    (D) Nephron

121. Crossing over is more likely to occur between genes that are

    (A) close together on the chromosome.
    (B) on different chromosomes.
    (C) located on the X chromosome.
    (D) far apart on a chromosome.

122. Human skin develops from

    (A) ectoderm.
    (B) mesoderm.
    (C) endoderm.
    (D) trophoderm.

123. Vitamin C deficiency problems include

    (A) scurvy.
    (B) burning feet syndrome.
    (C) hair loss.
    (D) toxemia.

124. In minks, the gene for brown fur (B) is dominant to the gene for silver fur (b). Which set of genotypes represents a cross that could produce offspring with silver fur from parents that both have brown fur?

    (A) Bb × Bb
    (B) BB × Bb
    (C) BB × bb
    (D) Bb × bb

125. HIV (human immunodeficiency virus) infects mostly

   (A) CT-cells
   (B) D-killer cells
   (C) T-helper cells
   (D) none of the above

126. Carbohydrate digestion begins in the _____ with the action of the enzyme _____.

   (A) mouth; amylase
   (B) stomach; pepsin
   (C) small intestine; cholecystokinin
   (D) large intestine; water

127. What are the basic nutrients the body must have?

   (A) Calcium, carbohydrates, protein, fats, vitamins, minerals, water
   (B) Carbohydrates, protein, fats, vitamins, minerals, water
   (C) Salt, carbohydrates, protein, fats, vitamins, minerals, water
   (D) None of the above

128. _____ is a condition where a person's concerns about dieting, food restriction, fear of becoming overweight, and dissatisfaction with body image interfere with normal daily life.

   (A) Binge-eating disorder
   (B) Bulimia nervosa
   (C) Affective-eating disorder
   (D) Disordered eating patterns

129. A major function of white blood cells is to fight

   (A) pain.
   (B) infections.
   (C) glucose intolerance.
   (D) None of the above

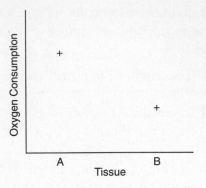

Figure 1.

130. In Figure 1, the oxygen consumption of tissues A and B were determined with the following results:

   (A) Tissue A has either a greater number of mitochondria, larger mitochondria, or more enzymatic activity.
   (B) Tissue A has a lesser number of mitochondria, smaller mitochondria, or less enzymatic activity.
   (C) Tissue A has a lesser number of mitochondria, medium-sized mitochondria, or less enzymatic activity.
   (D) Tissue A has to have a smaller nucleus.

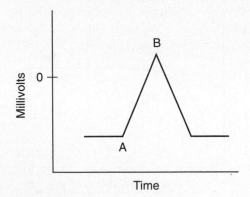

Figure 2.

131. In Figure 2, the ascending portion of the action potential observed in the cell in the graph is caused by

   (A) fluoride efflux out of the cell.
   (B) potassium influx into the cell.
   (C) sodium efflux out of the cell.
   (D) sodium influx into the cell.

132. The pancreas produces which two hormones?

    (A) Melatonin and serotonin
    (B) Adrenalin and noradrenaline
    (C) Insulin and glucagon
    (D) None of the above

133. Hormones are distributed throughout the body by means of the

    (A) gallbladder.
    (B) blood.
    (C) pancreas.
    (D) stomach.

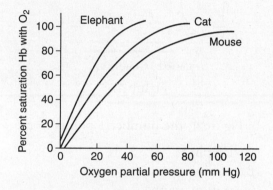

Figure 3.

134. In Figure 3, for an animal's hemoglobin to unload more readily it must

    (A) have a high metabolic rate and high oxygen requirements.
    (B) have a low metabolic rate and low oxygen requirements.
    (C) have an intermediate oxygen requirement.
    (D) not require oxygen.

135. According to the CDC, which hand hygiene method is best for killing bacteria?

    (A) Plain soap and water
    (B) Antimicrobial soap and water
    (C) Alcohol-based handrub
    (D) None of the above

136. Transmission across a synapse is slower than impulse conduction along a neuron because

    (A) there is more surface area in a synapse than a neuron.
    (B) synaptic vesicles clog the neural pathways and the signal takes longer.
    (C) it involves a series of events.
    (D) partial depolarization requires more time to accomplish.

137. Neurological drugs alter synaptic function in which ways?

    (A) Interferes with synthesis of the appropriate transmitter
    (B) Blocks uptake of the transmitter into synaptic vesicles
    (C) Prevents the release of transmitter from the vesicles into the cleft
    (D) All of the above

138. Which statement is NOT characteristic of red blood cells?

    (A) Red blood cells carry oxygen from the lungs to the tissues.
    (B) Mature red blood cells lack a nucleus.
    (C) The normal life span of a red blood cell is about 30 days.
    (D) Hemoglobin is present in red blood cells.

139. In neurons, dendrites

    (A) send signals to other neurons.
    (B) secret neurotransmitters.
    (C) secrete hormones.
    (D) receive signals from other neurons.

140. Which form of diabetes may not require insulin injections for disease management?

    (A) Type 1
    (B) Type 2
    (C) Both A and B
    (D) Neither A nor B

141. This process occurs when double strands of a DNA segment separate and RNA nucleotides pair with DNA nucleotides.

    (A) Transcription
    (B) Translation
    (C) Transduction
    (D) Transmetric

142. Apoptosis describes a process of

    (A) cell specialization.
    (B) cell death.
    (C) cell differentiation.
    (D) cell proliferation.

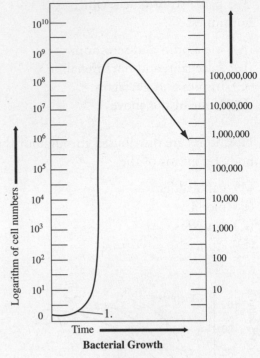

Figure 4.

143. In Figure 4, the number 1 points to the

    (A) lag phase.
    (B) decline phase.
    (C) stationary phase.
    (D) logarithmic phase.

144. One bacterial cell is placed in a nutrient broth test tube at 12 noon. Its generation time is 30 minutes, and its growth occurs by binary fission. By 2:00 P.M., the size of the population of bacteria in the test tube is

    (A) 4.
    (B) 8.
    (C) 16.
    (D) 32.

STOP

End of Biology section. If you have any time left, you may go over your work in this section only.

READING COMPREHENSION

48 QUESTIONS (#145–#192)

TIME: 50 MINUTES

> **Directions:** Read each of the following passages, and choose the **best** answer to each of the questions that follows each passage.

Passage 1

As many as 50 million Americans have high blood pressure, defined as a systolic blood pressure ≥140 mm Hg and a diastolic blood pressure ≥90 mm Hg. Although blood pressure generally increases with age, the onset of hypertension most often occurs in the third, fourth, or fifth decade of life. The prevalence of hypertension in the elderly population (age ≥65 years) is approximately 63% in whites and 76% in blacks. In younger generations (35 to 45 years of age), the prevalence is markedly different with 44% among black men, 37% among black women, 26% among white men, and 17% among white women.

A specific cause of sustained hypertension cannot be found in the vast majority of individuals with high blood pressure. Genetic factors have been suggested to play a role in essential hypertension due to the fact that high blood pressure may be hereditary. Evidence that a single gene may account for specific subtypes of hypertension has also been suggested. Genetic traits include high angiotensin levels, increased aldosterone and other adrenal steroids, and high sodium-lithium countertransport. More direct approaches for preventing or treating hypertension could be achieved by identifying individuals with these traits. Factors such as sodium excretion and transport rates, blood pressure response to plasma volume expansion, electrolyte homeostasis, and glomerular filtration rate help explain the predisposition for a person to develop hypertension.

Anti-hypertensive drug therapy should be individualized according to various patient characteristics and fundamental pathophysiologic circumstances. Dietary intake has been shown to be similar in all races but blacks ingest less potassium and calcium than whites. Supplemental potassium and calcium has shown to cause a modest reduction in blood pressure in some studies. Therefore, it would seem reasonable to ascertain the affects of increasing the amount of potassium and calcium in the diet as part of the non-pharmacologic regulation of hypertension. The initial treatment for hypertension is lifestyle changes unless target-organ damage is present. These changes include sodium restriction, weight reduction, increased physical activity, and ethanol reduction or abstinence. In terms of target-organ damage, diuretics and beta-blockers are first-line therapy. Control of blood pressure and prevention of cardiovascular morbidity and mortality are the goals of antihypertensive therapy. By maintaining arterial blood pressure below 140 mm Hg systolic and 90 mm Hg diastolic and by controlling other risk factors such as smoking, hyperlipidemia, and diabetes, morbidity and mortality may be averted.

145. The onset of hypertension most often occurs in which decades?

(A) Third and fifth
(B) Third, fourth, and fifth
(C) Fourth, fifth, and sixth
(D) Fifth, sixth, and seventh

146. Which of the following statements is false?

(A) It has been suggested that genetic factors may play a role in essential hypertension.
(B) Unless target-organ damage is present, the initial treatment for hypertension should be lifestyle changes.
(C) The prevalence of hypertension in younger white men is higher than the prevalence of hypertension in elderly blacks.
(D) Some studies have shown blood pressure reduction with the use of supplemental calcium and potassium.

147. According to the passage, initial treatment for hypertension is lifestyle changes which include

    (A) smoking cessation, weight reduction, decreased physical activity, and ethanol restriction.
    (B) sodium restriction, weight reduction, increased physical activity, and ethanol reduction or abstinence.
    (C) ethanol reduction or abstinence, sodium restriction, reduced mental activity or stress, and gaining weight.
    (D) weight reduction, increase sodium intake, ethanol reduction, and increase stress.

148. Two of the factors that help provide an explanation of hypertensive development are centered around

    (A) diuretic usage and abstinence.
    (B) electrolyte homeostasis and sodium excretion.
    (C) increased calcium intake and proper medication adherence.
    (D) decreased medication therapy costs and decreased steroid usage.

149. Genetic factors have been suggested to play a role in essential hypertension based on the fact that

    (A) parents can get it from their children.
    (B) if ancestors have high angiotensin levels they have a higher rate of morbidity.
    (C) geneticists know which gene causes hypertension.
    (D) high blood pressure may be hereditary.

150. Anti-hypertensive therapy should be individualized according to

    (A) patient characteristics and fundamental pathophysiologic circumstances.
    (B) number of offspring and dietary habits stemming from care of those offspring.
    (C) features found in their family tree.
    (D) the climate of the state where the patient lives.

151. Morbidity and mortality associated with hypertension may be averted if an individual can maintain an arterial blood pressure of

    (A) 155 mm Hg systolic and 77 mm Hg diastolic.
    (B) 136 mm Hg systolic and 99 mm Hg diastolic.
    (C) 160 mm Hg systolic and 98 mm Hg diastolic.
    (D) 135 mm Hg systolic and 85 mm Hg diastolic.

152. How many Americans currently suffer from high blood pressure?

    (A) As many as 60 billion
    (B) As many as 50 billion
    (C) As many as 50 million
    (D) As many as 40 million

Passage 2

Non-adherence to medication therapy results in numerous adverse effects such as increased hospitalizations and even death. Additionally, it costs the U.S. healthcare system billions of dollars each year. It is important to assess patients' adherence to medications.

Improper medication adherence encompasses an assortment of behaviors. These include not having a prescription filled, forgetting or intentionally not taking a medication, consuming an incorrect amount of a medication, taking a medication at the wrong time, ceasing therapy too soon, or continuing therapy after advised to discontinue. All forms of improper medication taking behavior may jeopardize health outcomes.

Measuring medication-taking behavior is often difficult. The ideal method of measurement should be simultaneously unobtrusive (to avoid patient sensitization and maximize cooperation), objective (to produce discrete and reproducible data for each subject), and practical (to maximize portability and minimize cost). Refill records, pill counts, electronic medication dispensers/caps, patient surveys (interviews), blood-drug level monitoring, and urine assay for drug metabolites can be used as clues to identify improper medication use.

Before altering therapy based on the assumption that a patient is taking a medication as prescribed, practitioners should ascertain patient's medication taking behavior. This becomes especially important when modifying dosages of medications. Due to the advantages and disadvantages of each measurement, it is important for practitioners to use a combination of methods to assess a patient's medication usage behavior and relate these findings to the patient's clinical presentation.

153. The ideal method of medication adherence measurement should be

   (A) simultaneously functional, easy, and reliable.
   (B) simultaneously fun, personalized, and fancy-free.
   (C) simultaneously practical, objective, and unobtrusive.
   (D) simultaneously advantageous, creative, and unpretentious.

154. According to the passage, current techniques for assessing a patient's medication usage include

   (A) blood-drug level monitoring, pill counts, refill records, and half-life tables.
   (B) refill records, patient interviews, electronic medication dispensers, and nucleic acid levels.
   (C) pill counts, electronic medication dispensers, patient interviews, x-ray, and refill records.
   (D) blood-level drug monitoring, refill records, electronic medication dispensers, and urine assays for drug metabolites.

155. Improper medication adherence encompasses

   (A) taking a medication too soon, not taking enough of the drug, and forgetting to take the medication.
   (B) not having the prescription filled, continuing to take the medication after therapy has been discontinued, forgetting or intentionally not taking the medication, and consuming the wrong amount of medication.
   (C) not having the prescription filled, taking the medication before therapy has been continued, forgetting or intentionally not taking the medication, and consuming too much medication.
   (D) all of the above

156. Before altering therapy based on the assumption that the medication is being taken as prescribed, practitioners should

   (A) assess the patient's behavior concerning taking their medication.
   (B) check the patient's blood glucose levels and ask about their dietary intake.
   (C) discern the patient's refill rate and whether they were on schedule.
   (D) decide if the patient is in the maintenance phase of adherence.

157. Which of the following statements is true?

    (A) Since patients always take their medications as prescribed, practitioners should never ascertain a patient's medication behavior.
    (B) Bad health outcomes and improper medication-taking behavior are unrelated.
    (C) It is not necessary to combine methods to identify improper medication use, since the advantages of each measurement used outweighs the disadvantages.
    (D) Discontinuing medication therapy after being advised to continue is a form of improper medication adherence.

158. It is important to assess patients' adherence to medication because

    (A) if they are not adherent then their medication will not work.
    (B) it can result in adverse effects such as increased hospitalizations and perhaps death.
    (C) it costs the U.S. government trillions in lawsuits each year.
    (D) maintenance of adherence contributes to an increase in suicides.

Passage 3

A dreaded disease is striking California's coast live oaks with the ferocity of an oak-tree Ebola virus, causing the trees to sprout sores, hemorrhage sap, and become infested with beetles and various fungi. The trees die within a few weeks of their first symptoms.

A pathologist at the University of California, Davis, announced that his team had found the cause of the disease dubbed "Sudden Oak Death." The tree-slayer is a new member of the genus Phytophthora, whose name means "plant destroyer." Its kin include pathogens responsible for the Irish potato famine and die-offs in Australian eucalyptus forests and European oak groves. "We don't know if (the new species) was just recently introduced, or if it has always been here and something else has changed that has allowed it to go crazy," one pathologist says.

The first trees to succumb to the plague 5 years ago were tan oaks, which often grow in the understory of redwood forests. Last year the disease began hitting large numbers of coast live oaks, the signature species in scenic coastal woodlands. Alarmingly, the pathogen has begun to blight another species, the black oak.

Knowing the culprit doesn't make the outlook much brighter. "Fungicides can save individual oaks," says one pathologist, "but we can't go to Mount Tamalpais and spray 10,000 trees." And prevention is largely limited to warning people not to carry oak firewood to uninfected areas. The Sierra Nevada hosts black oaks, and pathologists fear the deadly spores could strike groves in beloved Yosemite Valley.

From "Culprit Named in Sudden Oak Death," *Science*, Vol 289, August 2000. Page 859. Reprinted with permission from AAAS.

159. "Sudden Oak Death" causes trees to

    (A) grow multiple trunks and become infested with mold.
    (B) sprout sores, hemorrhage sap, and become infested with beetles and various fungi.
    (C) lose all leaves, branches and wilt.
    (D) hemorrhage at the tips, spout new branches, and become infested with termites.

160. This plague began

    (A) 5 years ago.
    (B) 10 years ago.
    (C) 15 years ago.
    (D) 2 years ago.

161. The cause of this disease is

    (A) phytohemagglutinin.
    (B) phytosterol.
    (C) phytophthora.
    (D) phytoalexin.

162. The first trees to succumb were

    (A) tan oaks.
    (B) coast live oaks.
    (C) black oaks.
    (D) European oaks.

163. The greatest fear of this plague is that it will strike

    (A) redwood forests.
    (B) Yosemite Valley.
    (C) Australian eucalyptus forests.
    (D) coastal woodlands.

164. The tree species that have been affected by the tree virus are

    (A) the tan oak, coast live oak, and the black oak.
    (B) the redwood oak, the tan oak, and the firewood oak.
    (C) the Mount St. Helen's live oak.
    (D) the Irish and Australian coastal oak.

165. Which of the following statements is true?

    (A) Pathologists know the exact origin of the oak pathogen species.
    (B) Tan oaks are often found growing in the under-story of redwood forests.
    (C) Sierra Nevada hosts both black and tan oaks.
    (D) Fungicides will save an estimated 10,000 trees in Mount Tamalpais.

166. Coast live oaks are a characteristic oak species in

    (A) redwood forests.
    (B) Yosemite Valley.
    (C) Sierra Nevada.
    (D) scenic coastal woodlands.

Passage 4

We humans sense old age through feeling those creaky joints or observing those graying hairs but, according to Apfeld and Kenyon reporting in a recent issue of Nature, the nematode worm senses its age by smelling and tasting the environment. These investigators show that worms with defective olfactory organs (that would normally detect odor molecules in the environment) live longer than their comrades with a keener sense of smell. By comparing these worms with other mutant nematodes that live an unusually long time, the researchers found clues to how a reduced ability to "smell the roses" might lengthen life-span.

The worm's olfactory sense organs—amphids on the head and plasmids on the tail—are composed of a cluster of nerve cells, the ends of which are modified into cilia. The cilia are encircled by a sheath and a socket cell that form a pore in the worm's skin through which the tips of the cilia protrude. Odor molecules and soluble compounds bind to G protein-coupled receptors (similar to the olfactory and taste receptors of mammals) located at the tip of each cilium. Worms with a poor sense of smell—because their olfactory organs have defective or absent cilia, blocked pores, or damaged sheaths—live much longer, yet are otherwise normal (for example, their feeding and reproductive behaviors are unchanged). Mutations in TAX-4—a channel regulated by cyclic GMP that sits under the G protein-coupled receptor and transduces the sensory signals into electrical impulses—also imbue the worm with a longer life.

But mutations in the worm's olfactory machinery are not the only defects that extend its life-span. In an earlier study, Kenyon's group found that defects in the reproductive system could prolong life by decreasing the activity of DAF-2 (a receptor for an insulin-like molecule) and increasing the activity of DAF-16 (a transcription factor). By looking at worms defective in both sensory perception and reproduction, Apfeld and Kenyon worked out a putative pathway through which smell might influence a worm's longevity.

An environmental signal, perhaps produced by bacteria (the worm's favorite food), binds to G protein-coupled olfactory receptors on sensory cilia activating TAX-4, which then incites electrical activity in the sensory neurons. This activity triggers secretory vesicles in the neurons to release insulin-like molecules, which bind to DAF-2 and activate the insulin-like signaling pathway. This then switches on genes that will ensure the worm dies at the usual age of 2 weeks. A reduced ability to sense olfactory cues would result in a decrease in DAF-2 activation and an increase in life-span.

This chain of events is not proven, but insulin-like molecules that might bind to DAF-2 have been identified in the nematode. Such a pathway would also make physiological sense. After all, if food is scarce it may behoove the worm to live longer to ensure that it has the chance to produce its full quota of offspring. A scarcity of food also promotes longevity in rodents and primates. But so far it seems that in these more complicated creatures a poor sense of smell is not a harbinger of a ripe old age.

From "Nota Bene: Sensing Old Age" by Orda Smith, *Science*, Vol 287, January 2000. Page 54. Reprinted with permission from AAAS.

167. A worm usually lives to the "old age" of

    (A) 3 weeks.
    (B) 5 weeks.
    (C) 1 week.
    (D) 2 weeks.

168. TAX-4 is

    (A) a channel regulated by cyclic GMP which sits beneath the G protein-coupled receptor and transduces the sensory signals into electrical impulses.
    (B) a cyclic regulated AMP which lies above the G protein-coupled receptor and transduces the neurological signals into electrical impulses.
    (C) a liability which the nematode has to deal with four times the amount of cyclic GMP next to the G protein-coupled receptor.
    (D) a receptor for an insulin-like molecule which activate the insulin-like pathway.

169. A nematode worm detects its age by

    (A) a biological stopwatch which notes sunrise and sunset.
    (B) burrowing through the soil at speeds up to 0.01 mph.
    (C) whether it has had the chance to produce its full quota of offspring.
    (D) smelling and tasting the environment.

170. The worm's olfactory sense organs are composed of

    (A) a cluster of nervous tissue surrounded by a sheath which protects it.
    (B) socket cells that are embedded in the head and tail of the worm.
    (C) a cluster of nerve cells of which the ends are modified into cilia.
    (D) their individual mouths and noses which are covered with cilia.

171. What other traits in the worm extend its lifespan?

    (A) Defects in the circulatory system.
    (B) Mutations in the excretory system.
    (C) Alterations in the lymphatic system.
    (D) Aberrations in the reproductive system.

172. DAF-2 is

    (A) a receptor for an insulin-like molecule.
    (B) a transcription factor.
    (C) a transduction factor.
    (D) a binding site for a glucose molecule.

173. A logical pathway by which smell might influence a worm's longevity was achieved by studying

    (A) worms flawed in both circulatory and sensory perception.
    (B) worms defective in both reproduction and sensory perception.
    (C) worms deficient in only the reproductive system.
    (D) worms impaired in the nervous and circulatory system.

174. Secretory vesicles in the neurons are stimulated by what to release insulin-like molecules?

    (A) TAX-4 excites electrical activity.
    (B) DAF-2 activates the insulin-like pathway.
    (C) DAF-16 regulates the electrical activity.
    (D) TAX-2 initiates the secretory vesicles.

175. A scarcity of food is known to promote longevity in

    (A) nematodes.
    (B) nematodes and rodents.
    (C) nonprimates and nematodes.
    (D) rodents and primates.

176. The reduced ability to sense olfactory cues results in

    (A) a decrease in life-span and an increase in DAF-2 activation.
    (B) a decrease in DAF-2 activation and an increase in lifespan.
    (C) a decrease in TAX-4 which incites electrical activity.
    (D) a decrease in DAF-16 which creates more gene activity.

Passage 5

Presidents of the United States are not like you and me. A new personality assessment presented this week at the American Psychological Association conference in Washington, D.C., shows that, compared to the public they serve, presidents are more likely to be extroverted, assertive, and disagreeable. They're also less modest and straightforward.

Says who? Historians who have written book-length biographies of Oval Office occupants. Psychologist Steve Rubenzer of the Mental Health and Mental Retardation Authority of Harris County in Houston, Texas, and colleagues asked the biographers to fill out three standard personality inventories on their subjects, basing answers on the presidents' behavior during the 5 years preceding their reigns. The researchers compared the presidents' scores to population norms and compared the profiles of successful commanders-in-chief with those history hasn't smiled upon.

"Great" presidents, such as Jefferson and Lincoln, they find, "are attentive to their emotions, willing to question traditional values ... imaginative, and more interested in art and beauty than less successful Chief Executives." They're also more assertive, stubborn, and "tender-minded," which is a measure of concern for the less fortunate. Rubenzer hasn't analyzed the current presidential contenders yet—he prefers to have at least three "unbiased" historians fill out the forms for each president or presidential wanna-be.

From "Presidential Personalities," *Science*, Vol 289, August 2000. Page 859. Reprinted with permission from AAAS.

177. This personality assessment was presented at a conference of which group?

    (A) The American Pharmacists Association
    (B) The Annual Physicians Association
    (C) The American Psychological Association
    (D) The Association of Practicing Psychiatrists

178. This data was collected from

    (A) historians.
    (B) presidents.
    (C) psychologists.
    (D) historiographers.

179. Steve Rubenzer and his team of researchers

    (A) are historians who write biographies.
    (B) are from Houston, Texas.
    (C) are from Washington, D.C.
    (D) work in the Oval Office.

180. The standard personality inventories that were completed by the biographers were based on

    (A) the comparisons of current presidential contenders.
    (B) the presidents' behaviors during the five years after their term of office.
    (C) biased population norms.
    (D) the presidents' behaviors during the five years before their term of office.

181. According to the passage, "great" presidents include those such as

    (A) Kennedy and Roosevelt.
    (B) Jefferson and Lincoln.
    (C) Bush and Wilson.
    (D) Adams and Carter.

182. In this article, use of the word *tender-minded* meant

    (A) less stubborn.
    (B) more concerned for the less-fortunate.
    (C) more apathetic toward the environment.
    (D) less concerned for the more-fortunate.

183. According to Rubenzer, how many historians should fill out the forms for each presidential contender or presidential wanna-be?

    (A) Three
    (B) Two
    (C) As many as possible, as long as they are biased.
    (D) One

184. Presidents are more likely to be

    (A) disagreeable, extroverted, and assertive.
    (B) agreeable, apathetic, and introverted.
    (C) unwilling to question traditional values.
    (D) less interested in art and beauty.

Passage 6

Drug interactions, a common type of drug-related problem, are categorized as pharmacokinetic, pharmacodynamic, or a combination of both. Pharmacokinetic drug interactions include changes in absorption, distribution, excretion, and metabolism; whereas, pharmacodynamic drug interactions may lead to antagonist or synergistic effects. Not all drug interactions are undesirable; in fact, many drug interactions are used to produce desirable effects. Patients who take drugs with narrow therapeutic indices and drugs that interfere with the pharmacokinetic properties of other drugs are at increased risk of experiencing a drug interaction. Also, patients who take multiple medications per day or take multiple doses of medications per day are at increased risk. Because renal transplant patients take immunosuppressive agents that have narrow therapeutic indices and are subjected to multiple medications per day, they are vulnerable to experiencing adverse drug events. To prevent adverse drug interactions, an alternative therapy should be considered when possible or the dose or schedule of the drugs should be adjusted to reduce the occurrence of an adverse experience. Additionally, adequate monitoring to prevent and detect adverse effects is an essential part of patient care.

A common pharmacokinetic interaction involves drugs that interfere with the absorption of other medications. Drugs that bind and decrease the gastrointestinal absorption of another drug, such as cholestyramine decreasing the absorption of tacrolimus, typically can be prevented by administering the agents two to three hours apart from each other. Prokinetic agents interfere with the rate of absorption. Since many transplant patients take prokinetic agents, such as metochlopromide, this may increase the bioavailability of other medications. This is of significant importance since immunosuppressive agents have narrow therapeutic indices and toxicity may result from this interaction. If the prokinetic agent cannot be avoided, careful monitoring (e.g., serum drug levels, clinical presentation of patient) and adjustments should be made to prevent immunosuppressant toxicity.

185. Prokinetic agents

 (A) interfere with the rate of metabolism.
 (B) affect all interactions in the gastrointestinal tract.
 (C) interfere with the rate of absorption.
 (D) should be monitored and adjusted.

186. Which of the following statements is true?

 (A) Renal transplant patients are less likely to experience adverse drug events due to the narrow therapeutic indices of their immunosuppressive agents.
 (B) There are three categories of drug interactions.
 (C) Drug interference with the absorption of other medications is a rare form of pharmacodynamic interaction.
 (D) Adequate monitoring is needed only to detect, not prevent, adverse events.

187. Toxicity can result from a prokinetic agent being administered with an immunosuppressive agent because

 (A) cholestyramine has a narrow therapeutic index.
 (B) patients have to take immunosuppressive agents multiple times per day.
 (C) the prokinetic agent may increase the bioavailability of the immunosuppressive agent.
 (D) all drug interactions are undesirable.

188. Pharmacokinetic drug interactions include

 (A) changes in allocation, circulation, and dispersion.
 (B) changes in absorption, distribution, excretion, and metabolism.
 (C) reactions which affect composition of other medications.
 (D) cumulative and additive effects.

189. Patients that are at increased risk of experiencing a drug interaction include

 (A) patients who take multiple medications per day or multiple doses of medications per day.
 (B) patients who take drugs with narrow therapeutic indices.
 (C) patients who take drugs that interfere with the pharmacokinetic properties of other drugs.
 (D) All of the above.

190. In this passage, an example of a drug that binds and decreases the gastrointestinal absorption of another drug is

    (A) tacrolimus.
    (B) metochlopromide.
    (C) sirolimus.
    (D) cholestyramine.

191. To prevent adverse drug reactions

    (A) consult neighbors regularly.
    (B) consider an alternate therapy or alter the dose or schedule of the drugs.
    (C) time medication regimens with meals.
    (D) increase water intake.

192. If the prokinetic agent cannot be avoided, to prevent immunosuppressant toxicity

    (A) carefully arrange the patients medication consumption schedule.
    (B) monitor compliance to see if the prokinetic factor is really necessary.
    (C) monitor serum levels and the clinical presentation of the patient and make appropriate adjustments.
    (D) educate the patient on the types of adverse drug reactions which may occur.

STOP

End of Reading Comprehension section. If you have any time left, you may go over your work in this section only.

QUANTITATIVE ABILITY

48 QUESTIONS (#193–#240)

TIME: 40 MINUTES

Directions: Choose the **best** answer to each of the following questions.

193. If a square plot of land 210 feet on one side contains one acre, approximately how many square feet are in the one acre of land?

(A) 44,100
(B) 28,400
(C) 2,860
(D) 840

194. Given the function $f(x) = \dfrac{x^2}{6-x}$,

compute $\dfrac{dy}{dx}$.

$x^2(6-x)^{-1}$

(A) $\dfrac{12x + x^2}{(6-x)^2}$

(B) $\dfrac{12x - x^2}{(6-x)^2}$

(C) $\dfrac{x^2 - 12x}{(6-x)^2}$

(D) $\dfrac{-12x - 3x^2}{(6-x)^2}$

195. What is the mean value for the sequence {4, 5, 11, 18, 20, 22, 34, 35, 38}?

(A) 20.77
(B) 25.77
(C) 30.77
(D) 35.77

196. One tablespoonful contains 15 mL of volume. If a patient takes one tablespoonful three times a day, how many days supply will be provided by a 12 ounce bottle? (One ounce = 30 mL)

(A) 6
(B) 8
(C) 12
(D) 16

197. Given that $\ln(a) = 6$ and $\ln(b) = 2$,

$\ln\left(\dfrac{a}{b}\right) =$

(A) 4
(B) 3
(C) $\ln(3)$
(D) $\ln(4)$

198. Eighty-six degrees Fahrenheit =

(A) 30 degrees Celsius
(B) 15 degrees Celsius
(C) 20 degrees Celsius
(D) 30 degrees Celsius

199. What is the median value for the sequence {4, 5, 39, 20, 18, 34, 35, 22, 38, 11}?

(A) 22
(B) 18
(C) 20
(D) 21

200. Evaluate the integral $\int\limits_{3}^{4}(9x^2)\,dx$.

(A) 273
(B) 63
(C) 18
(D) 111

201. Lisa's gas tank is 4/5 full. She completely filled the tank by putting in an additional 7 gallons. What is the capacity of the gas tank?

(A) 30 gallons
(B) 35 gallons
(C) 25 gallons
(D) 40 gallons

202. $10^2 + 9^2 =$

    (A) 90^4
    (B) 19^4
    (C) 1.81×10^2
    (D) 1^4

203. Determine the length of the line segment with endpoints $(5, 7)$ and $(3, -1)$.

    (A) $\sqrt{66}$

    (B) $\sqrt{62}$

    (C) $\sqrt{68}$

    (D) $\sqrt{60}$

204. John has $6.60 in quarters and dimes. He has twice as many quarters as dimes. How many quarters does he have?

    (A) 11
    (B) 20
    (C) 18
    (D) 22

205. Simplify the expression $\dfrac{1}{x} + \dfrac{1}{y}$.

    (A) $\dfrac{2}{xy}$

    (B) $\dfrac{y + x}{xy}$

    (C) $\dfrac{2}{x + y}$

    (D) None of these

206. Given the function $f(x) = 2x + 5$, what is $f^{-1}(x)$?

    (A) $\dfrac{x - 5}{2}$

    (B) $5x - 2$

    (C) $\dfrac{1}{2x + 5}$

    (D) $2x - 5$

For problems 207–209, consider the given graph of the function $y = f(x)$.

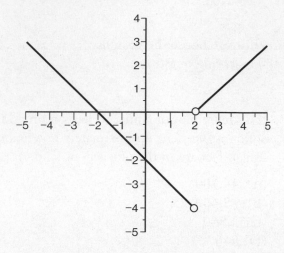

207. $\displaystyle\lim_{x \to 2^+} f(x) =$

    (A) 0 and −4
    (B) Does not exist
    (C) 0 or −4
    (D) 0

208. $\displaystyle\lim_{x \to 2^-} f(x) =$

    (A) −4
    (B) Does not exist
    (C) 0 or −4
    (D) 0 and −4

209. $\displaystyle\lim_{x \to 2} f(x) =$

    (A) −4
    (B) Does not exist
    (C) 0
    (D) 0 and −4

210. $\log(mn) =$

    (A) $\log(m) - \log(n)$
    (B) $\log(m) + \log(n)$

    (C) $\log\left(\dfrac{m}{n}\right)$

    (D) $\dfrac{\log(m)}{\log(n)}$

211. A truck travels at a steady speed of 100 kilometers per hour from 12 noon until 6 P.M. How many miles will be driven?

    (A) 968
    (B) 600
    (C) 372
    (D) 106

212. Thirty-two percent of 800 equals

    (A) 256
    (B) 266
    (C) 246
    (D) 236

For questions 213 and 214, consider the given graph.

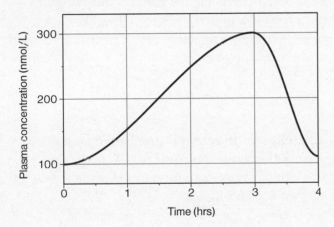

213. What is the maximum plasma concentration?

    (A) 100 nmol/L
    (B) None of these
    (C) 200 nmol/L
    (D) 300 nmol/L

214. When does the maximum plasma concentration occur?

    (A) After 3 hours
    (B) After 1 hour
    (C) After 4 hours
    (D) None of the above

215. $\lim\limits_{x \to \infty} \left(\dfrac{5x^4 + 2x^3 - x + 7}{3x^4 + 8x^2 - 10} \right) =$

    (A) ∞
    (B) Undefined
    (C) 1
    (D) $\dfrac{5}{3}$

216. A man is tossing a coin. The first three tosses have been heads. What are the chances that heads will occur on the fourth toss?

    (A) 50%
    (B) 25%
    (C) 12.5%
    (D) 6.25%

217. The height h of a projectile is given by $h(x) = -0.008x^2 + x$, where x is the horizontal distance the projectile travels. The projectile hits the ground after it has traveled a horizontal distance of

    (A) 140 feet
    (B) 200 feet
    (C) 250 feet
    (D) 125 feet

218. A store reduces the selling price of an item by 30%. The new price is $210. What was the original price?

    (A) $320
    (B) $240
    (C) $300
    (D) $280

219. Event A has a probability of $\frac{5}{9}$. What is the probability that event A does NOT occur?

    (A) $\frac{4}{9}$

    (B) $\frac{9}{5}$

    (C) $-\frac{5}{9}$

    (D) Not enough information

220. Calculate the value of x in the expression $4x = \frac{1}{2}$.

    (A) $\frac{1}{42}$

    (B) $\frac{1}{24}$

    (C) $\frac{1}{16}$

    (D) $\frac{1}{8}$

For questions 221 and 222, consider the data shown in the table below.

Drug Prescribed	# of patients
Drug A	730
Drug B	185
Drug C	90
Drug D	466
Other	29

221. What percentage of patients received prescriptions for Drug A or Drug B?

    (A) 40%
    (B) 65%
    (C) 60%
    (D) 75%

222. What percentage of patients did NOT receive a prescription for Drug D?

    (A) 69%
    (B) 31%
    (C) 47%
    (D) 53%

223. Digoxin Injection is supplied in ampules of 500 micrograms per 2 mL. What quantity must a nurse administer to provide a dose of 0.25 milligrams?

    (A) 0.2 mL
    (B) 0.5 mL
    (C) 1.0 mL
    (D) 2.0 ml

224. Determine the slope of the line passing through the points (9, 4) and (–5, 1).

    (A) $\frac{3}{14}$

    (B) $-\frac{3}{14}$

    (C) $\frac{14}{3}$

    (D) $-\frac{14}{3}$

For question 225, consider the given graph of the function $y = f(x)$.

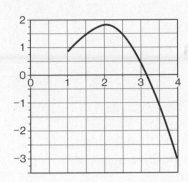

225. Identify the graph of the function $y = f(x + 3)$.

(A)

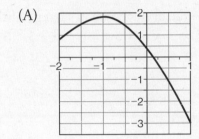

(B)

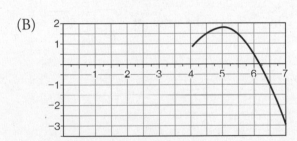

(C)

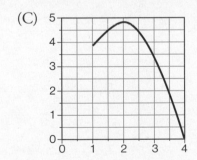

(D)

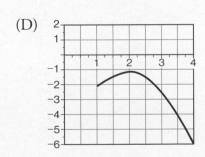

226. A patient's creatine clearance rate (CrCl) can be calculated by using the following formula:

$$CrCl = \frac{140 - \text{age in years}}{72 \cdot SCr} \cdot (\text{ideal body weight in kilograms})$$

What is the CrCl for a 58-year-old patient who has a SCr of 2.6 and an ideal body weight of 76 kg?

(A) 23
(B) 33
(C) 30
(D) 37

227. If the domain of f is $(-\infty, 5)$, what is the range of f^{-1}?

(A) $(5, \infty)$

(B) $(-\infty, \frac{1}{5})$

(C) $(-\infty, 5)$

(D) $(\frac{1}{5}, \infty)$

For questions 228–231, consider the given graph of the function $y = f(x)$.

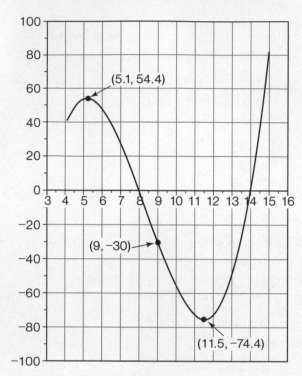

228. Identify the x value(s) for which $f'(x) < 0$.

    (A) $5.1 < x < 11.5$
    (B) $5.1 > x > 11.5$
    (C) $8 < x < 14$
    (D) $8 > x > 14$

229. Identify the x value(s) for which $f''(x) > 0$.

    (A) $9 > x > \infty$
    (B) $-\infty < x < 9$
    (C) $9 < x < \infty$
    (D) $-\infty > x > 9$

230. Identify the relative minima (if any).

    (A) $(5.1, 11.4)$
    (B) $(9, -30)$
    (C) None
    (D) $(11.5, -74.4)$

231. $\lim\limits_{x \to 14} \left(\dfrac{f(x) - f(14)}{x - 14} \right) =$

    (A) a negative number
    (B) a positive number
    (C) 0
    (D) Not enough information

232. Determine the average rate of change of the function $f(x) = x^3$ on the interval $2 \leq x \leq 4$.

    (A) 28
    (B) 56
    (C) 36
    (D) 38

233. What is the value of $\sqrt{45} + \sqrt{80}$?

    (A) $4\sqrt{125}$
    (B) $5\sqrt{35}$
    (C) $4\sqrt{9}$
    (D) $7\sqrt{5}$

Practice Test 2

234. What is the slope of the line shown in the graph below?

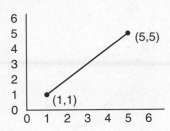

    (A) 1
    (B) 2
    (C) 4
    (D) 10

235. What is the median of the following values:

    10, 12, 9, 10, 11, 9, 9, 10, 8, 12?

    (A) 2
    (B) 9.5
    (C) 10
    (D) 12

236. How many three-letter codes can be formed from the set {*A, B, C, D, E,*}? Repeated letters are allowed.

    (A) 60
    (B) 120
    (C) 80
    (D) 125

237. Determine the *x*-coordinate of the points,

    if any, where the graph of $f(x) = \dfrac{x}{x+1}$ has

    a horizontal tangent line.

    (A) −1
    (B) none
    (C) 1
    (D) 0

238. Identify the graph that demonstrates a quadratic relationship between the variables *x* and *y*.

    (A)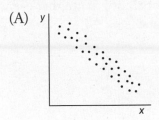

    (B)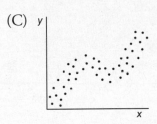

    (C)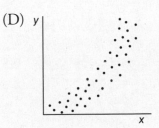

    (D)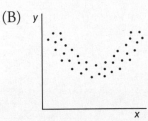

239. Event *A* has a probability of 0.35. Event *B* has a probability of 0.22. The probability that events *A* and *B* both occur is 0.09. What is the probability that either event *A* or event *B* occurs?

(A) 0.57
(B) 0.52
(C) 0.48
(D) 0.66

240. Find the exact value of the shaded area.

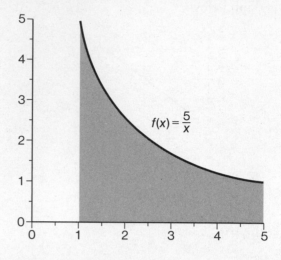

(A) $\ln(5)$
(B) $\ln(25)$
(C) $5 \cdot \ln(5)$
(D) $\dfrac{1}{5} \cdot \ln(5)$

STOP

End of Quantitative Ability section. If you have any time left, you may go over your work in this section only.

Practice Test 2

ESSAY

TIME: 30 MINUTES

Directions: Write a well-constructed essay addressing the statement below.

"Discuss solutions to the problem of graphic and violent television programming."

_____

_____

_____

_____

_____

_____

_____

_____

_____

_____

_____

_____

_____

_____

_____

_____

_____

_____

_____

_____

ESSAY

TIME: 30 MINUTES

Directions: Write a well-constructed essay addressing the statement below.

"Discuss solutions to the problem of illegal immigration in the United States."

_____

_____

_____

_____

_____

_____

_____

_____

_____

_____

_____

_____

_____

_____

_____

_____

_____

_____

_____

_____

_____

_____

Practice Test 2

Answer Key
PRACTICE TEST 2

VERBAL ABILITY

1. D	13. A	25. D	37. D
2. C	14. A	26. A	38. C
3. A	15. D	27. C	39. A
4. B	16. B	28. D	40. B
5. D	17. B	29. B	41. A
6. A	18. B	30. C	42. C
7. C	19. C	31. B	43. D
8. D	20. A	32. A	44. A
9. A	21. A	33. C	45. B
10. B	22. B	34. D	46. C
11. D	23. D	35. A	47. D
12. B	24. A	36. C	48. C

CHEMISTRY

49. B	61. D	73. D	85. C
50. A	62. B	74. A	86. B
51. A	63. B	75. C	87. B
52. A	64. B	76. D	88. D
53. D	65. D	77. C	89. B
54. A	66. A	78. C	90. D
55. C	67. B	79. C	91. A
56. B	68. C	80. A	92. D
57. C	69. B	81. C	93. B
58. D	70. D	82. B	94. A
59. C	71. A	83. B	95. A
60. B	72. A	84. A	96. C

BIOLOGY

97. B	109. A	121. D	133. B
98. D	110. D	122. A	134. A
99. D	111. D	123. A	135. C
100. A	112. B	124. A	136. C
101. A	113. B	125. C	137. D
102. B	114. D	126. A	138. C
103. A	115. D	127. B	139. D
104. C	116. A	128. D	140. B
105. D	117. D	129. B	141. A
106. B	118. C	130. A	142. B
107. D	119. C	131. D	143. A
108. C	120. B	132. C	144. C

Answer Key
PRACTICE TEST 2

READING COMPREHENSION

145.	B	157.	D	169.	D	181.	B
146.	C	158.	B	170.	C	182.	B
147.	B	159.	B	171.	D	183.	A
148.	B	160.	A	172.	A	184.	A
149.	D	161.	C	173.	B	185.	C
150.	A	162.	A	174.	A	186.	B
151.	D	163.	B	175.	D	187.	C
152.	C	164.	A	176.	B	188.	B
153.	C	165.	B	177.	C	189.	D
154.	D	166.	D	178.	A	190.	D
155.	D	167.	D	179.	B	191.	B
156.	A	168.	A	180.	D	192.	C

QUANTITATIVE ABILITY

193.	A	205.	B	217.	D	229.	C
194.	B	206.	A	218.	C	230.	D
195.	A	207.	D	219.	A	231.	B
196.	B	208.	A	220.	D	232.	A
197.	A	209.	B	221.	C	233.	D
198.	A	210.	B	222.	A	234.	A
199.	D	211.	C	223.	C	235.	C
200.	D	212.	A	224.	A	236.	D
201.	B	213.	D	225.	A	237.	B
202.	C	214.	A	226.	B	238.	B
203.	C	215.	D	227.	C	239.	C
204.	D	216.	A	228.	A	240.	C

EXPLANATORY ANSWERS

1. **(D)** This is an analogy of a "lack of" or "without" relationship where one word means lack of or without the other. Shallow is lack of depth and apathetic is lack of caring.

2. **(C)** This is an analogy of "used to" or "serves to" relationship. Glue is used to fasten and an elevator is used to lift.

3. **(A)** This is an analogy of characteristics or description. An oracle by definition has foresight and a sage has wisdom.

4. **(B)** This is an analogy of characteristic or description. A florist sells flowers and a jeweler sells rings.

5. **(D)** In this worker-to-tool analogy, the gardener uses a trowel just as the mechanic uses a wrench. (If you chose A, you may have mistaken this for an analogy of association, but you need to select the name of a specific tool instead.)

6. **(A)** This is an analogy of characteristic or description in which the blueprint is the plan of the building and the outline is the plan of a report.

7. **(C)** This is an analogy of characteristic or description. An antiseptic helps to eliminate germs, water helps to eliminate thirst.

8. **(D)** This is an analogy of a "lack of" or "without" relationship. Sluggish means lack of energy and satiated means lack of hunger.

9. **(A)** This is an analogy of characteristic or description. A book can be located in a library and a horse can be found in a stable.

10. **(B)** This is an analogy of a "lack of" or "without" relationship. A neophyte is without experience and an invalid is not healthy.

11. **(D)** This is an analogy of characteristic or description. A bus carries passengers and a freighter carries cargo.

12. **(B)** This is an analogy of synonyms. To verify is to confirm and conciliation is to appease.

13. **(A)** This is an analogy of characteristic or description. An embargo prevents trade and a helmet prevents injury.

14. **(A)** This is an analogy of synonyms. To be resolute means to be full of determination and to be skeptical means to be full of doubt.

15. **(D)** This is an analogy of "used to" or "serves to" relationship. A meter is used to measure length and a pound is used to measure weight.

16. **(B)** This is an analogy of characteristic or description. A rose is a type of flower and an elm is a type of tree.

17. **(B)** This may also be considered an analogy of description or characteristic. A swamp is associated with humidity and a desert is associated with aridity (which means dryness).

18. **(B)** This is a part-to-whole analogy. An anaconda is a type of snake and basketball is a type of sport. To help clarify this kind of analogy, think of the group of all snakes and the group of all sports as "wholes," of which the anaconda and basketball are merely parts.

19. **(C)** This is an analogy of characteristics or description. A bruise is a mark on the skin and a stain is a mark on fabric.

20. **(A)** This is an analogy of purpose or use. A sphygmomanometer is used to measure blood pressure, and a thermometer is used to measure temperature.

21. **(A)** In this analogy of antonyms, "ebb" and "flow" have opposite meanings, and the opposite of "regress" is "advance."

22. **(B)** This is an analogy of association. The Oedipus complex is associated with Freud, and the uncertainty principle is associated with the physicist Heisenberg.

23. **(D)** In this part-to-whole analogy, the Hindenberg is an example of a blimp, and the Titanic is an example of an ocean liner. (The fact that both met tragic fates is not relevant here.)

24. **(A)** In this geographical analogy, Phoenix is the capital city of Arizona, and Atlanta is the capital city of Georgia.

25. **(D)** The word anthropomorphic means having a human shape or human characteristics; theriomorphic means having an animal shape or animal characteristics. This analogy is based on the definitions of words.

26. **(A)** This is an analogy of association. The blues are associated with Mississippi, and bluegrass music is associated with Kentucky.

27. **(C)** In this analogy of part to whole, the nuclear membrane is part of a cell, and the hypotenuse is part of a triangle.

28. **(D)** Since bass and treble represent opposite ends of a portion of the spectrum of sound, this can be considered either an analogy of antonyms or an analogy of degree. Acme and nadir also represent opposites.

29. **(B)** This analogy may be considered one of antonyms or of degree, since the pairs of terms (imperceptible and tangible, mild and severe) represent opposite extremes.

30. **(C)** The correct word that will complete the blank in this sentence describes a pond that has green surface film or residue resulting from several years of lifelessness. Accordingly, if the pond is characterized as "lifeless"—meaning dormant, inactive, or motionless—then the correct answer for the blank should also have the same meanings. The correct answer is Answer C—stagnant.

31. **(B)** The correct word for the blank in this sentence will have a meaning that is related to two concepts—"both" and "handedness." Since the prefix "ambi" means "both" or "combined," we can assume that the correct word will have this prefix also. "Dexterous" generally describes a person who has the skill, coordination, or agility to use their hands and/or body. Answer B (ambidextrous) is the result of combining these two word parts, and it is the correct answer in this sentence.

32. **(A)** "Planning ahead" is the key phrase that connects the correct word for the first blank and the type of events that may occur and spoil a camping trip (the correct word for the second blank). Generally speaking, a camping trip can be characterized as an informal, improvised event. Planning ahead is typically done to try to avoid or bypass some of the unpredictable events that may happen. Thus, based on the answer choices provided, Answer A is the correct choice for this sentence completion.

33. **(C)** The correct word for the blank in this sentence describes a particular type of proportional or parallel relationship where something happens as a result of something else. In this sentence, the relationship is further described as lowered or decreased blood pressure, resulting in an increased or accelerated heart rate. When blood pressure goes down, then the reverse or direct opposite happens for the heart rate—it goes up. Answer C (inversely) best describes this specific type of relationship.

34. **(D)** In this sentence, managing the financial costs of college in an independent fashion may have been difficult or impossible had it not been for something or someone—the correct word that completes the blank. Whatever or whomever this may be provided substantial monetary support or sponsorship, because they are further described as generous. A person who contributes or donates money toward the best interests or "benefit" (containing the word prefix "bene" meaning "good") of another is called a patron or philanthropist. Of the words listed in the answer choices, only Answer D is synonymous with this type of person; therefore, Answer D (benefactor) is the correct response.

35. **(A)** An example of the correct word for the first blank in this sentence completion is Greek mythology, which is somehow related to the concept or theory of the existence of multiple gods or holy beings (religion). Since the prefix "poly" means "many" or "much," we can conclude that the word for the first blank will describe something that is founded or based (synonymous with the correct word for the second blank) on the idea of numerous gods. Based on the answer choices listed and by reading each of the choices into both blanks in the sentence, Answer A is the best match and makes the most sense, given the sentence's context.

36. **(C)** The correct word for the first blank in this sentence will further describe the type of existence where the tree and fungi live together or cohabitate; however, we must also look closely at the two parts that make up this sentence. The first part of this sentence tells us that not all fungi are detrimental to trees, that is, harmful, hurtful, or damaging. The second

part provides an alternative or counter-example to what has been stated in the first part. Thus, the correct word for the second blank will contradict what was said previously, meaning "advantageous" or "helpful." Answer C is the correct response for both blanks in this sentence completion. "Symbiotic" is made up of the words "sym" (meaning "together") and "bio" (meaning "life" or "living"), and "benefit" is synonymous with "good contributions" and "valuable."

37. **(D)** Most babies cry when they are upset or in distress. If the baby in this sentence "may start crying again," then this most likely means that the baby may become agitated or uncomfortable after a period of time when he/she was not crying. During this peaceful time, which was brought about by the new toy, the baby was calm and appeased. Answer D (pacify) is the correct answer to complete this sentence.

38. **(C)** The prefix "super" denotes "over," "surpassing," or "excessive." If 50 pages is defined as the maximum page limit previously required for manuscripts, then 150 pages more than exceeds and surpasses this limit. One hundred and fifty pages goes above and beyond the previous maximum page limit. Based on the sentence's context and by looking at the answer choices listed, only Answer C (superceded) provides the best word to correctly complete the sentence.

39. **(A)** In this sentence the listener has made some action associated with a question directed toward the presentation's speaker. Since the listener is described as both puzzled and impatient, we can assume that the listener could not wait to ask his or her question, and therefore interrupted the speaker in order to do so. Typically, questions are solicited and answered by a speaker when their presentation has finished or been completed. Thus, Answer A (interjected and conclude) is the correct answer.

40. **(B)** In this sentence, the correct word will relate to an action regarding the message where it does not have to be "exactly as it was spoken." Since the express purpose of taking a message is so that it can be given, meaning "relayed" or "disclosed to a designated recipient," we can assume that the correct word for the first blank will also have the same meaning. Continuing on in the sentence, there are additional instructions that may be done for this message (the second blank's correct word): "in your own words." If a verbal communication is not worded "exactly as spoken," then it is typically said to be "rephrased" or "reworded." Based on this, to "disclose" the message means to "communicate" it, and if the message was not exactly as spoken, then it was "paraphrased," and Answer B is the correct answer for this sentence.

41. **(A)** The phrase "one-way" is a clue that lets us know that this sentence is centered on motion or movement. Here, "one-way" describes the direction or pathway of the impulses in the nervous system. Of the answer choices listed, Answer A—"conduction," meaning "to direct, convey, or transmit"—is the best response for the blank in this sentence, based on the sentence's context.

42. **(C)** By reading each of the answer choices into this sentence, Answer C makes the most sense, given the sentence's context. "Impromptu" remarks are ones that are improvised or unrehearsed. The unexpected and spontaneous nature of the facilitator's request most likely caught this woman off guard and unready, which best matches the word "unprepared" given in this answer choice. Answer C is the best response to complete both blanks in this sentence.

43. **(D)** The correct word for the blank directly connects the unavailability of theater seating with the manager hanging the "Standing Room Only" sign. There was no verbal or physical interaction with the manager, so this conclusion or deduction of a filled seating capacity was based simply on seeing the manager hang the sign. To have an understanding, reasoning, or conclusion based on an assumption or something that is not directly communicated means to "infer." Accordingly, Answer D (inferred) is the correct response.

44. **(A)** In most cases, rain that falls onto the ground will be absorbed into the soil. If the soil below cannot hold any more water because it is already filled with all the water it can hold, then rainwater will form puddles above ground. This typically occurs after a heavy rainfall. Words that are synonymous with being "thoroughly soaked or overfilled with water" caused by an "excess or deluge" of rain are found in Answer A—"saturated" and "overabundance."

45. **(B)** The correct word for the first blank will describe a negative attitude characterized by contempt, disdain, and superiority. This is further compounded by the thought of the volunteers as "inferior," meaning "underneath" or "lowly" (indicated by the correct response for the second blank). Looking closer at the word parts in the answers listed can provide additional clues that lead to the correct responses. The word prefix "con" means "against" or "opposing." To "condescend" means to be "against lowering oneself," and in this sentence's context, it means to have a high or elevated attitude. The prefix "sub" means "below" or "lesser." The word "substandard" means "of a lesser quality" or to be "below acceptable levels." Based on this, the best matches for both of the sentence blanks are found in Answer B—condescending and substandard.

46. **(C)** In this sentence, information that should not be included in the report will be synonymous with "irrelevant" (meaning "nonessential" or "without bearing or importance"). Generally speaking, you would NOT include information that is unimportant or not pertinent if you want to make the report as short and concise as possible, instead of long and verbose. Accordingly, Answer C—extraneous and succinct—provides the best answer choices for both blanks in this sentence.

47. **(D)** The correct word that will complete the first blank in this sentence will describe one of the obvious, distinct, or prominent aspects of a charismatic and vivacious presentation. Furthermore, there is something so appealing about the man's presentation ability that he was able to engage or

stimulate the interest of apathetic and lethargic children (indicated by the word that will complete the second blank). This presenter brought about a significant change in the children's demeanor to the point where they wanted to fully participate. Based on these conclusions, Answer D (salient and captivate) provides the best match for both blanks in this sentence.

48. **(C)** In this sentence, the completion of the initial class is characterized as "imperative"—vital, crucial, or non-negotiable. Oftentimes, an initial or preliminary class can provide such fundamental and essential information that it is deemed to be required. Furthermore, classes such as these must be completed in order to move on, progress, or proceed to any subsequent classes. Based on this, Answer C (mandatory and advance) provides the best match for both blanks in this sentence.

49. **(B)** In translation or protein synthesis, the nucleotide sequence (or base sequence) in a messenger RNA (mRNA) determines the order of amino acids in the resulting protein. Each three nucleotides or bases is called a codon and each codon "codes" for the incorporation of a specific amino acid in the growing protein. The term *anticodon* refers to the corresponding nucleotide sequence in the tRNA that carries the particular amino acid to the ribosome where protein synthesis occurs.

50. **(A)** When a solute is dissolved in a solvent some of the physical properties of the solvent are affected—the boiling point, the freezing point, and the osmotic pressure. The impact on these properties is a function of the number of solute particles dissolved and not the specific identity of the particles themselves and are called colligative properties. Dissolved solutes raise the boiling point, lower the freezing point, and raise the osmotic pressure. The conduction of electricity by a solution is dependent on the presence of ions in solutions. If a given solute dissolves in the solvent resulting in the presence of ions, then the solution will conduct electricity and the solute is said to be an electrolyte.

51. **(A)** In the symbol for the lithium ion, $^7_3\text{Li}^{+1}$, the bottom number, 3, is the number of protons. One could obtain the number of neutrons, 4, by subtracting the number of protons, 3, from the number of protons plus neutrons, 7.

52. **(A)** Nucleotides, which are polymerized in both DNA and RNA, consist of a purine or pyrimidine (base), a ribose or deoxyribose sugar, and a phosphate.

53. **(D)** Of the major classes of biomolecules, the lipids are characterized by their hydrophobicity (or lipophilicity) due to their structural nonpolarity. The other biomolecular classes (proteins, carbohydrates, and nucleic acids) have more polar features (like carbon-oxygen bonds, carbon-nitrogen bonds, oxygen-hyrogen bonds, and nitrogen-hydrogen bonds) and are therefore more hydrophilic (lipophobic).

54. **(A)** This molecule has two chiral centers. The one with the chlorine has chlorine as priority 1, the side of the ring closest to the methyl as priority 2, the other side of the ring as priority 3, and the hydrogen as priority 4. Positioning the hydrogen away from you gives 1, 2, 3 as counterclockwise and thus S at that chiral center. The other chiral center has priority 1 as the side of the ring closest to the chlorine, priority 2 as the other side of the ring, priority 3 as the methyl group, and priority 4 as the hydrogen. Again, positioning the hydrogen away from you (which it already is in the structure given), the other three are arranged as 1, 2, 3 in a counterclockwise manner and thus also S.

55. **(C)** When $KMnO_4$ is reacted with any alkyl benzene having at least one benzylic hydrogen (the benzylic position is the carbon adjacent to the ring), benzoic acid results.

56. **(B)** Moles may be defined as grams/molar mass.

$$\text{Moles} = \frac{\text{Grams}}{\text{Molar Mass}}$$

The molar mass of carbon dioxide, CO_2, is

$$1\ C = 1(12) = 12$$

$$2\ O = 2(16) = 32$$

$$12 + 32 = 44\ \frac{\text{grams}}{\text{mole}}$$

Dividing 22 grams by $44\ \frac{\text{grams}}{\text{mole}}$ gives 0.50 mole.

57. **(C)** Percentage yield is defined as $100 \times \dfrac{\text{actual yield}}{\text{theoretical yield}}$.

Theoretical yield is the number of grams calculated as being possible to produce in a reaction. Actual yield is the number of grams actually isolated in a reaction.

$$H_2 + Cl_2 \rightarrow 2\ HCl$$

From the balanced equation above it can be seen that 1 mole of hydrogen reacts with 1 mole of chlorine to produce 2 moles of hydrogen chloride. In the problem, grams of hydrogen are given and they react with excess chlorine. Therefore, hydrogen is the limiting reagent and is used to calculate the theoretical yield. Theoretical yield may be calculated as follows:

$$\text{grams } H_2 \rightarrow \text{moles } H_2 \rightarrow \text{moles } Cl_2 \rightarrow \text{grams } HCl$$

Refer to explanation to question 56 for definition of moles.

Grams H_2

1.0

Moles H_2

$$\frac{1.0 \text{ gram}}{2 \text{ grams per mole}} = 0.5 \text{ moles } H_2$$

Moles HCl

$$0.5 \text{ moles } H_2 \times \frac{2 \text{ moles HCl}}{1 \text{ mole } H_2} = 1.0 \text{ mole HCl}$$

Grams HCl

$$1.0 \text{ mole HCl} \times \frac{36.5 \text{ grams HCl}}{1 \text{ mole HCl}} = 36.5 \text{ grams HCl} \left(\text{theoretical yield} \right)$$

$$\text{Percentage yield} = \frac{\text{Actual Yield}}{\text{Theoretical Yield}} \times 100 = \frac{18.3 \text{ grams HCl}}{36.5 \text{ grams HCl}} \times 100$$

$$= 50\%$$

58. **(D)** There are 6×10^{23} atoms, Avogadro's number, present in one mole of any element. To calculate the number of moles in 1.2×10^6 atoms of copper, divide the number of atoms by the number of atoms in one mole.

$$\frac{1.2 \times 10^6 \text{ atoms Cu}}{6 \times 10^{23} \text{ atoms/mole}} = 0.2 \times 10^{-17} = 2.0 \times 10^{-18} \text{ mole}$$

59. **(C)** When an amine reacts with an acid halide, a nucleophilic acyl substitution reaction occurs in which the amine substitutes for the halogen of the acid halide producing an amide. It may help to see what functional groups are involved by first drawing out each line bond structure.

60. **(B)** A neutralization reaction is one in which an acid and a base react to produce a salt and water. In equation B, the acid, HCl, reacts with the base, $CaCO_3$, to produce the salt, $CaCl_2$ and initially H_2CO_3, carbonic acid.

$$2HCl + CaCO_3 \rightarrow CaCl_2 + H_2CO_3$$

However, carbonic acid is unstable and decomposes to carbon dioxide, CO_2, and water, H_2O.

$$H_2CO_3 \rightarrow CO_2 + H_2O$$

Equation A is a single displacement reaction, displacement of the H in HCl by Mg.

$$Mg + 2HCl \rightarrow MgCl_2 + H_2$$

Equation C is a double displacement reaction, in which the positive and negative ions change partners. The Ba replaces the Na and the Na replaces the Ba.

$$BaCl_2 + Na_2SO_4 \rightarrow BaSO_4 + 2NaCl$$

Equation D is a decomposition reaction, in which $KClO_3$ decomposes to KCl and O_2.

$$2KClO_3 \rightarrow 2KCl + 3O_2$$

61. **(D)** In order to determine the oxidation number of an element in a formula, it is necessary to assign oxidation numbers to all the other elements in the formula. For example, in PO_4^{-3}, oxygen has an oxidation number of -2. There are four atoms of oxygen in the formula, so the total oxidation value of oxygen is $4(-2) = -8$. Since the ion has a charge of -3, the oxidation number of phosphorus should be such that when it is combined with -8, a charge of -3 remains. Therefore, the oxidation number of phosphorus is $-3 = -8 + ?$. The value of $+5 = ?$. Oxygen is assigned an oxidation number of -2, except when it is present in a peroxide, eg. H_2O_2, when the oxidation number is -1.

62. **(B)** Denaturation involves the disruption of noncovalent intermolecular forces (in particular, hydrogen bonding, dipole-dipole interactions). Peptide bonds are covalent, and digestion involves the cleavage of these.

63. **(B)** Molarity is defined as moles of solute divided by liters of solution.

$$M = \frac{\text{moles solute}}{\text{liters solution}} = \frac{\text{grams/molar mass}}{\text{liters solution}}$$

Substituting the given values for sodium hydroxide, NaOH, (molar mass = 40 grams/mole) into the above formula gives

$$2.0\ M = \frac{x/40 \text{ gm per mole}}{0.8 \text{ liter}}$$

Solving for x gives a value of 64 grams.

64. **(B)** Since volume is constant in an autoclave, the equation

$$\frac{P_1V_1}{T_1} = \frac{P_2V_2}{T_2} \text{ reduces to } \frac{P_1}{T_1} = \frac{P_2}{T_2}$$

Temperature in the gas equations is always in Kelvin. Substituting the values given in the problem into the above equation gives

$$\frac{1 \text{ atm}}{27 + 273} = \frac{5.0 \text{ atm}}{x} \qquad x = 1500 \text{ K}$$

$$1500 - 273 = 1227°C$$

65. **(D)** The major biomolecular classes are carbohydrates (have multiple alcohol groups), nucleic acids (have phosphates, carbohydrates, and aromatic heterocycles), proteins (have amide/peptide bonds), and lipids (have long carbon chains).

66. **(A)** The correct electron configuration for magnesium, Mg, is $1s^2 2s^2 2p^6 3s^2$. Magnesium is the 12th element in counting the elements from left to right across each row. Therefore, the atomic number, the number of protons, is 12 and the number of electrons is 12 for the neutral atom. The letters s, p, d, and f indicate the type of orbital. The number in front of the symbols, as in 1s, indicates the number of the orbital, in this case 1. The superscript, as in $1s^2$, indicates the number of electrons present in the orbital, in this case 2. The electron configuration of Mg, $1s^2 2s^2 2p^6 3s^2$, shows the 12 electrons in the neutral atom.

67. **(B)** When an alkyl halide is converted to an alkene, a base is used. If the halide is primary or secondary, a strong base is required to accomplish an E2 elimination. NH_3 is a weak base but potassium t-butoxide is a strong base.

68. **(C)** $NaBH_4$ is a hydride-reducing agent that reduces aldehydes and ketones to alcohols.

69. **(B)** Compounds formed from elements located close together in the periodic table are generally covalently bonded, for example ICl. Compounds formed from elements located far apart in the periodic table are generally ionically bonded. The element hydrogen, H, is an exception to this general rule. Sometimes hydrogen is covalently bonded, as in CH_4, other times hydrogen is ionically bonded as in hydrochloric acid, HCl.

70. **(D)** ^1H NMR gives information about the hydrogens in a molecule. Since there are three signals, there are three kinds of hydrogen in the molecule. Choice (A) can be excluded since the molecule has only four kinds of hydrogen, and choice (C) can be excluded since the molecule has five kinds of hydrogen. After comparing the number of signals in the spectrum to the number of different kinds of hydrogen in the molecule, look at the splitting pattern and integration information. Simple splitting patterns follow the n + 1 rule, meaning that the splitting pattern for a group of hydrogens will be equal to the number of neighboring hydrogens (those on an adjacent carbon) plus one. A doublet indicates that the hydrogens represented by that signal have one neighboring hydrogen, a singlet indicates that the hydrogens represented by that signal have no neighboring hydrogens, and a septet indicates that the hydrogens represented by that signal have six neighboring hydrogens. Both remaining choices (B) and (D) are consistent with the observed splitting pattern. The next level of comparison should be the chemical shifts of the signals. Since the septet is farthest downfield, the hydrogen represented by the signal must be the most deshielded in the molecule. In choice (B), the signal for the methyl hydrogens (represented by the singlet since there are no neighboring hydrogens) would be farthest downfield (due to the adjacent oxygen)—the singlet is not the signal far-

thest downfield so (B) can be excluded. That leaves (D) as the correct answer, and indeed the hydrogen represented by the septet (since it has six neighboring hydrogens) is expected to be the signal farthest downfield.

71. **(A)** Resonance structures do not have atoms in different places, only pi and unshared electrons. The only structure for which this is true is choice (A).

72. **(A)** A nonpolar covalent bond is a bond in which electrons are equally shared between the two atoms forming the bond, i.e. both atoms have the same electronegativity. Atoms have identical electronegativities only when they are the same element. Therefore, the C — C bond is nonpolar. The bond between lithium and chlorine, Li — Cl, is ionic, answer B. The bond between hydrogen and fluorine, H — F, answer C, is polar. The electrons comprising the bond between the two atoms are unequally shared, with fluorine, which has the higher electronegativity, having more electron density around itself than does hydrogen. The bond between boron and carbon, B — C, answer D is slightly polar, with the electrons being drawn slightly more toward carbon than toward boron, B. Electronegativity increases from left to right across the rows of the periodic table and decreases from top to bottom in the columns or families. The closer elements are to each other, the more likely their electronegativities are to be close in value. The following statement is an important relationship. Generally, as the size of the atom decreases, electronegativity increases.

73. **(D)** Ionic compounds boil at higher temperatures than do covalent compounds, because positive and negative ions are strongly attracted to each other and much energy (high boiling point) is needed to separate them. Sodium chloride, NaCl, is the only ionic compound indicated in the problem.

74. **(A)** The solution is 12 M, which means 12 moles of solute per liter of solution. Molality is the number of moles of solute per kilogram of solvent. The density of the solution is 1.2 g/mL, which means that 1 L of solution would have a mass of 1,200 g. Since the solution is 12 M, there would be 12 moles of solute (total mass of solute is 12 moles × 33 g/mol = 406 g) in 1 L or 1,200 g of solution. That means there is about 800 g of solvent. Molality would be 12 moles solute/0.800 kg of solvent.

75. **(C)** Cell membranes contain phospholipids, steroid hormones are lipids, and triglycerides in adipose tissue are lipids that store carbon chains for later oxidation through beta oxidation.

76. **(D)** A 1.5 M NaBr solution would contain 1.5 moles of NaBr per liter of solution. Since 100 mL is 0.100 L, then 0.15 moles of NaBr are needed (0.100 L × 1.5 moles/1 L). The formula weight of NaBr is 103 g/mol so 0.15 moles would have a mass of 15.45 g or 15.5 g. To make 100 mL of solution, water would be added to reach a total volume of 100 mL (adding 100 mL of water may result in less than 100 mL of solution because solutes can result in a contraction of volume).

77. **(C)** Phospholipids are esters of glycerol with one or more fatty acids (long-chain carboxylic acids) and a phosphate (at physiological pH, phosphate groups are negatively charged and therefore polar). The phospholipids contain a hydrophilic region (the phosphate groups) and a hydrophobic region (the long-chain fatty acids) and, when in an aqueous environment, will form a bilayer in which their hydrophobic regions are facing each other with their hydrophilic regions along the edges of the bilayer.

78. **(C)** The conformation of a protein is driven by its amino acid sequence that determines the kinds of amino acid side chains present. The hydrophilic side chains will be oriented toward the exterior of the conformation (where the polar water molecules are) and the hydrophobic side chains oriented toward the interior of the conformation (where water is excluded).

79. **(C)** Boiling point is based on molecular weight (the heavier the molecule, the higher the boiling point) and strength of intermolecular attractions. For the options available, choices (A) and (C) have the lowest molecular weight. For those two, the only intermolecular force possible is van der Waal's force (also known as London force). The more extended molecule in (A) would have more available sites for this type of force, but the more compact molecule in (C) would have fewer available sites (less surface area) so the intermolecular forces among molecules of (C) would be less extensive and it would boil at a lower temperature.

80. **(A)** The shape of a molecule is believed to be determined by the number of electron pairs around the central atom. In the molecule BCl_3, the central B atom is bonded to three Cl atoms by three bonds which are made up of three electron pairs. Three electron pairs around the central atom equates to a trigonal planar shape. Two electron pairs around the central atom gives a linear shape. Four electron pairs around the central atom gives a tetrahedral shape.

81. **(C)** The ammonium ion, NH_4^{+1}, has four bonds, four electron pairs around the central atom, and therefore the ion has a tetrahedral shape. On the other hand, the ammonia molecule, NH_3, has three bonding pairs of electrons and one nonbonding pair of electrons around the central nitrogen, N, atom. Ammonia has a trigonal pyramid shape.

82. **(B)** To hydrate an alkene, there are two major options: oxymercuration-demercuration (the reagents in (A)) and hydroboration-oxidation (the reagents in (B)). Oxymercuration-demercuration yields the Markovnikov alcohol (the new H goes on the least highly substituted carbon of the alkene and the OH goes on the more highly substituted carbon of the alkene) and hydroboration-oxidation yields the anti-Markovnikov alcohol (the reverse orientation).

83. **(B)** Each carbon atom in $H_2C = CH_2$ is bonded to three other atoms, bonded by two single bonds to two hydrogen atoms and bonded by a double bond to the other carbon atom. To determine the shape of the molecule, the double bond is considered to be one pair of electrons. Therefore, each carbon is assumed to have three electron pairs around itself and the shape of the molecule around each carbon atom is trigonal planar with a 120° bond angle. The hybridization of the trigonal planar carbon atom is sp^2.

84. **(A)** The value of the pH measures the acidity or basicity of a solution and is defined as $pH = -\log[H^{+1}]$. Substituting $[H^{+1}] = 1 \times 10^{-5}$ into the pH equation gives a pH = 5.

85. **(C)** The reason why there are "gas laws" or equations that describe the behavior of gases in general is because gases behave similarly. One of the gas laws is Boyle's law which states that as the volume of a gas is increased, its pressure will decrease (or $P_1V_1 = P_2V_2$). The Kinetic Molecular Theory of gases (the theory that summarizes our understanding of gases as a result of the observations of the gas laws) states that the kinetic energy of gas particles increases with increased Kelvin temperature (i.e., they are directly proportional).

86. **(B)** The acetate ion, CH_3COO^{-1} or Ac^{-1}, reacts with water to produce hydroxide ion and consequently the solution is basic.

$$Ac^{-1} + H_2O \rightarrow HAc + OH^{-1}$$

87. **(B)** A buffer solution is one in which the pH remains constant even when small amounts of acid or base are added to the solution. A buffer solution consists of a weak acid and its salt, or a weak base and its salt. Acetic acid, CH_3COOH, is the only weak acid present, along with its salt sodium acetate, CH_3COONa. The other acids, HCl, HNO_3, H_2SO_4, are all strong acids.

88. **(D)** Molecular orbital, MO, theory includes both sigma and pi bonds. Sigma bonds have a symmetrical concentration of electron density along the bond between the two bonded atoms. Pi bonds have electron density both above and below the plane of the bond. Single bonds in molecules are sigma bonds. The double bond, $C = C$, in the ethylene molecule consists of one sigma bond and one pi bond. A triple bond, for example, consists of one sigma and two pi bonds.

89. **(B)** According to the Kinetic Molecular Theory of Matter, the molecules in a solid are close together, the molecules of a liquid are farther apart, and the molecules of a gas are farthest apart. The farther apart molecules are, the more freely they can move.

90. **(D)** Grignard reagents attack carbonyl carbons. The reaction of ethyl Grignard with the ketone in choice (A) would give ethyl cyclopentanol whereas its reaction with choice (C) would give 3-ethyl-3-pentanol. Reaction of ethyl Grignard with the aldehyde in choice (D) gives 3-pentanol.

91. **(A)** To name esters, name the alkyl group attached to the oxygen first (in this case, methyl) and then name the rest of the molecule as if its a carboxylate. Choice (B) is not even an ester (it would be named 2,3-dimethylbutanoate), choice (C) is named 2-methylbutyl ethanoate, and choice (D) is also not an ester (and named 2,2-dimethylbutanoate).

92. **(D)** Protein synthesis or translation involves mRNA (the nucleotide sequence that determines the amino acid sequence in the protein synthesized), rRNA (that combines with specific proteins to form the ribosome on which protein synthesis occurs), and various tRNAs (that bring the appropriate amino acids to the ribosome for incorporation into the growing protein).

93. **(B)** The change in free energy, ΔG, represents the energy which can be used to do work in a reaction. The change in free energy may be used to determine whether a reaction will take place as written or not.

    If $\Delta G < 0$, the reaction occurs spontaneously in the direction written.

    If $\Delta G > 0$, the reaction does not occur spontaneously in the direction written, but does occur spontaneously in the opposite direction.

    If $\Delta G = 0$, the reaction is at equilibrium and no change occurs.

94. **(A)** Entropy is a measure of the amount of disorder in a reaction system. More freedom of movement, or disorder, of molecules is possible in a gas than in a liquid than in a solid. In equation A, a solid is converted to a solid and a gas. More disorder can be present in the reaction system in the products, where a gas is produced, than in the reactants, where a solid is used. Disorder increases. In equation B, a gas is converted to a liquid. Disorder decreases. In equation C, two different gases are converted to a liquid. Disorder decreases. In equation D, a liquid and a gas are converted to a solid. Disorder decreases.

95. **(A)** Only a change in temperature can cause a change in the equilibrium constant of a reaction. An increase in temperature causes the reaction to shift toward the direction that absorbs heat, i.e. the endothermic reaction. A decrease in temperature causes the reaction to shift toward the direction that evolves heat, i.e. the exothermic reaction. Changes in either the volume, answer B, or concentration, answer C, of one of the components in the reaction system will cause a corresponding change in the volume or concentration of another component in the system to maintain a constant equilibrium constant. A catalyst, answer D, will cause a change in the mechanism and the activation energy of a reaction but has no effect upon the equilibrium constant.

96. **(C)** Gamma rays have the highest energy of the three forms of radiation listed. Therefore, the gamma rays can penetrate shields which would stop the other two forms of radiation. Beta particles are the next most energetic, and hence dangerous. Alpha particles are the least energetic and the least dangerous.

97. **(B)** RNA polymerase I transcribes genes encoding ribosomal RNA, RNA polymerase II transcribes protein-coding genes into messenger RNAs and RNA polymerase III transcribes genes that encode transfer RNA.

98. **(D)** The plasma membrane controls exchange of materials between the inside and outside of cell, regulates cell's chemical composition, and is the outermost layer of animal cells. The mitochondrion is the power plant of the cell and it provides energy in the form of ATP through oxidative phosphorylation.

99. **(D)** No explanation needed.

100. **(A)** 0% will have white hair color.

	B	B
b	Bb	Bb
b	Bb	Bb

101. **(A)** Meiosis is a special process in cell division comprising two nuclear divisions in rapid succession that result in four gametocytes, each containing half the number of chromosomes found in somatic cells. When the two gametes unite in fertilization, the fusion reconstitutes the diploid number of chromosomes.

102. **(B)** No explanation needed.

103. **(A)** The proper sequencing is prophase, metaphase, anaphase, and telophase. During prophase, the chromosomes condense, the nuclear membrane deteriorates, and the spindle microtubules attach to the chromosomes. During metaphase, the chromosomes move to the center of the cell. During anaphase, each kinetochore divides and the chromosomes separate. During telophase, the nuclear membrane reforms around each new daughter cell's nucleus.

104. **(C)** Both tooth abrasion and gum recession are serious health conditions associated with smokeless tobacco.

105. **(D)** An endocrine gland has no ducts, releases its secretion into the surrounding interstitial fluid, and depends on the circulatory system to transport the secreted hormone to its target tissue.

106. **(B)** Oxytocin is responsible for causing contractions of the uterus and ejecting milk from the mammary glands.

107. **(D)** Each cell contains a complete set of genes. The differentiation status of a cell is determined by the subset of the gene expressed in that cell.

108. **(C)** Calcitonin causes blood calcium levels to decrease. It is produced by the parafollicular cells of the thyroid gland, and it increases in response to increased blood calcium level. Low blood calcium may result in weak bones and tetany.

109. **(A)** No explanation needed.

110. **(D)** The medulla is a modified portion of the sympathetic nervous system. Its major secretory products are epinephrine and small amounts of norepinephrine, which are released during stress, exercise, injury, emotional excitement, or in response to low blood glucose.

111. **(D)** No explanation needed.

112. **(B)** The Tricuspid valve is the valve closing the orifice between the right atrium and the right ventricle of the heart. The Bicuspid valve is the valve closing the orifice between the left atrium and left ventricle of the heart. Choices C and D are not heart valves.

113. **(B)** The red blood cell would enter the right atrium through the inferior vena cava and pass into the right ventricle. The red blood cell would exit the right ventricle through the pulmonary trunk, pass through the lungs, and return to the left atrium through the pulmonary vein. From the left atrium, the red blood cell would enter the left ventricle and leave the heart through the aorta.

114. **(D)** About 97% of the oxygen transported in blood is bound to the heme portion of hemoglobin inside erythrocytes. About 3% is transported dissolved in plasma.

115. **(D)** All of the structures listed increase the mucosal surface area of the small intestine.

116. **(A)** Vitamins function as coenzymes, parts of coenzymes, or parts of enzymes. Most vitamins cannot be synthesized by the body, and they are not broken down before use. Vitamins A, D, E, and K are fat-soluble vitamins.

117. **(D)** The kidney performs all of these functions.

118. **(C)** A reaction in which the enzyme is the catalyst may be written as follows:

Enzyme + Substrate – Enzyme-Substrate complex – Enzyme + Product

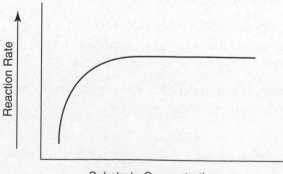

The substrate binds to a specific site on the surface of the enzyme, known as the active site, after which product and enzyme are released. The enzyme is then available to bind another substrate. At low substrate concentration, the reaction rate increases sharply with increasing substrate concentration because there are abundant free enzyme molecules available to bind to an added substrate. At high substrate concentration, the reaction rate reaches a plateau as the enzyme active sites become saturated with substrate. The enzyme-substrate complex and no free enzymes are available to bind the added substrate.

119. **(C)** In a heterozygous cross-height, for example, when T represents the dominant, tall, trait and t represents the recessive, short, trait. Tt represents both parents. A cross between Tt × Tt would produce an occurrence of the dominant trait 75 percent of the time.

	T	t
T	TT	Tt
t	Tt	tt

Tall: 3 (75%)   Short: 1 (25%)

120. **(B)** The villi are specialized, finger-shaped structures in the lower intestine that are designed for absorption of digested nutrients. The alveoli are structures that allow the passage of carbon dioxide and oxygen into the lungs. Nephrons are the functional unit of the kidney. Bowman's capsule is where the filtration of the blood occurs in the nephrons of the kidney.

121. **(D)** The probability is that crossing over increases for genes far apart in a chromosome.

122. **(A)** Skin develops from the ectoderm.

123. **(A)** No explanation needed.

124. **(A)** One-fourth of their offspring, on average, will have silver fur. Choices C and D are not a possibility because none of the parents have silver fur.

	B	b
B	BB	Bb
b	Bb	bb

125. **(C)** The T-helper cells (T_4) cells are the most infected.

126. **(A)** Digestion begins in the mouth and salivary amylase breaks down starches.

127. **(B)** No explanation needed.

128. **(D)** Disordered eating patterns occur when concerns about dieting, food restriction, fear of becoming overweight, and dissatisfaction with body image interfere with normal daily life. Bulimia nervosa is an eating

disorder in which a person eats a great deal of food and then vomits or uses other purging methods. Individuals with binge-eating disorder eat large amounts of food frequently and repeatedly. Choice (C) is a nonsense answer.

129. **(B)** A major function of white blood cells (WBC) is to fight infections.

130. **(A)** Because mitochondria use oxygen to produce ATP, the greater oxygen consumption indicates that tissue A has either a greater number of mitochondria, larger mitochondria, or more enzymatic activity then tissue B.

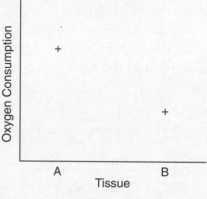

Figure 1.

131. **(D)** A large sodium (Na⁺) influx into the cell results in the resting potential becoming more positive. An action potential is produced when the charge difference across the plasma membrane reverses and then returns to the resting condition which requires the movement of sodium (Na⁺) ions into the cell. There is generally a higher concentration of potassium (K⁺) ions inside the cell than outside, and conversely a higher concentration of sodium (Na⁺) ions outside the cell than inside. Following the action potential, the sodium-potassium exchange pump restores ion concentrations by moving sodium (Na⁺) ions out of the cell and potassium (K⁺) ions into the cell.

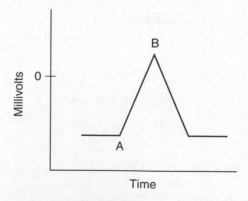

Figure 2.

132. **(C)** The pancreas produces insulin and glucagon. The adrenal glands produce adrenaline and noradrenaline. The pineal gland produces melatonin and serotonin.

133. **(B)** Hormones are secreted in the blood from a specific gland and are distributed by the blood to a specific target site. Blood (answer B) plays a role in the general distribution of hormones.

134. **(A)** In general, the smaller the animal, the farther to the right its curve will be. Therefore, small animals with high metabolic rates and correspondingly high oxygen requirements tend to have hemoglobin that unloads more readily.

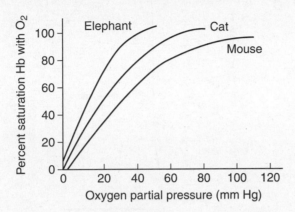

Figure 3.

135. **(C)** No explanation needed.

136. **(C)** Transmission across a synapse involves an influx of Ca+ ions into the terminal, followed by movement of transmitter vesicles, exocytosis, diffusion of the transmitter across the cleft, and finally the diffusion of ions through the postsynaptic channels.

137. **(D)** Neurological drugs alter synaptic function by many different methods including: interfering with synthesis of the appropriate transmitter, blocking uptake of the transmitter into synaptic vesicles, preventing release of transmitter from vesicles into the cleft, or blocking the receptor sites on the postsynaptic membrane so that the transmitter has no effect even when released.

138. **(C)** Statements A, B, and D are correct. The only false statement is C. The normal life span of red blood cells is approximately 120 days, not 30 days.

139. **(D)** Neuronal dendrites receive signals from other neurons.

140. **(B)** No explanation needed.

141. **(A)** No explanation needed.

142. **(B)** Apoptosis refers to programmed cell death.

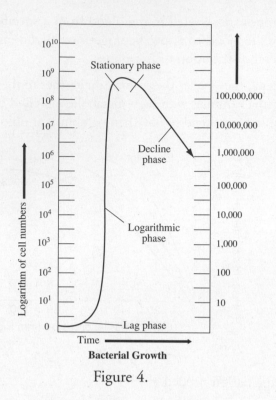

Figure 4.

143. **(A)** See Figure 4.

144. **(C)** Since it multiplies by binary fission at a generation time of 30 minutes, the population within 2 hours (12 noon–2:00 P.M.) is 2 at 12:30, 4 at 1 P.M., 8 at 1:30 P.M., and 16 at 2:00 P.M.

Passage 1

152   As many as 50 million Americans have high blood pressure, defined as a systolic blood pressure ≥140 mm Hg and a diastolic blood pressure ≥90 mm Hg. Although blood pressure generally increases with age, the onset of hypertension most often
145   occurs in the third, fourth, or fifth decade of life. The prevalence of hypertension
146   in the elderly population (age ≥ 65 years) is approximately 63% in whites and 76% in blacks. In younger generations (35 to 45 years of age), the prevalence is markedly different with 44% among black men, 37% among black women, 26% among white men, and 17% among white women.

A specific cause of sustained hypertension cannot be found in the vast majority of individuals with high blood pressure. Genetic factors have been suggested to play
149   a role in essential hypertension due to the fact that high blood pressure may be hereditary. Evidence that a single gene may account for specific subtypes of hypertension has also been suggested. Genetic traits include high angiotensin levels,

increased aldosterone and other adrenal steroids, and high sodium-lithium counter-transport. More direct approaches for preventing or treating hypertension could be achieved by identifying individuals with these traits. <u>Factors such as sodium excretion and transport rates, blood pressure response to plasma volume expansion, electrolyte homeostasis, and glomerular filtration rate help explain the predisposition for a person to develop hypertension.</u>   148

<u>Anti-hypertensive drug therapy should be individualized according to various patient characteristics and fundamental pathophysiologic circumstances.</u> Dietary   150
intake has been shown to be similar in all races but blacks ingest less potassium and calcium than whites. Supplemental potassium and calcium has shown to cause a modest reduction in blood pressure in some studies. Therefore, it would seem reasonable to ascertain the affects of increasing the amount of potassium and calcium in the diet as part of the non-pharmacologic regulation of hypertension. The initial treatment for hypertension is life-style unless target-organ damage is present. <u>These changes include sodium reduction, weight reduction, increased physical activity, and ethanol reduction or abstinence.</u> In terms of target-organ damage, diuretics and   147
beta-blockers are first-line therapy. Control of blood pressure and prevention of cardiovascular morbidity and mortality are the goals of antihypertensive therapy. <u>By maintaining arterial blood pressure below 140 mm Hg systolic and 90 mm Hg diastolic and by controlling other risk factors such as smoking, hyperlipidemia, and diabetes, morbidity and mortality may be averted.</u>   151

145. **(B)** No explanation needed.

146. **(C)** The passage states that, in the younger generation, the prevalence of hypertension in white men is 26%. The prevalence of hypertension in elderly blacks is 76%.

147. **(B)** Although all choices may represent life-style changes, according to the passage life-style changes that are suggested to lower blood pressure include sodium restriction, weight reduction, increased physical activity, and ethanol reduction or abstinence. Weight gain and increased stress may increase blood pressure.

148. **(B)** No explanation needed.

149. **(D)** No explanation needed.

150. **(A)** No explanation needed.

151. **(D)** The passage states that by maintaining arterial blood pressure below 140 mm Hg systolic and 90 mm Hg diastolic and by controlling other risk factors, morbidity and mortality may be averted.

152. **(C)** No explanation needed.

Passage 2

158 Non-adherence to medication therapy results in numerous adverse effects such as increased hospitalizations and even death. Additionally, it costs the U.S. healthcare system billions of dollars each year. It is important to assess patients' adherence to medications.

Improper medication adherence encompasses an assortment of behaviors. These
155 include not having a prescription filled, forgetting or intentionally not taking a
157 medication, consuming an incorrect amount of a medication, taking a medication at the wrong time, ceasing therapy too soon, or continuing therapy after advised to discontinue. All forms of improper medication-taking behavior may jeopardize health outcomes.

153 Measuring medication-taking behavior is often difficult. The ideal method of measurement should be simultaneously unobtrusive (to avoid patient sensitization and maximize cooperation), objective (to produce discrete and reproducible data
154 for each subject), and practical (to maximize portability and minimize cost). Refill records, pill counts, electronic medication dispensers/caps, patient surveys (interviews), blood-drug level monitoring, and urine assay for drug metabolites can be used as clues to identify improper medication use.

156 Before altering therapy based on the assumption that a patient is taking a medication as prescribed, practitioners should ascertain patient's medication-taking behavior. This becomes especially important when modifying dosages of medications. Due to the advantages and disadvantages of each measurement, it is important for practitioners to use a combination of methods to assess a patient's medication-usage behavior and relate these findings to the patient's clinical presentation.

153. **(C)** The passage specifically states that the ideal method of measurement should be simultaneously unobtrusive (to avoid patient sensitization and maximize cooperation), objective (to produce discrete and reproducible data for each subject), and practical (to maximize portability and minimize cost).

154. **(D)** According to the passage, half-life tables, nucleic acid levels, and patient examinations are not techniques for assessing patient's medication usage. Answer D lists techniques used to assess medication usage.

155. **(D)** Choices A, B, and C are all forms of improper medication adherence.

156. **(A)** No explanation needed.

157. **(D)** No explanation needed.

158. **(B)** Medications may still work even if the patient does not take it as advised, therefore ruling out A. C is not the answer because the passage specifically stated billions and not trillions, and no mention of lawsuits was made. Also, no mention of suicides was made. The first sentence of the passage discussed that non-adherence to medication therapy results in numerous adverse effects such as increased hospitalizations and even death. Therefore, the answer is B.

Passage 3

A dreaded disease is striking California's coast live oaks with the ferocity of an oak-tree Ebola virus, <u>causing the trees to sprout sores, hemorrhage sap, and become 159 infested with beetles and various fungi.</u> The trees die within a few weeks of their first symptoms.

A pathologist at the University of California, Davis, announced that his team had found the cause of the disease dubbed "Sudden Oak Death". <u>The tree-slayer is a new member of the genus Phytophthora,</u> whose name means "plant destroyer". Its kin 161 include pathogens responsible for the Irish potato famine and die-offs in Australian eucalyptus forests and European oak groves. "We don't know if (the new species) was just recently introduced, or if it has always been here and something else has changed that has allowed it to go crazy," one pathologist says.

<u>The first trees to succumb to the plague 5 years ago were tan oaks, which often 160; 162 grow in the understory of redwood forests. Last year the disease began hitting large 164–166 numbers of coast live oaks, the signature species in scenic coastal woodlands. Alarmingly, the pathogen has begun to blight another species, the black oak.</u>

Knowing the culprit doesn't make the outlook much brighter. "Fungicides can save individual oaks," says one pathologist, "but we can't go to Mount Tamalpais and spray 10,000 trees." And prevention is largely limited to warning people not to carry oak firewood to uninfected areas. The Sierra Nevada hosts black oaks, and <u>pathologists fear deadly spores could strike groves in beloved Yosemite Valley.</u> 163

Reprinted with permission from *Science*, Vol 289, August 2000. Page 859.

159. **(B)** No explanation needed.

160. **(A)** No explanation needed.

161. **(C)** No explanation needed.

162. **(A)** No explanation needed.

163. **(B)** No explanation needed.

164. **(A)** No explanation needed.

165. **(B)** No explanation needed.

166. **(D)** No explanation needed.

Passage 4

We humans sense old age through feeling those creaky joints or observing those graying hairs but, according to Apfeld and Kenyon reporting in a recent issue of Nature, <u>the nematode worm senses its age by smelling and tasting the environment.</u> 169 These investigators show that worms with defective olfactory organs (that would normally detect odor molecules in the environment) live longer than their comrades with a keener sense of smell. By comparing these worms with other mutant nematodes that live an unusually long time, the researchers found clues to how a reduced ability to "smell the roses" might lengthen lifespan.

170   The worm's <u>olfactory sense organs—amphids on the head and plasmids on the tail—are composed of a cluster of nerve cells, the ends of which are modified into cilia.</u> The cilia are encircled by a sheath and a socket cell that form a pore in the worm's skin through which the tips of the cilia protrude. Odor molecules and soluble compounds bind to G protein-coupled receptors (similar to the olfactory and taste receptors of mammals) located at the tip of each cilium. Worms with a poor sense of smell—because their olfactory organs have defective or absent cilia, blocked pores, or damaged sheaths—live much longer, yet are otherwise normal (for example, their feeding and reproductive behaviors are unchanged). <u>Mutations in TAX-4—a channel regulated by cyclic GMP that sits under the G-protein-coupled receptor and transduces the sensory signals into electrical impulses</u>—also imbue the worm with a longer life.

But mutations in the worms olfactory machinery are not the only defects that extend its lifespan. In an earlier study, Kenyon's group found that <u>defects in the reproductive system could prolong life by decreasing the activity of DAF-2 (a receptor for an insulin-like molecule) and increasing the activity of DAF-16 (a transcription factor). By looking at worms defective in both sensory perception and reproduction, Apfeld and Kenyon worked out a putative pathway through which smell might influence a worm's longevity.</u>

An environmental signal, perhaps produced by bacteria (the worm's favorite food), binds to G protein-coupled olfactory receptors on sensory cilia <u>activating TAX-4, which then incites electrical activity in the sensory neurons. This activity triggers secretory vesicles in the neurons to release insulin-like molecules,</u> which bind to DAF-2 and activate the insulin-like signaling pathway. <u>This then switches on genes that will ensure the worm dies at the usual age of 2 weeks. A reduced ability to sense olfactory cues would result in a decrease in DAF-2 activation and an increase in life-span.</u>

This chain of events is not proven, but insulin-like molecules that might bind to DAF-2 have been identified in the nematode. Such a pathway would also make physiological sense. After all, if food is scarce it may behoove the worm to live longer to ensure that it has the chance to produce its full quota of offspring. <u>A scarcity of food also promotes longevity in rodents and primates).</u> But so far it seems that in these more complicated creatures a poor sense of smell is not a harbinger of a ripe old age.

168

171
172

173

174

167
176

175

Reprinted with permission from *Science*, Vol 287, January 2000. Page 54.

167. **(D)** No explanation needed.

168. **(A)** No explanation needed.

169. **(D)** No explanation needed.

170. **(C)** No explanation needed.

171. **(D)** No explanation needed.

172. **(A)** No explanation needed.

173. **(B)** No explanation needed.

174. **(A)** No explanation needed.

175. **(D)** No explanation needed.

176. **(B)** No explanation needed.

Passage 5

Presidents of the United States are not like you and me. A new personality assessment <u>presented this week at the American Psychological Association</u> conference in   177
Washington, D.C., shows that, compared to the public they serve, <u>presidents are</u>
<u>more likely to be extroverted, assertive, and disagreeable</u>. They're also less modest   184
and straightforward.

    Says who? <u>Historians who have written book-length biographies of Oval Office</u>   178
<u>occupants</u>. <u>Psychologist Steve Rubenzer of the Mental Health and Mental</u>   179
<u>Retardation Authority of Harris County in Houston, Texas,</u> and colleagues asked the
biographers to fill out three standard personality inventories on their subjects, <u>basing</u>   180
<u>answers on the presidents' behavior during the 5 years preceding their reigns</u>. The
researchers compared the presidents' scores to population norms and compared the
profiles of successful commanders-in-chief with those history hasn't smiled upon.

    "<u>Great" presidents, such as Jefferson and Lincoln</u>, they find, "are attentive to their   181
emotions, willing to question traditional values ... imaginative, and more interested
in art and beauty than less successful Chief Executives." They're also more assertive,
stubborn, and "<u>tender-minded," which is a measure of concern for the less fortu-</u>   182
<u>nate</u>. Rubenzer hasn't analyzed the current presidential contenders yet—<u>he prefers</u>
<u>to have at least three "unbiased" historians fill out the forms for each president or</u>   183
presidential wanna-be.

———————————
Reprinted with permission from *Science*, Vol 289, August 2000. Page 859.

177. **(C)** No explanation needed.

178. **(A)** No explanation needed.

179. **(B)** No explanation needed.

180. **(D)** No explanation needed.

181. **(B)** No explanation needed.

182. **(B)** No explanation needed.

183. **(A)** No explanation needed.

184. **(A)** No explanation needed.

Passage 6

186 Drug interactions, a common type of drug-related problem, are categorized as pharmacokinetic, pharmacodynamic, or a combination of both. Pharmacokinetic drug
188 interactions include changes in absorption, distribution, excretion, and metabolism; whereas, pharmacodynamic drug interactions may lead to antagonistic or synergistic effects. Not all drug interactions are undesirable, in fact, many drug interactions are used to produce desirable effects. Patients who take drugs with narrow therapeu-
189 tic indices and drugs that interfere with the pharmacokinetic properties of other drugs are at increased risk of experiencing a drug interaction. Also, patients who take multiple medications per day or take multiple doses of medications per day are at increased risk. Because renal transplant patients take immunosuppressive agents that have narrow therapeutic indices and are subjected to multiple medications per day, they are vulnerable to experiencing adverse drug events. To prevent adverse
191 drug interactions, an alternative therapy should be considered when possible or the dose or schedule of the drugs should be adjusted to reduce the occurrence of an adverse experience. Additionally, adequate monitoring to prevent and detect adverse effects is an essential part of patient care.

A common pharmacokinetic interaction involves drugs that interfere with the
190 absorption of other medications. Drugs that bind and decrease the gastrointestinal absorption of another drug, such as cholestyramine decreasing the absorption of tacrolimus, typically can be prevented by administering the agents two to three hours
185 apart from each other. Prokinetic agents interfere with the rate of absorption. Since
187 many transplant patients take prokinetic agents, such as metochlopromide, this may increase the bioavailability of other medications. This is of significant importance since immunosuppressive agents have narrow therapeutic indices and toxicity may
192 result from this interaction. If the prokinetic agent cannot be avoided, careful monitoring (e.g., serum drug levels, clinical presentation of patient) and adjustments should be made to prevent immunosuppressant toxicity.

185. **(C)** No explanation needed.

186. **(B)** The passage states that drug interactions are characterized as (1) pharmacokinetic, (2) pharmacodynamic, or (3) a combination of both.

187. **(C)** No explanation needed.

188. **(B)** No explanation needed.

189. **(D)** No explanation needed.

190. **(D)** No explanation needed.

191. **(B)** No explanation needed.

192. **(C)** No explanation needed.

193. **(A)** A square has the same dimensions on all four sides. Area is calculated by multiplying two sides together. Thus, 210 feet · 210 feet = 44,100 square feet.

   Two other lessons should be learned from this question. (1) Since 210 · 210 means the one digit will be a zero, any answer without a zero in the ones place cannot be a correct answer. (2) Estimation can be a means of identifying possible answers. In this case, one can multiply 200 · 200 to get 40,000. Since 210 is greater than 200, the answer must be greater than 40,000. Any number smaller than that cannot be the correct answer.

194. **(B)** We use the Quotient Rule for derivatives.

$$\frac{d}{dx}\left(\frac{f(x)}{g(x)}\right) = \frac{g(x)\cdot f'(x) - g'(x)\cdot f(x)}{\left(g(x)\right)^2} = \frac{(6-x)(2x)-(x^2)(-1)}{(6-x)^2} = \frac{12x - x^2}{(6-x)^2}$$

195. **(A)** We compute $\dfrac{4+5+11+18+20+22+34+35+38}{9} = \dfrac{187}{9} \approx 20.77$.

196. **(B)** 12 ounces times 30 mL per ounce = 360 mL total volume

   15 mL (x) 3 doses per day = 45 mL per day; 360 mL divided by 45 mL = 8 days

   An alternative solution: Since 30 mL = one ounce and 15 mL = one dose, then each ounce has two doses. Twelve ounces times two doses per ounce = 24 doses; divide by 3 doses per day to obtain 8 days.

197. **(A)** We use the Quotient Rule for logarithms.

$$\ln\left(\frac{a}{b}\right) = \ln(a) - \ln(b) = 6 - 2 = 4$$

198. **(A)** Use the conversion formula

$$\text{Celsius Temp} = \frac{5}{9}\cdot(\text{Fahrenheit Temp} - 32) = \frac{5}{9}\cdot(86 - 32) = \frac{5}{9}\cdot(54) = 30.$$

199. **(D)** We list the values in increasing order: 4, 5, 11, 18, 20, 22, 34, 35, 38, 39.

   Because there are an even number of values in the list, the median value is the average of the two values in the middle of the list (20 and 22). Add 20 + 22 = 42. Then, divide 42 by 2: 42 ÷ 2 = 21, that is, the median = 21.

200. **(D)** We use the Fundamental Theorem of Calculus for integrals.

$$\int_{3}^{4}\left(9x^2\right)dx = \frac{9x^3}{3}\bigg|_{3}^{4} = 3x^3\bigg|_{3}^{4} = 3\cdot 4^3 - 3\cdot 3^3 = 192 - 81 = 111$$

201. **(B)** Since the tank is already 4/5 full, the additional 7 gallons equals 1/5 of the tank's capacity. Thus, $7 = \frac{1}{5}x \Rightarrow x = 35$.

202. **(C)** Calculate each number separately such that $10^2 = 100$ and $9^2 = 81$. Added together they equal 181. 181 can also be expressed as 1.81×10^2.

203. **(C)** We calculate the distance using the formula

$$\sqrt{\left(x_2 - x_1\right)^2 + \left(y_2 - y_1\right)^2} = \sqrt{\left(3-5\right)^2 + \left(-1-7\right)^2} = \sqrt{4+64} = \sqrt{68}.$$

204. **(D)** Let x = the number of dimes, and $2x$ = the number of quarters. This yields the equation $10 \cdot x + 25 \cdot 2x$ = total money in cents. So, we solve the equation

$10 \cdot x + 25 \cdot 2x = 660$

$$60x = 660 \Rightarrow x = \frac{660}{60} = 11$$

Thus, John has 11 dimes, so $11 \cdot 2 = 22$, which means he has 22 quarters.

205. **(B)** We add the expressions by finding a common denominator.

206. **(A)** To determine $f^{-1}(x)$, interchange the x and y values in the formula for f, then solve for y.

$$f(x) = 2x + 5 \Rightarrow y = 2x + 5$$
$$x = 2y + 5$$
$$x - 5 = 2y$$
$$y = \frac{x-5}{2}$$

207. **(D)** As x approaches 2 from the right-hand side, the values of $f(x)$ approach 0.

208. **(A)** As x approaches 2 from the left-hand side, the values of $f(x)$ approach -4.

209. **(B)** The left-hand and right-hand limits are not equal.

210. **(B)** The *Product Rule* for logarithms states that

$$\log(M) + \log(N) = \log(M \cdot N)$$

211. **(C)** From 12 Noon to 6 P.M. is 6 hours. At a speed of 100 kilometers (km) per hour, the truck will travel 600 kilometers. Several conversions can be used to change kilometers to miles. One mile = 1.6 kilometers; one kilometer = 0.62 miles

For this problem 600 km (x) 0.62 miles per km = 372 miles.

212. **(A)** We compute $(0.32) \cdot (800) = 256$.

213. **(D)** The highest point on the graph has a y coordinate equal to 300.

214. **(A)** The highest point on the graph occurs when the x coordinate equals 3.

215. **(D)** Note that $\lim\limits_{x \to \infty}\left(\dfrac{5x^4 + 2x^3 - x + 7}{3x^4 + 8x^2 - 10}\right) \to \dfrac{5x^4}{3x^4} = \dfrac{5}{3}$.

216. **(A)** When a coin is tossed only two outcomes are possible, heads or tails. No matter how many times a coin has been tossed, the probability on any one toss is 50 : 50 or 1 chance out of 2 for either heads or tails. Thus, there is a 50% chance for heads (or tails) on this toss.

217. **(D)** The projectile hits the ground when the height equals zero. So we solve the equation $-0.008x^2 + x = 0$.

$$-0.008x^2 + x = 0$$

$$x(-0.008x^2 + 1) = 0$$

$$x = 0, \; -0.008x + 1 = 0 \Rightarrow x = \dfrac{-1}{-0.008} = 125$$

218. **(C)** Let x = the original price in dollars. The sale price is given by the original price minus the percent discount. Thus, we have the equation

$$210 = x - 0.30x \Rightarrow 210 = 0.7x \Rightarrow x = \dfrac{210}{0.7} = 300.$$

219. **(A)** We use the formula $P(\overline{A}) = 1 - P(A) = 1 - \dfrac{5}{9} = \dfrac{4}{9}$.

220. **(D)** The expression $4x = \dfrac{1}{2}$ can be solved by dividing both sides of the equation by four to provide the new equation $x = \dfrac{1}{2} \div 4$.

The four can become $\dfrac{4}{1}$. Now the equation is $x = \dfrac{1}{2} \div \dfrac{4}{1}$.

This rearranges for the purpose of division to become $x = \dfrac{1}{2} \times \dfrac{1}{4}$.

Solving yields $x = \dfrac{1}{8}$.

221. **(C)** There were 730 + 185 = 915 patients who had Drug A or Drug B. There were 1,500 total patients.

Thus, probability $\dfrac{915}{1,500}$ = 0.61 = 61% ≈ 60%.

222. **(A)** The percentage of patients prescribed Drug D was

$\dfrac{466}{1,500}$ ≈ 0.31 = 31%.

Thus, the percentage of patients who did NOT have a prescription for Drug D was 1 − 0.31 = 0.69 = 69%.

223. **(C)** 1 milligram (mg) = 1000 micrograms (mcg). You must convert either the concentration of the Digoxin Injection (500 mcg/2 mL = 0.5 mg/2 mL) or the dose desired (0.25 mg = 250 mcg) so that you are working with numbers that have the same dimension.

$$\frac{2 \text{ mL}}{500 \text{ mcg}} \cdot \frac{1,000 \text{ mcg}}{1 \text{ mg}} = \frac{4 \text{ mL}}{1 \text{ mg}}$$

So we have the ratio $\dfrac{4 \text{ mL}}{1 \text{ mg}} \cdot \dfrac{0.25}{0.25} = \dfrac{1 \text{ mL}}{0.25 \text{ mg}}$

224. **(A)** We calculate the slope using the formula $\dfrac{\Delta y}{\Delta x} = \dfrac{4-1}{9-(-5)} = \dfrac{3}{14}$.

225. **(A)** The original graph is shifted 3 units to the left.

226. **(B)** We plug into the given formula

$$\text{CrCl} = \left(\frac{(140-58)}{(72 \cdot 2.6)} \right) \cdot (76) = \left(\frac{82}{187} \right) \cdot (76) \approx 33.$$

227. **(C)** A fundamental property of inverse functions states that the domain of the function f is equal to the range of the inverse function f^{-1}.

228. **(A)** The graph has a negative slope when $5.1 < x < 11.5$.

229. **(C)** The graph is concave up when $9 < x < \infty$.

230. **(D)** No explanation needed.

231. **(B)** Note that $\lim\limits_{x \to 14} \left(\dfrac{f(x) - f(14)}{x - 14} \right) = f'(14)$ = the slope of the graph

when $x = 14$.

232. **(A)** We compute $\dfrac{f(4) - f(2)}{4 - 2} = \dfrac{64 - 8}{2} = 28$.

233. **(D)**
$$\sqrt{45} = \sqrt{9 \cdot 5} = 3\sqrt{5}$$
$$\sqrt{80} = \sqrt{16 \cdot 5} = 4\sqrt{5}$$
$$3\sqrt{5} + 4\sqrt{5} = 7\sqrt{5}$$

234. **(A)** The formula for slope (m) of a line is $m = \dfrac{y_2 - y_1}{x_2 - x_1}$.

Substituting the values into the formula yields $m = \dfrac{5-1}{5-1} = 1$.

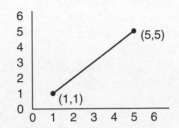

235. **(C)** Arrange the values in order from least to highest: 8, 9, 9, 9, <u>10</u>, <u>10</u>, 10, 11, 12, 12. Because there are an even number of values, you will need to find the average of the two values that fall in the middle of the list (10 and 10 as underlined). Add 10 + 10 = 20. Then, divide 20 by 2, 20 ÷ 2 = 10. The median value is 10.

236. **(D)** There are 5 options for each of the 3 letters. Total = $5^3 = 125$.

237. **(B)** The graph of $f(x) = \dfrac{x}{x+1}$ has a horizontal tangent line at the points where $f'(x) = 0$.

The Quotient Rule for derivatives states that the derivative of $\dfrac{p(x)}{q(x)}$ is

given by $\dfrac{q(x) \cdot p'(x) - p(x) \cdot q'(x)}{\left(q(x)\right)^2}$.

$$f(x) = \frac{x}{x+1}$$

$$f'(x) = \frac{(x+1)(1) - x(1)}{(x+1)^2} = \frac{x+1-x}{(x+1)^2} = \frac{1}{(x+1)^2}$$

Since this expression never equals 0, the graph has no horizontal tangent lines.

238. **(B)** A quadratic relationship between two variables yields a graph that is a parabola, which is represented in choice (B). The relationships represented in the answer choices are as follows: (A) linear, (B) quadratic, (C) polynomial, and (D) exponential.

239. **(C)** With the understanding that the symbol $\cup$ means the set of elements either in A or B or in both, and the symbol $\cap$ means the set that contains all those elements that A and B have in common, we use the formula

$$P(A \cup B) = P(A) + P(B) - P(A \cap B) = 0.35 + 0.22 - 0.09 = 0.48.$$

240. **(C)** We compute the definite integral

$$\int_{1}^{x} \frac{5}{x}\,dx = 5 \cdot \ln{(x)}\Big|_{1}^{5} = 5 \cdot \ln{(5)} - 5 \cdot \ln{(1)} = 5 \cdot \ln{(5)}$$

Appendix: Weights, Measures, and Conversions

LENGTH

1 inch (in.)		= 2.54 cm
1 foot (ft.)	= 12 in.	= 0.3048 m
1 yard (yd.)	= 3 ft.	= 0.9144 m
1 mile (mi.)	= 1,760 yd.	= 1.6093 km
1 millimeter (mm)		= 0.0394 in.
1 centimeter (cm)	= 10 mm	= 0.3937 in.
1 meter (m)	= 1,000 mm	= 1.0936 yd.
1 kilometer (km)	= 1,000 m	= 0.6214 mi.

AREA

1 square inch (in^2)		= 6.4516 cm^2
1 square foot (ft^2)	= 144 in^2	= 0.093 m^2
1 square yard (yd^2)	= 9 ft^2	= 0.8361 m^2
1 acre	= 4840 yd^2	= 4046.86 m^2
1 square mile (mi^2)	= 640 acres	= 2.59 km^2
1 square centimeter (cm^2)	= 100 mm^2	= 0.155 in^2
1 square meter (m^2)	= 10,000 cm^2	= 1.196 yd^2
1 hectare (ha)	= 10,000 m^2	= 2.4711 acres
1 square kilometer (km^2)	= 100 ha	= 0.3861 mi^2

WEIGHT

1 ounce (oz.)	= 437.5 grains	= 28.35 g
1 pound (lb.)	= 16 oz.	= 0.4536 kg
1 kilogram (kg)	= 1,000 g	= 2.2 lb.
1 short ton	= 2,000 lb.	= 0.9072 metric ton
1 long ton	= 2,240 lb.	= 1.0161 metric ton
1 milligram (mg)		= 0.0154 grain
1 gram (g)	= 1,000 mg	= 0.0353 oz.
1 tonne	= 1,000 kg	= 1.1023 short tons
1 tonne		= 0.9842 long ton

VOLUME

1 cubic inch (in^3)		= 16.387 cm^3
1 cubic foot (ft^3)	= 1,728 in.^{3}	= 0.028 m^3
1 cubic yard (yd^3)	= 27 ft.^{3}	= 0.7646 m^3
1 cubic centimeter (cm^3)		= 0.061 in^3
1 cubic decimeter (dm^3)	= 1,000 cm^3	= 0.0353 ft^3
1 cubic meter (m^3)	= 1,000 dm^3	= 1.3079 yd^3
1 liter (L)	= 1 dm^3	= 0.2642 gal.
1 hectoliter (hL)	= 100 L	= 2.8378 bushel (bu.)
1 fluid ounce (fl. oz.)		= 29.573 mL
1 liquid pint (pt.)	= 16 fl. oz.	= 0.4732 L
1 liquid quart (qt.)	= 2 pt.	= 0.946 L
1 gallon (gal.)	= 4 qt.	= 3.7853 L

TEMPERATURE

$$\text{Celsius}° = \frac{5}{9}(\text{F}° - 32°)$$

$$\text{Fahrenheit}° = \frac{9}{5}(\text{C}°) + 32$$

$$\text{Kelvin} = 273.15 + \text{C}°$$

Index